Immunology and Rheumatology in Questions

Haralampos M. Moutsopoulos
Evangelia Zampeli
Editors

Immunology and Rheumatology in Questions

Second Edition

Springer

Editors
Haralampos M. Moutsopoulos
Academy of Athens
Athens
Greece

Evangelia Zampeli
Bioclinic General Hospital of Athens
and Institute for Autoimmune Systemic
and Neurological Disorders
Athens
Greece

ISBN 978-3-030-56669-2 ISBN 978-3-030-56670-8 (eBook)
https://doi.org/10.1007/978-3-030-56670-8

This Springer imprint is published by the registered company Springer Nature Switzerland AG
The registered company address is: Gewerbestrasse 11, 6330 Cham, Switzerland

Preface

Rheumatology is a medical specialty which provides diagnosis, treatment, and follow-up of patients suffering from diseases which can affect, in addition to the musculoskeletal system, every organ of the human body. The etiology of these disorders is diverse, expanding from immune-mediated to genetic, degenerative, and metabolic disorders. Therefore, the specialists of this medical field should be adequately trained in all internal medicine fields. On the other hand, physicians from almost all medical domains should be able to recognize manifestations of rheumatic disorders and refer the patient to a rheumatology specialist in order to categorize the disease process and to institute the appropriate therapeutic scheme. In addition, rheumatologists should understand in depth the pathogenetic mechanisms of diseases so as to request necessary and appropriate laboratory and molecular tests which will aim at diagnosis and proper therapy.

The progress of molecular immunobiology has aided the comprehension of the pathogenetic aspects of autoimmune/connective tissue diseases and the identification of critical molecules in the arena of immune-mediated tissue damage in these disorders. Biotechnological development of inhibitors of specific pathogenetic molecules has significantly improved the therapeutic armamentarium of rheumatologists.

The necessity to present the second edition of our book entitled *Immunology and Rheumatology in Questions* has been driven not only by the great response of the readers to the first edition, but mostly by the commitment to keep up with the evolving and increasing knowledge in the field of rheumatology. In our days, medical knowledge expands faster than the ability of physicians to assimilate and apply it effectively, and this holds true in education, patient care, and research. On the other hand, it is of paramount importance that this newly emerging knowledge should be carefully and critically assessed before being incorporated in a didactic manual.

Although the manual you hold in your hands cannot replace the knowledge that rheumatologists should gain from reading rheumatology textbooks or from continuous education through every day studying of scientific journals of the field, we hope and believe that this handbook will be a useful tool for education and self-assessment of physicians' knowledge and anticipate that it will fulfill an unmet need in the rheumatology literature.

Athens, Greece — Haralampos M. Moutsopoulos
Athens, Greece — Evangelia Zampeli

Introduction

As in the first edition, the goal of this second edition of our book *Immunology and Rheumatology in Questions* is primarily to serve as an educative and self-evaluation manual of rheumatology knowledge for medical students; physicians in internal medicine, rheumatology, physical/rehabilitation medicine, family practice, and orthopedic surgery training; and specialists in practice who desire to refresh their knowledge in the field.

In this second edition, keeping the short, concise questions-and-answers format of the first edition, we made a great effort to critically incorporate all new knowledge generated in the past 3 years in the field of rheumatology and to bridge classical and current evidence-based knowledge, so as to present didactic and credible information. All the questions and their corresponding answers constituting the second edition of this handbook are divided into four main parts comprising fourteen chapters in total. More than 120 new questions and answers and more than 25 new images have been added to the second edition, while the answers to more than 90 questions of the first edition have been modified according to current evidence-based knowledge.

In this manual, laconic questions and answers address manifestations of the musculoskeletal system as well as of other organs, differential diagnosis, laboratory and imaging tests, pathology pictures, therapeutic interventions, drug mode of action, and undesired side effects. Since the etiology of inflammatory/autoimmune (connective tissue) diseases is mediated through the attack of the immune system against self-antigens, two sections with relative questions and answers are included in the manual. One summarizes basic immunology knowledge and the other presents pathogenetic and laboratory aspects of the inflammatory/autoimmune diseases. We believe that the information given in these chapters will help the readers to better comprehend immune-pathogenic mechanisms operating in the expression of inflammatory/autoimmune diseases. A spherical approach of the different autoimmune rheumatic (connective tissue) diseases is presented in respective chapters. Since manifestations of rheumatic diseases are often expressed in the skin, oral mucosa, eyes, and ears, or are associated with metabolic, endocrine, and hematological diseases, separate sections are devoted to these manifestations. Updated references are given only for answers providing information which cannot be found in the classical textbooks of rheumatology. To further reinforce the didactic goal of this manual, representative photos showing clinical manifestations, imaging findings, and histopathologic features are presented close to the corresponding questions.

Closing this short note, we would like to thank Professor Jacques-Olivier Pers for going thoroughly through Chaps. 1 and 2 in order to add, correct, and update the respective questions and answers. Furthermore, we would like to express our gratitude to Professors M. C. Dalakas, A. A. Drosos, E. Seyahi, F. N. Skopouli, A. G. Tzioufas, and P. V. Voulgari and Drs. C. Kampolis and S. Plastiras for providing photos of their patients and/or their biological materials. Last but not least, we would like to thank our patients who gave us permission to take photos of their clinical manifestations.

Contents

Part I

An Introductory Approach to Autoimmune Disorders

Basic Immunology

1

Jacques-Olivier Pers,
Panayiotis G. Vlachoyiannopoulos,
Evangelia Zampeli,
and Haralampos M. Moutsopoulos

Abstract

Immune system provides the mechanisms for attacking foreign invaders, eliminating autologous toxic substances and offering self-tolerance.

A reductionist approach of the immune system components and their interactions as provided in this chapter will offer knowledge important to better understand the core mechanisms of autoimmune diseases and design therapies targeting their pathogenic mechanisms.

Immunity is divided into (a) innate (or natural), implemented by macrophages, dendritic cells, granulocytes (neutrophils, basophils, and eosinophils), natural killer cells, the complement system, and the acute-phase proteins, and (b) adaptive, implemented by B and T cells. Immune cells express sensors on cytoplasmic or endosomal membranes or in the cytoplasm, called "pathogen-associated molecular pattern receptors" (PAMPRs), also called pattern recognition receptors (PRRs), and damage-associated molecular pattern receptors (DAMPRs) to sense foreign invaders or damaged tissues and provide defense against them. Natural immunity cells provide the first line of defense, usually successful in eliminating pathogens, but also they limber up the adaptive immune system to take action in case of any failure of defense. The sensors of B and T cells are their antigen receptors (membrane immunoglobulins and T-cell receptors, respectively) which are dissimilar to each other in terms of specificity; each receptor recognizes very specifically one antigen and especially a few peptide residues on it (epitope). However, by taking as a whole the pool of lymphocytes, their receptors offer a vast array of specificities exceeding 10^{11} that is more than the genes of the human body. This implies that not particular genes but rather gene fragments are spontaneously rearranged to make an immunoglobulin or a T-cell receptor gene. One such rearrangement for each peptide chain of the receptor is allowed, so

J.-O. Pers
UMR1227, Lymphocytes B et Autoimmunité, Université de Brest, Inserm, Brest, France
e-mail: pers@univ-brest.fr

P. G. Vlachoyiannopoulos
Department of Pathophysiology, School of Medicine, National University of Athens, Athens, Greece
e-mail: pvlah@med.uoa.gr

E. Zampeli
Bioclinic General Hospital of Athens and Institute for Autoimmune Systemic and Neurological Disorders, Athens, Greece
e-mail: ezampeli@bioclinic.gr

H. M. Moutsopoulos (✉)
Academy of Athens, Athens, Greece
e-mail: hmoutsop@med.uoa.gr

H. M. Moutsopoulos, E. Zampeli (eds.), *Immunology and Rheumatology in Questions*,
https://doi.org/10.1007/978-3-030-56670-8_1

the cells will retain their antigenic specificity as long as they live. Immune cells communicate with each other and approach their targets, either by cell-to-cell contact using adhesion molecules or by soluble mediators known as cytokines or chemokines, respectively.

Mechanisms like central (taking place in bone marrow and thymus) and peripheral (taking place in the lymph nodes) tolerance ensure that the immune system will not attack self. Braking of tolerance initiates autoimmune reactivity which may be subclinical but, under certain circumstances, may obtain a clinical phenotype.

1. Which are the main Cluster of Differentiation (CD) molecules on the surface of immunocytes?

CD molecules are cell surface markers that characterize different immune cell subtypes. In a simplistic way some CD molecules characterize the main immune cell subsets:

- CD4: T cells (helper/inducer), monocytes, macrophages, dendritic cells
- CD8: T cells (cytotoxic), NK cells
- CD14: monocytes
- CD15: granulocytes
- CD16: granulocytes and NK cells
- CD19: B cells (a component of the B cell receptor)
- CD20: B cells (type III transmembrane protein)
- CD22: B cells
- CD28: all T cells (co-stimulatory receptor)
- CD34: myeloblasts, lymphoblasts, endothelial cells
- CD38: plasma cells, B cells, T cells
- CD40: antigen-presenting cells (co-stimulatory protein)
- CD45: all leukocytes, all hemopoietic cells (except erythrocytes)
- CD57: T cells, NK cells, B cells, monocytes

2. Which are the primary and secondary lymphoid organs?

Primary or central lymphoid organs are those where lymphocytes are originally generated and educated to discriminate self from non-self; these include the bone marrow and thymus. *Secondary or peripheral lymphoid organs* are the lymph nodes, the spleen, and the lymphoid tissues of the gut, upper and lower respiratory tract, urogenital system, other mucosae, and arteries. Lymphocytes in these tissues are educated to react appropriately to foreign antigens in specific areas called germinal centers.

3. Which are the components of the innate immune system?

The innate immune system is constituted from:

- Physical barriers: Epithelial surfaces of skin, eye, oral, nasopharyngeal, respiratory, and gastrointestinal tracts, epithelial and phagocytic cell enzymes (i.e., lysozyme)
- Mucosal secretions: Sweat, tears, saliva, and gastric acid
- Antimicrobial peptides: For example, defensins, Pathogen-associated molecular pattern receptors (PAMPRs)
- Damage-associated molecular pattern receptors (DAMPRs)
- Cell receptors that sense microorganisms and signal a defensive response (e.g., Toll-like receptors)
- Cells: Polymorphonuclear leukocytes, macrophages, dendritic cells, natural killer cells, and mast cells
- Proteins: Acute-phase proteins, e.g., complement proteins and C-reactive protein
- The release of cytokines and chemokines

4. Which are the main functions of the innate immune system?

The innate immune system is evolutionary the oldest defense body mechanism. The immune response that it generates is rapid, yet not highly specific, and does not generate an immunological memory.

Its main functions are:

- Removal of dead cells and foreign invaders via phagocytosis (macrophages, polymorphonuclear leukocytes, etc.)
- Recruitment of immune cells of the adaptive immune response
- Activation of the complement system cascade which promotes clearance of the foreign invaders, necrotic cells, as well as antigen–antibody complexes
- As long as the cells of the innate immune system phagocytose foreign invaders, they present antigens, acting as antigen-presenting cells, to the cells of the adaptive immunity and initiate specific immune responses

5. How do innate immune cells recognize foreign invaders?

Cells of the innate immune system following exposure to bacterial or viral antigens ingest the foreign pathogen by phagocytosis. Structurally conserved microbe-associated molecules, known as pathogen-associated molecular patterns (PAMPs), are recognized by an array of specific sensors present in the plasma, plasma membranes, and host cytosol termed pattern recognition receptors (PRRs). The first classes of cellular PRRs to be identified were the transmembrane sensors called Toll-like receptors (TLRs). The nucleotide oligomerization domain (Nod)-like receptors (NLRs) and the retinoid acid-inducible gene-I (RIG-I)-like receptors (RLRs) are intracellular cytosolic sensors of PAMPs and danger-associated molecular patterns (DAMPs). RLRs are helicases that sense primarily viruses. NLRs can cooperate with TLRs and orchestrate the inflammatory and apoptotic response. TLRs are expressed on macrophages, dendritic cells, natural killer (NK) cells, B and T lymphocytes, as well as on non-immune cells like epithelial and endothelial cells as well as on fibroblasts. Of the 10 human TLRs, six of them are located on the cell surface (TLR1, 2, 4, 5, 6, and 10) where they bind a diversity of molecule types, whereas TLR3, 7, 8, and 9 are in endosomes and sense nucleic acids. Each TLR recognizes different ligands:

- TLR1: Bacterial lipoproteins
- TLR2: Bacterial peptidoglycans and porins, virus envelope glycoproteins
- TLR3: Viral double-stranded RNA
- TLR4: Gram-negative bacteria (LPS) and host-derived HMGB1 and HSPs
- TLR5: Bacterial flagellin
- TLR6: Bacterial diacyl lipopeptides and lipoteichoic acid
- TLRs 7 and 8: Virus single-stranded RNA
- TRL9: Unmethylated CpG DNA of viruses and bacteria
- TLR10: Triacylated lipopeptides

6. What is the function of natural killer cells?

Natural killer (NK) cells control the spread of several types of tumors and viral infections and thus limit the tissue damage. NK cells can also play a regulatory role by interacting with dendritic cells, macrophages, endothelial cells, and T cells. NK cells can thus limit or exacerbate immune responses. NK cells have the ability to distinguish the normal host cells through the killer cell immunoglobulin-like receptor (KIR) and CD94-NKG2A inhibitory receptors which recognize the Major histocompatibility complex (MHC) class I expressed on the surface of these normal cells. The binding of these receptors inhibits lysis and cytokine secretion by NK cells. In addition, NK cells have granules with perforins and granzymes that act on target cells inducing lysis or apoptosis and also express PRRs including TLR-2, -3, -4, -5, -7, and -8. Once activated, NK cells secrete interferon (IFN)-γ, tumor necrosis factor (TNF)-α growth factors, interleukin (IL)-5, IL-10, IL-13, and chemokines.

7. Which are the subsets and functions of innate lymphoid cells?

Innate lymphoid cells (ILCs) were described as a branch of lymphoid lineage. They reside in tissues and are found in abundance in the intestinal lamina propria.

ILCs have been categorized into five subsets on the basis of their developmental pathways. In addition to NK cells and lymphoid tissue inducer cells, these are ILC1, ILC2, and ILC3. The characterization of the three ILC subsets was based on their cytokine production profile. ILC1 subset depends on the transcription factor T-bet, but not eomesodermin (EOMES) and, as well as NK cells, produces interferon (IFN)-γ and is non-cytotoxic; ILC2 depends on GATA-binding protein 3 (GATA3) and produces IL-4, IL-5, and IL-13; and ILC3 depends on retinoic acid receptor-related orphan receptor-γt (RORγt), and comprises subsets that can be distinguished on the basis of expression of the natural cytotoxicity receptors NKp46 (also known as NCR1) and NKp44 (also known as NCR2) and produces IL-17 and IL-22. Thus, their cytokine profile is similar to cytokine profiles of T helper (Th)1, Th2, and Th17/22 lymphocytes. Unlike T and B cells, ILCs do not express antigen-specific receptors derived from recombination-activating gene (RAG)-dependent gene rearrangements but are activated by cytokines produced by other innate immune cells as well as epithelial cells. ILCs exist in three differentiation stages as immature, naive, and primed. The immature ILCs express the CD5 molecule, the naive ILCs express the CD45RA molecule, while the primed ILCs express the CD45RO molecule. The ILC subsets have a huge plasticity with the ability to change phenotype and function according to the signals they encounter in the tissue they reside. The ILCs in addition to their traditional function as antimicrobial cell population play a significant role in maintaining tissue homeostasis and in regulating metabolic processes.

8. Which are the maturation, differentiation, and function of human mast cells?

Mast cells develop in the bone marrow but migrate as immature precursors that mature in peripheral tissues, especially in the skin, the intestines, and the mucosae of the airways. This cell population is part of the first-line host defense against pathogens that enter the body across epithelial barriers. They are also involved in IgE-mediated allergic responses, since they carry a high-affinity Fc receptor for IgE immunoglobulin but remain inactive until at least two molecules of surface IgE will be cross-linked by binding the antigenic determinants of an allergen.

Mast cells are thought to serve at least three important functions in host defense. First, due to their location near body surfaces, they are able to recruit antigen-specific lymphocytes and non-specific effector cells, such as neutrophils, macrophages, basophils, and eosinophils, to sites where infectious agents are most likely to be encountered by the host. Second, by recruiting inflammatory cells, they cause intense inflammation which results in increasing the flow of lymph from sites of infection to the regional lymph nodes, where naive lymphocytes are first activated. Third, mast cell-derived leukotrienes (LTs) such as LTC4, LTD4, and LTE4 trigger muscular contraction and contribute to the physical elimination of pathogens from the lungs or the gut.

9. Which mediators are released from human mast cells?

- Reactive oxygen species (ROS)
- Preformed mediators stocked in their granules: serine proteases (chymase and tryptase), histamine, heparin, serotonin, and ATP
- Lysosomal enzymes: β-hexosaminidase, β-glucuronidase, and arylsulfatases
- Newly formed lipid mediators (eicosanoids): prostaglandin D2, leukotriene C4, thromboxane, and platelet-activating factor (PAF)
- Cytokines: Tumor necrosis factor-α (TNF-α) and IL-1β, basic fibroblast growth factor (BFGF), stem cell factor (SCF), IL-4, and chemokines

10. Which are the complement proteins, their production and function?

The complement system includes over 30 proteins and/or protein fragments. These proteins or their fragments are in the serum, serosal cavities, and cell membranes. They are generally synthesized by the liver and normally circulate as inactive precursors (pro-proteins). They constitute around 10% of the serum γ-globulins.

At sites of infection or inflammation, the complement system is sequentially activated through an enzyme-triggered cascade. The complement system, in order to perform its actions, is activated on large surfaces such as pathogen walls or large immune complexes, through three different ways: the *classical*, the *alternative*, and the *lectin pathways*. These pathways depend on different molecules for their initiation:

- The *classical* pathway involves complement components C1, C2, and C4 and is activated from antigen-antibody complexes binding to C1, which itself has three subcomponents C1q, C1r, and C1s. The pathway forms a C3 convertase (C4b2a), which splits C3 into two fragments: C3b (attaches to the surface of microbial pathogens and opsonizes them) and C3a (activates mast cells to release vasoactive substances such as histamine)
- The *alternative* complement pathway is activated by lipopolysaccharides on microbial cell surfaces in the absence of an antibody. It can also be triggered by foreign materials and damaged tissues. IgA complexes and the C3 nephritic factor (an autoantibody of C3 convertase) can also activate this pathway. It involves different factors (B, D, H, and I) that interact with each other and with C3b, to form a C3 convertase (C3bBb), which in turn activates more C3, leading to an amplification loop
- The *lectin* pathway is activated by the binding of mannose-binding lectin (MBL) to mannose residues on the pathogen surface. This further activates MBL-associated serine proteases, which activate C4 and C2, to form a C3 convertase (C4b2a)
- The final *lytic* pathway is initiated by the splitting of C5 into C5b. C6, C7, C8, and C9 unite with C5b forming the membrane attack complex (MAC), a multimolecular structure that inserts into the membrane creating a functional pore leading to cell lysis

11. When do antibody complexes lead to complement activation?

Large complexes are formed in great antibody excess and are rapidly removed from the circulation by the mononuclear phagocyte system and are therefore relatively harmless. The pathogenic complexes are of small or intermediate size (formed in slight antigen excess), which bind less avidly to phagocytic cells and therefore circulate longer. The mononuclear phagocyte system normally filters out the circulating immune complexes. Persistence of immune complexes in the circulation and increased tissue deposition occurs when macrophages are overloaded or have an intrinsic dysfunction. In addition, several other factors, such as charge of the immune complexes (anionic versus cationic), valence of the antigen, avidity of the antibody, affinity of the antigen to various tissue components, three-dimensional (lattice) structure of the complexes, and hemodynamic factors, influence the tissue deposition of complexes. A number of antibody-intrinsic factors are known to impact the ability of a given immunoglobulin to exhibit Antibody-Mediated Complement Activation (AMCA). The four subclasses of IgG (IgG1, IgG2, IgG3, and IgG4) display distinct complement activation profiles. In general, IgG1 and IgG3 are considered to be the most efficient activators, while IgG2 can be weakly activating, and IgG4 is often considered to be somewhat incapable of driving complement activation. Additionally, IgG Fc domains contain a conserved N-linked glycan in the vicinity of the C1q binding interface, which is required for efficient C1 activation.

12. Which are the key regulators of the complement system?

- C1 inhibitor: inactivates the proteases that associate with the recognition molecules of the *classical* and *lectin* pathways
- Complement receptor type 1 (CR1) (also referred to as CD35): is a membrane-bound complement inhibitor that can facilitate C3b/C4b degradation
- C4bBP: blocks the formation of C3 convertase in the *classical* pathway

- Membrane cofactor protein: blocks C3 convertase in both *classical* and *alternative* pathways
- Decay-accelerating factor: is anchored on cell membranes and promotes C3 convertase dissociation in both *classical* and *alternative* pathways
- Factor H: is the main regulator of the activity of the *alternative* complement pathway. Together with its splice variant factor H-like protein 1 (FHL-1), it inhibits complement activation at the level of the central C3b molecule, thus also blocks the amplification loop and the terminal pathway

13. Which one of the activated complement components acts as vasodilator and which as chemoattractant?

Proteins C3a, C4a, and C5a act as "anaphylatoxins." They can trigger the degranulation of mast cells and basophils to release histamine resulting in increased vascular permeability and augmented inflammation. In addition, C5a is a powerful chemoattractant for neutrophils and stimulates their degranulation. C5a and C3a also upregulate adhesion molecule expression on endothelial cells.

14. What is opsonization?

Opsonization is an immune process through which specific IgG antibodies or the C3b complement component (acting as an opsonin) bind to the surface of the foreign invader or the necrotic parts of host cells and the complex is being uptaken from the phagocytes through their Fc or C3b receptors (Fig. 1.1).

15. Which cells can act as antigen-presenting cells (APCs)?

Macrophages, dendritic cells, and B lymphocytes can act as professional APCs. The expression of MHC class II molecules along with co-stimulatory molecules and pattern recognition receptors (PRRs) is a defining feature of professional APCs. The non-professional APCs include

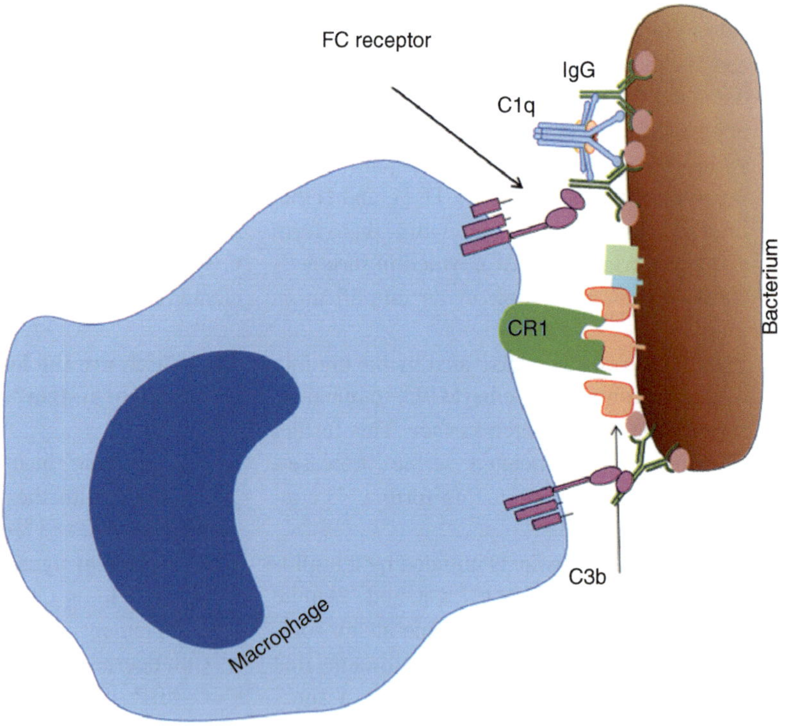

Fig. 1.1 Opsonization: Bacteria opsonized by immunoglobulins and C3b complement component are phagocytosed when the Fc portion of antibody and C3b bind to their receptors on the surface of phagocytes (*Figure created by Professor Panayiotis G. Vlachoyiannopoulos, MD*)

all nucleated cell types in the body and typically express MHC class I molecules. However, it has been observed that antigen presentation to $CD4^+$ cells via MHC class II is not restricted to the classically professional APCs. Other leukocytes, including granulocytes, such as mast cells and neutrophils, can be induced to do so, as can endothelial and epithelial cells under certain circumstances, especially in autoimmunity.

16. What are the different subsets of monocytes?

Monocytes are innate blood cells that maintain vascular homeostasis and are early responders to pathogens in acute infections. There are three well-characterized classes of monocytes: classical ($CD14^+CD16^-$), intermediate ($CD14^+CD16^+$), and non-classical ($CD14^-CD16^+$). Classical monocytes are critical for the initial inflammatory response, can differentiate into macrophages in tissues and can contribute to chronic disease. Intermediate monocytes are highly phagocytic cells that produce high levels of reactive oxygen species (ROS) and inflammatory mediators. Non-classical monocytes have been widely viewed as anti-inflammatory, as they maintain vascular homeostasis and constitute a first line of defense in recognition and clearance of pathogens.

17. What are neutrophil extracellular traps?

Upon interaction with an invading microbe or cytokine discharge (IL-1β, TNFα, and IL-8), neutrophils release their chromatin material together with a wide range of granular enzymes to form net-like structures known as neutrophil extracellular traps (NETs). NETs cannot only trap the invading pathogen but also degrade them with NET-associated proteolytic enzymes. NETs accelerate the inflammatory processes by releasing a wide range of active molecules like danger-associated molecular patterns (DAMPs), histones, as well as active lytic enzymes in extracellular space, leading to further immune responses. Several of the molecules forming the NETs (e.g., myeloperoxidase, double-stranded DNA, and histones) serve as autoantigens in systemic autoimmune diseases such as anti-neutrophil cytoplasmic antigen (ANCA)-positive vasculitis and systemic lupus erythematosus (SLE). Thus, several groups have proposed that in predisposed individuals aberrant NET formation plays a role in the generation of autoimmune responses. This hypothesis is supported by the observation that initiation or exacerbation of autoimmune responses often occurs following microbial infections.

18. How is tumor progression locus 2 (TPL2) kinase implicated in controlling inflammation?

TPL2 is a mitogen-activated protein kinase (MAP3K). Recent evidence suggests that TPL2 positively regulates the isoforms p38α and p38δ of p38 MAPK on neutrophils.

p38 MAPK is a ubiquitous protein kinase that plays an important role in the inflammatory response. Stimulation of inflammatory cells, such as neutrophils, macrophages, and T lymphocytes, leads ultimately to a cascade of protein phosphorylation resulting in phosphorylation of p38. Phosphorylated p38 in turn causes production and secretion of pro-inflammatory cytokines such as interleukin 1β (IL-1β) and tumor necrosis factor-alpha (TNF-α).

In the absence of TLP2, macrophages have impaired production of inflammatory mediators such as IL-1β, TNF-α, IL-6, and IL-10. TLP2 has been shown to facilitate the migration of neutrophils into inflamed sites. In neutrophils, pharmacological inhibition of TPL2 selectively inhibits pro-inflammatory cytokines and chemokines via the MAPK and p38 pathways. In addition, TPL2 signaling is linked to the regulation of the adaptive immune system. In TPL2 knockout mice, it has been seen that TPL2 plays a role in Th1 differentiation and regulation of the inflammatory response in a T cell transfer model of colitis. TPL2 is also needed for MAPK signaling in B cells mediated by CD40 and/or BCR stimulation, which is important for immunoglobulin production.

19. Which cell populations express the human leukocyte antigen (HLA) class I alloantigens and which the HLA class II?

HLA class I molecules: are expressed on nearly all nucleated cells of the body. The antigens they present are peptide fragments endogenous to the cytoplasm of the cells expressing the MHC molecule, and they present them to $CD8^+$ T cells. The resultant T-cell response is cell-mediated killing or suppression of the MHC class I-presenting cell. Dendritic cells (DCs) and macrophages, can present exogenous antigens on MHC-I in a process called cross-presentation. This pathway plays a key role in antimicrobial and antitumor immunity, and also in immune tolerance.

HLA class II molecules: are expressed on professional APCs such as DCs, B cells, monocytes/macrophages, and any other activated APCs. In humans, HLA-DR, HLA-DQ, and HLA-DP molecules are the three classical and highly polymorphic MHC-II molecules. The antigens they present are peptide fragments present in lysosomal compartments as a result of phagocytosis or receptor-mediated endocytosis (e.g., bacterial material), and they present them to $CD4^+$ helper T cells. The resultant T-cell response is phagocytic and/or antibody response to eradicate the antigen presented.

20. Which are the components of the adaptive immune system?

Main components of the adaptive immune system are two subsets of leukocytes; the T and B lymphocytes. B cells and T cells are derived from the same multipotent hematopoietic stem cells and are morphologically indistinguishable from one another until after they are activated. These cell populations constitute the 20–40% of white blood cells (WBCs); their total mass is about the same with that of the brain or the liver. The majority of lymphocytes are in the lymphoid organs and in the tissues. B lymphocytes, through their products, the immunoglobulins, play a major role in humoral immune responses and can also function as APCs. T lymphocytes are the major players in cell-mediated immune responses. The adaptive immune response is relatively slow yet highly specific, and additionally it creates immunological memory; in other words, after an initial response to a specific pathogen, the next encounter with the same antigen leads to an enhanced response to that antigen.

21. Which are the steps of T-lymphocyte maturation and differentiation?

T lymphocytes mature and differentiate in the thymus during an antigen-independent stage and later in the peripheral lymphoid organs during an antigen-dependent stage. Distinct stages of maturation and differentiation of T cells in the thymus are marked by the presence of surface molecules, namely, T-cell antigen receptor, CD3 protein complex (which acts as an adaptor to T-cell receptor), and the co-receptors, CD4, and CD8. More details on the developmental stages of T cells are the following:

(a) Upon arrival from the bone marrow, T cells are negative for the T-cell antigen receptor and also negative for CD3, CD4, and CD8 surface molecules; these are called "double-negative T cells" or "double-negative thymocytes." These T cells are still pluripotent
(b) The double-negative thymocytes give rise to two different cell populations that can be distinguished from each other on the basis of the type of T-cell antigen receptor: the $CD3^+$ $CD4^-CD8^-\gamma\delta$ T cells, which are a minority; these cells possess a T-cell receptor constituted of γ- and δ-chains (the repertoire of these chains is limited); however, the majority of thymocytes become $CD3^+$ $CD4^+$ $CD8^+\alpha\beta$ T cells ("double-positive" αβ T cells)
(c) The $CD3^+$ $CD4^-CD8^-\gamma\delta$ T cells move to the mucosal tissues. The double-positive αβ T cells remain in the thymus, enlarge, and continue to divide
(d) The large double-positive αβ T cells undergo a stage of small, resting double-positive αβ T cells. These cells initially express low levels of αβ T-cell antigen receptors. Most of these

cells fail to recognize molecular complexes constituted of self-peptides bound to self-MHCs, and they die in the thymus. This process is called “positive selection”

(e) The small double-positive αβ T cells whose receptors recognize molecular complexes constituted of self-peptides bound to self-MHCs (“positively selected” cells), lose either the CD4 or the CD8 co-receptors, and become “single-positive αβ T cells”

(f) During the double-positive stage, but also after that, thymocytes which recognize with high-affinity molecular complexes of self-peptides bound to self-MHCs die, and the surviving cells are capable of responding to foreign antigens. This process is called “negative selection”

(g) At this stage rearrangement of α-chain locus begins and the level of expression, and the repertoire of surface αβ T-cell receptor increases. Thymocytes are now either $CD3^+$ $CD4^+$ $CD8^-$αβ T cells or $CD3^+$ $CD8^+$ $CD4^-$αβ T cells, which continue to mature inside the thymus for a while and then exit to periphery. These cells are called naive cells since they have not yet recognized an antigen

(h) Upon recognition of foreign antigen in peripheral lymphoid organs, $CD4^+$, as well as $CD8^+$T cells, are differentiated to effector T cells; these are capable of leaving peripheral lymphoid organs and act within tissues

22. Which are the main subsets and functions of T lymphocytes?

T-lymphocyte subsets are:

(a) *$CD3^+$ $CD4^-$ $CD8^-$ γδ T cells* home to mucosal tissues. They serve as an early-stage defense mechanism in mucosal surfaces. The actual diversity of γδ T-cell receptor is very limited. They are triggered by alarm signals such as heat shock proteins and several metabolites of pathogenic bacteria. Some subsets of $CD3^+CD4^-CD8^-$ γδ T cells do not require antigen presentation through MHC, resembling thus cells of the innate immune system. Yet, they have functions, particularly related to tissue homeostasis and wound healing

(b) *$CD8^+$ T cells*. These cells are also called “cytotoxic T lymphocytes (CTLs).” They recognize cells infected by viruses (target cells). The target cells express MHC class I molecules in complex with viral antigens. CTLs kill them through a process called apoptosis. $CD8^+$ T cells in order to kill the target cell and reduce the burden of virus, release molecules such as perforins, granzymes, interferon-γ (IFN-γ), and tumor necrosis factor-α (TNF-α) and express on their surface Fas ligand (Fas-L). Perforins are molecules which penetrate the membrane of infected cells; they are polymerized making holes in the membrane, while granzymes pass through these holes and enter the target cell; within the target cell, granzymes activate the caspase cascade, which eventually leads to programmed cell death known as “apoptosis”

(c) *T helper (Th) 1 cells*. They recognize foreign antigens in complex with MHC class II molecules expressed on the surfaces of professional antigen-presenting cells (APCs). These cells contribute to killing of exclusively intracellular pathogens, such as bacteria entrapped into the phagosomes (*Mycobacterium tuberculosis* is a paradigm), as well as some viruses. The differentiation of naive T cells to Th1 phenotype is controlled by the cytokine interleukin (IL)-12. Cytokine signals combined with recognition of foreign antigens drive Th1 cells to secrete IFN-γ. IFN-γ will stimulate phagocytes to fuse the phagosomes with the lysosomes making the so-called phagolysosomes and thus destroy intracellular parasites

(d) *Th2 cells*. They primarily stimulate immune responses against extracellular pathogens but also contribute to allergic reactions through stimulation of B cells. They provide help to certain B cells in order to produce IgE antibodies. They also secrete IL-4 and IL-13. Differentiation of Th2 cells largely depends on APCs which produce IL-4 that differentiates naive T cells to the Th2 phenotype

(e) *Regulatory T cells (T_{regs})*. These cells are generated when naive cells encounter antigen presented by cells that release transforming growth factor-β (TGF-β). These cells produce also TGF-β and IL-10 and downregulate immune responses. T_{regs} express cytotoxic T-lymphocyte-associated protein 4 (CTLA-4) and CD25 molecules on their surface as well as the intracellular protein FOXP3, which is a transcription factor

(f) *Th17 cells*. These cells secrete IL-17, IL-22, and Granulocyte-macrophage colony-stimulating factor (GM-CSF). They participate in surveillance of fungi and extracellular bacteria as well as in the maintenance of barrier integrity. However, Th17 cells can become a pro-inflammatory cell subpopulation. Th17 cells are generated by $CD4^+$ naive T lymphocytes when they recognize an antigen expressed by a dendritic cell that produces TGF-β and IL-6. In addition to IL-6 and TGF-β, they are also stimulated by the cytokines IL-23 and IL-1β. Th17 cells contribute to autoinflammatory diseases such as rheumatoid arthritis, systemic lupus erythematosus, psoriasis, and multiple sclerosis

(g) *T follicular helper (T_{fh}) cells*. These are $CD4^+$ T cells found within B-cell follicles of secondary lymphoid organs. T_{fh} cells are identified by their B-cell follicle-homing receptor CXCR5, which is constitutively expressed on their surface. T_{fh} cells express CD40L and secrete IL-21 and IL-4. Using the above molecules, T_{fh} cells trigger the formation and maintenance of germinal centers and contribute to the differentiation of antigen-stimulated B cells to plasma cells in order to enhance antibody production

(h) *Th9 cells*. Th9 cells, a subset initially associated with the Th2 phenotype, are the primary source of IL-9. The production of IL-9 in Th9 cells is stimulated by TGFβ and IL-4 and inhibited by IFN-γ. The production of IL-9 requires transcription factors that include STAT6 (signal transducer and activator of transcription 6), PU.1, IRF4 (interferon response factor 4), and GATA3. Th9 cells promote inflammation in a variety of models but seem to be particularly capable of promoting allergic inflammation. Some of the effects of Th9 cells could be mediated through mast cells, but others are likely direct effects on tissue-resident cells

(i) *Th22 cells*. Th22 cells are unique in that they express IL-22 but not IL-17 and IFN-γ, and express the master transcription factor aryl hydrocarbon receptor. In addition to the production of IL-22, Th22 cells are characterized by surface expression of the chemokine receptors CCR4, CCR6, and CCR10 that are associated with cutaneous T cell homing. The major known functions of IL-22 are to regulate innate defense programs (e.g., antibacterial protein production), induce chemokine production, inhibit differentiation of some epithelial cells in the gastrointestinal and respiratory tracts, and stimulate tissue remodeling (Fig. 1.2)

23. What are MAIT cells?

Mucosal-associated invariant T (MAIT) cells are unconventional T cells that recognize microbial riboflavin-derivative antigens presented by the major histocompatibility complex (MHC) class I-like protein MR1. MAIT cells use a limited T cell antigen receptor (TCR) repertoire with public antigen specificities that are conserved across species. They can be activated by TCR-dependent and TCR-independent mechanisms and exhibit rapid, innate-like effector responses. In humans, peripheral MAIT cells are predominantly $CD8^+$ (~80%) or double negative (~20%) with a minor CD4-expressing population (~1%). MAIT cells are universally $CD161^{hi}$ (KLRB1, a C-type lectin-like receptor) and $CD26^{hi}$ (DPP4). The functioning of MAIT cells includes the potential for cytotoxicity, but they are especially known for their potent cytokine response. Stimulated MAIT cells rapidly release TNF, IFN-ɣ, and IL-17, but most studies have reported that they do not produce Th2 cytokines.

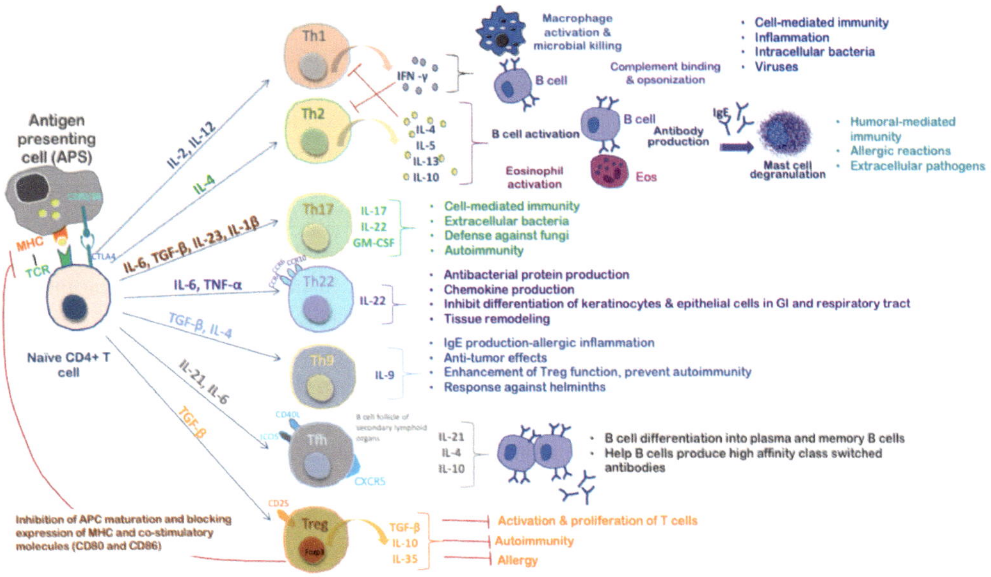

Fig. 1.2 Naïve CD4^{+} T cells, after antigen presentation, depending on the cytokine milieu, differentiate to distinct types of T helper (Th) cells. Each of these subsets of Th cells has different functions implicated in adaptive immune responses. On the other hand, regulatory T (T_{reg}) cells use several mechanisms to suppress the activation, proliferation, and cytokine production of T cells thereby promoting homeostasis and self-tolerance, essential for preventing autoimmunity (*Figure created by Evangelia Zampeli, MD*)

24. What are exhausted T lymphocytes?

Exhausted T cells (T_{ex}) are characterized by progressive loss of effector functions, high and sustained inhibitory receptor expression, metabolic dysregulation, poor memory recall and homeostatic self-renewal, and distinct transcriptional and epigenetic programs. Therefore, T_{ex} are distinct from effector (T_{eff}) and memory (T_{mem}) T cells. The development of T cell exhaustion is driven by persistent antigen stimulation, altered co-stimulation versus co-inhibition by cell surface receptors, and chronic inflammation. A sustained high expression of inhibitory receptors is a key feature of T_{ex} cells. T_{ex} cells can be, at least partially, reinvigorated through inhibitory receptor blockade, such as anti-Programmed cell death protein 1 (PD-1), and/or stimulating T cells using exhaustion-antagonizing soluble molecules such as cytokines. Although exhaustion has been best studied for CD8^{+} T cells, exhaustion can also occur in CD4^{+} T cells.

25. Which are the B-lymphocyte subsets and their functions?

B-lymphocyte subsets are as follows:

Transitional B cells (Tr B cells) represent a crucial link between immature B cells in the bone marrow and mature peripheral B cells. They are present in human bone marrow, peripheral blood, cord blood, and secondary lymphoid tissues. Accumulating evidence has suggested Tr B cells to be part of the integrated immune system. Since they are associated with several inflammatory diseases and are also found in circulation as well as tissues of healthy individuals, Tr B cells are thought to perform distinct functions in immune defense mechanisms including regulatory functions. BCR-mediated negative selection occurs at the T1 B cell stage, which serves to remove the self-reactive B cells; the remaining T1 B cells give rise to the late transitional B cells (T2/T3 B cells). These gradually develop into naïve follicular mature (FM) or marginal zone (MZ) B cells and eventually into mature naïve B cells.

Follicular B cells constitute the majority of B cells in the blood, lymph node, and spleen and are antibody-producing cells with a great array of specificities. They express surface immunoglobulins with a highly diverse array of specificities; they express also Fc receptors, MHC class II, as well as the surface molecules CD19 (a cell surface molecule in close junction with B-cell antigen receptor which decreases the threshold for antigen receptor-dependent stimulation) and CD23 (also known as FcεRII—a low-affinity receptor for IgE).

Marginal zone B cells constitute the minority of B cells in the blood, lymph nodes, and spleen and are also antibody-producing cells; they serve as the first line of defense against blood-borne pathogens, which reach the marginal zones through the circulation. They express surface immunoglobulin with limited receptor repertoire. These cells exhibit mainly antigen-independent stimulation, but they are also capable of undergoing antigen-dependent stimulation.

B-1 cells predominantly reside in the peritoneal and pleural cavity, produce natural antibodies, and exhibit T cell-independent activation. B-1 cells have been described in mice, and they overlap partially with $CD5^+$ B cells. B-1 cells have not been described in humans, but $CD5^+$ B cells exist. CD5 is a protein which reduces the severity of the activating signals derived from the B-cell receptors and makes B-1 cells to be activated by exogenous strong signals and not by signals derived from autologous tissues.

Regulatory B cells stop the expansion of pro-inflammatory lymphocytes through the secretion of IL-10, IL-35, and TGF-β while they promote the generation of T_{regs}. The specificity of regulatory B cells and the exact way they differentiate are not known.

Age-associated B cells (ABCs) are a novel B lymphocyte subset whose numbers increase continuously with age and are refractory to B cell receptor (BCR) ligation but activated by TLR7 or TLR9 signals. ABCs can be generated from naive follicular B cells and possibly other pre-immune B cell subsets, such as marginal zone, B1, and transitional B cells. Their differentiation requires TLR9 or TLR7 signals in the context of Th1 cytokines, particularly IFN-γ and IL-21. In contrast, Th2 cytokines such as IL-4 can impede ABC differentiation. ABCs contribute to immunological features of aging, including damped B cell genesis, altered immune responses to both primary and recall antigen challenges, and an increasing overall inflammatory climate. ABCs are elevated in autoimmune and autoinflammatory diseases (Fig. 1.3).

26. Which are the maturation and differentiation steps of B lymphocytes? Which stage is antigen independent and which one is antigen dependent? What is antibody class switching and how is it achieved by B cells?

The stages of maturation and differentiation of B lymphocytes (Fig. 1.3) are recognized by (a) distinct cell surface markers, (b) a specific pattern of immunoglobulin gene expression, and (c) cytoplasmic expression of transcription factors.

Pro-B cells express CD19 and CD10 surface molecules, while they retain the CD43 surface molecule expressed during the stem cell stage. CD43 is a transmembrane cell surface sialoglycoprotein on cells from hematologic lineage and contributes to ligand–receptor-induced T-cell activation. CD10 is a zinc-dependent metalloproteinase that cleaves and inactivates several hormones. During this stage, initiation of the expression of Rag-1 and Rag-2 (recombination-activating gene) proteins and the first recombination of immunoglobulin genes at the heavy-chain locus involving the D-J segment rearrangement take place. Rag-1 and Rag-2 proteins are important factors for the V-D-J rearrangement of immunoglobulin genes. The terminal deoxynucleotidyl transferase (TdT) that catalyzes the non-templated addition of junctional N nucleotides is also mainly expressed during the pro-B stage. Finally, the first C μ-exon of the C locus of the immunoglobulin heavy chain is rearranged with the VDJ segment, and a functional mRNA for the

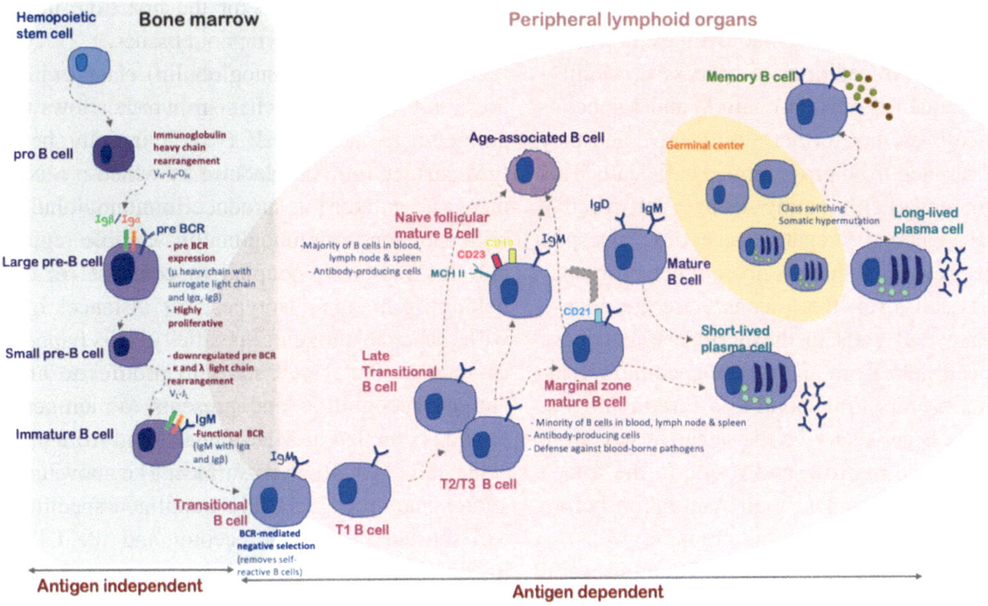

Fig. 1.3 Antigen-independent and antigen-dependent B cell developmental stages generating the distinct B lymphocyte subsets (*Figure created by Evangelia Zampeli, MD*)

heavy μ-chain is produced and translated to immunoglobulin μ-heavy chain. Only cells that achieve heavy-chain gene rearrangements survive. Pro-B cells do not respond to antigen.

Pre-B cells are the cells which have achieved a productive immunoglobulin μ-gene rearrangement. These cells express immunoglobulin μ-chain on their surface, but they have not rearranged gene segments of the immunoglobulin light chain. The immunoglobulin μ-chain is covalently linked to surrogate light chains, which are invariant; that means they are the same in all pre-B cells. Pre-B cells synthesize also the Igα and Igβ chains of the B-cell receptor. Pre-B cells undergo tremendous proliferation and expansion of thc B-ccll lineage. The signal for proliferation is not known, but this is probably the process of linking of the surrogate light chains to the immunoglobulin μ-chain. Activation of pre-B cell receptor leads to activation of Bruton's tyrosine kinase (BTK) which delivers signals for survival, proliferation, and maturation of pre-B cells, as well as of the B cells existing beyond this stage. At the pre-B-cell stage, three additional phenomena take place: (a) allelic exclusion, which means any individual B cell expresses an immunoglobulin heavy-chain protein encoded only by one of the two inherited alleles, (b) stimulation of the κ-light-chain recombination, and (c) discontinuation of the surrogate light-chain transcription. Pre-B cell expresses also two surface markers, the CD43 protein (presented previously) as well as the CD220 protein—an insulin receptor with tyrosine protein kinase activity.

Immature B cells: these cells have already rearranged a κ-light-chain gene, and the κ-light chain associates with the μ-protein; thus, immature B cells express fully assembled IgM immunoglobulin linked to the Igα and Igβ chains of the B-cell receptor, on their surface. Production of κ-protein prevents λ-rearrangement; therefore, λ-rearrangement occurs only in case κ-rearrangement was not productive. This phenomenon is called "light-chain isotype exclusion." If both alleles of κ- and λ-chains fail to rearrange successfully, the B cell will die. The *RAG* gene expression is discontinued, and the cell prevents further rearrangement of the immunoglobulin genes. Immature B cells do not respond to antigens. In case their receptors bind strongly to multivalent antigens in the bone marrow, the cells will die or sometimes they may undergo receptor editing—a process of modifying the sequence of light-chain V and J genes—so the cells are not further autoreactive and they can be rescued from programmed cell death. This phenomenon of eliminating strongly self-reactive B cells is called "negative selection." Despite negative selection, there is no complete tolerance at the B-cell level; that means there are always autoreactive B cells in the periphery, but these cells need help from an antigen-specific T lymphocyte in order to respond to a certain antigen. Immature B cells survive the negative selection, leave the bone marrow, and reside in the spleen for a while to complete their maturation before reaching peripheral lymphoid organs.

Mature B cells: these cells divide into several subsets as described previously: follicular B cells, marginal zone B cells, B1/CD5$^+$ B cells, regulatory B cells, and age-associated B cells (ABCs).

Mature B cells that belong to the follicular B-cell subset produce high levels of IgM as well as IgD immunoglobulin using the same VDJ exon and the same κ- or λ-chain to express IgM and IgD surface receptors with the same antigenic specificity. These cells still have not encountered an antigen but have the armamentarium to respond to antigen and are called "mature-naive B cells." Follicular B cells receive survival signals delivered by BAFF (called also BLyS) (B-cell activator or B-lymphocyte stimulator).

Marginal zone B cells are similar to B-1 cells described in mice; they express IgM and the CD21, which is the complement C3d receptor, identical to Epstein-Barr virus receptor. Unlike to what happens in mice, CD5$^+$ B cells in humans reside in both the spleen and the lymph nodes.

The stages of maturation of pro-B cells and pre-B cells are antigen independent. One could consider the negative selection observed at the immature B-cell stage as antigen dependent since these cells mature by encountering self-antigens in the bone marrow. However, immunologists agree that the word "antigen" in this context is used for exogenous antigens. Therefore, antigen dependent is only the maturation of naive B cells as soon as they encounter antigens for the first time in the lymph nodes or other lymphoid tissues.

Antibody (or immunoglobulin) class switching is a biological mechanism which allows the antigen-activated B cell (which initially bears IgM surface immunoglobulin by which it recognizes the antigen), to produce immunoglobulins with the same immunoglobulin variable region, but this region is coupled to constant regions belonging to other isotypes, for instance, IgG, with the same antigenic specificity. This happens as soon as the B cell starts to proliferate after antigen recognition and presents (a) antigenic peptides coupled to MHC class II and (b) a molecule called CD40 on its surface. The above constituents are recognized by an antigen-specific T cell through its T-cell receptor and the CD40 ligand, respectively. T cell then releases a mixture of IL-4 and IL-5 which regulates immunoglobulin class switching by the B cell.

27. In which stages of B-lymphocyte maturation and differentiation is the CD20 molecule expressed?

The CD20 molecule is expressed on the surface of late pro-B cells and continues to be expressed through all the stages of B-cell development (pre-B, immature B, mature B cells, as well as memory B cells) but not in plasmablasts or in plasma cells. Plasmablasts are immature plasma cells, and plasma cells are the effector B cells, which have been transformed into antibody-producing cells.

28. Which initial observations led to the postulation that antibodies are generated by "constant" and "variant" genes?

Analysis of amino acid sequence of various immunoglobulins, nearly 50 years ago, revealed that many antibodies of the same isotype shared identical sequences at their C-terminal ends, but they varied considerably at their N-terminal ends, which, as we know today, correspond to the antigen-binding sites of antibodies. This finding led to the postulation that each antibody chain is encoded by at least two genes, one for the "constant" and one for the "variant" region and these genes are combined at the DNA or RNA level constituting a "new" gene. DNA analysis in various tissues using markers of the "variant" (V) and "constant" (C) region revealed that in cells of any other origin except B lymphocytes, these regions were far away from each other within the genome and only in the B-cell DNA the V and C regions were closed, implying that during B-cell maturation and differentiation, a rearrangement of the immunoglobulin genes takes place and V and D regions are physically joint and translated to protein.

29. Which is the organization of immunoglobulin genes and what are the mechanisms for gene rearrangement for the production of the entire immunoglobulin chains? (Fig. 1.4)

We know today that three separate loci encode the immunoglobulin gene segments as follows: one locus for all the heavy-chain gene segments (located on chromosome 14), one for the κ-light-chain gene segments (located on chromosome 2), and one for λ-light-chain gene segments (located on chromosome 22). Gene segments lie in series at each locus from the 5′ end to 3′ end, encoding the variable (V) regions; at the 3′ end of the series of the V gene segments, there are series of gene segments encoding the so-called diversity region (D); at the 3′ end of them lie a series of gene segments encoding the so-called joining region (J); and at the 3′ end of them lie a series of gene segments encoding the constant region (C). Light chains lack D regions, but their gene segments are organized

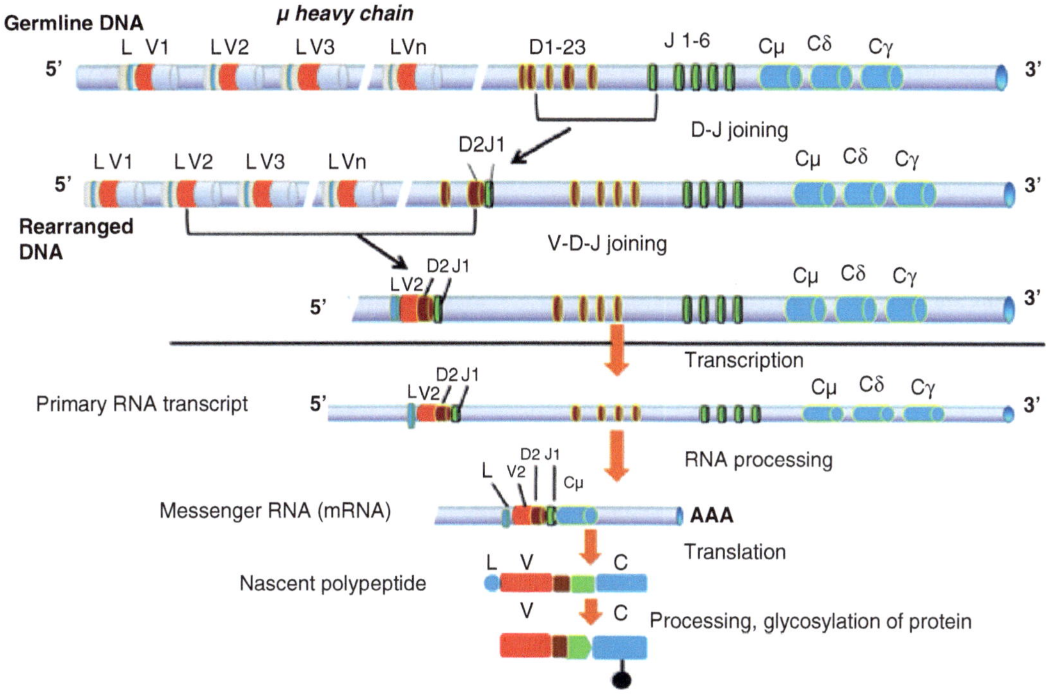

Fig. 1.4 Organization of immunoglobulin genes and mechanisms for gene rearrangement: The organization of the μ-chain gene segments is presented. Gene segments lie in series from the 5′ end to 3′ end, encoding the variable (V) regions; at the 3′ end of the series of the V gene segments, there are series of gene segments encoding the so-called diversity region (D); at the 3′ end of them lie series of gene segments encoding the so-called joining region (J); and at the 3′ end of them lie series of gene segments encoding the constant region. The VDJ recombination in every individual B cell involves a random selection of one V segment, one D segment (which is absent within the gene segments of the light chains), and one J gene segment to produce the VDJ exon. Therefore, a B cell may rearrange V1D2J2, another B cell may rearrange V2D3J5, etc. Every cell is capable of doing one gene rearrangement for the heavy and one for the light chain. Please note that after the VDJ gene segment rearrangement, the remaining rearrangements are performed at the primary RNA transcript level in order to produce a complete messenger RNA for the entire μ-heavy chain (*Figure created by Professor Panayiotis G. Vlachoyiannopoulos, MD*)

in the same fashion, as that of the heavy chains. The heavy-chain locus contains nearly 45 V gene segments each of about 300 base pairs long, the κ-locus contains 30 V gene segments, and the λ-locus contains 45 V gene segments. The κ-light-chain locus has only one C gene segment, and the λ-light-chain locus has four C gene segments; the heavy-chain locus has nine C gene segments each encoding one immunoglobulin isotype (IgG1, IgG2, IgG3, IgG4, IgA1, IgA2, IgM, IgE, and IgD). Each of the nine C gene segments is composed of five or six exons.

The VDJ recombination in every individual B cell involves a random selection of one V segment, one D segment (which is absent within the gene segments of the light chains), and one J gene segment to produce the VDJ exon. Therefore, a B cell may rearrange V1D2J2, another B cell may rearrange V2D3J5, etc. To complete the antigen-binding site, a VJ rearrangement among the light-chain gene segments should be also performed. Every cell is capable of doing one gene rearrangement for the heavy and one for the light chain; however, by taking together the whole B-cell population, a huge diversity of antigen receptors is generated. The C regions are located downstream of the rearranged VDJ exon (VJ exon for light chains) lying thousands of base pairs away. This part of the DNA is transcribed to RNA; RNA splicing contributes to deletion of the intervening RNA sequences and eventually brings together the VDJ exon (VJ exon for the light chains) with the C region exons; therefore, an mRNA is formed, which can be translated in the ribosomes to a complete immunoglobulin chain.

30. Which is the molecular mechanism through which the gene rearrangement for immunoglobulin production operates?

A thorough understanding of the mechanism of generation of antibody molecules needs to know the following: (a) the nature of recognition signals that drive VDJ recombination, (b) the enzymes involved in this process, and (c) the physical meaning of junctional diversity.

(a) Certain DNA sequences called "recombination signal sequences" (RSSs) are located at the 3′ end of V gene segments, at the 5′ end of each J segment, and at both ends of each D segment. RSSs are highly conserved stretches of seven nucleotides (heptamers) located close to the coding sequence followed by a spacer of 12 or 23 nucleotides also highly conserved; this is followed by a highly conserved stretch of nine nucleotides rich in AT (nonamer). Double-stranded brakes are generated between the heptamer of RSS and the adjacent V, D, or J coding sequence. For the heavy chain, for instance, a DJ recombination occurs first by properly aligning the 3′ end of one D and the 5′ end of one J segment. This happens because two distinct heptamers come to the right position to be aligned with each other in a way that bridges the gap between the two gene segments. The intervening double-stranded DNA is removed in the form of a circular DNA. Same mechanism operates for recombination of the V with the DJ exon

The process of VDJ recombination can be divided into four distinct stages:

- *Synapsis*: this is the phenomenon of bringing together two selected coding segments and their adjacent RSSs by a chromosomal looping process; thus, the coding sequences are held appropriately for a recombination event
- *Cleavage* is the generation of double-stranded brakes at the RSS-coding sequence junctions by enzymatic cleavage. This is implemented by a complex of two enzymes in which one is activated by the other and both act together; these enzymes are the products of the recombination-activating genes 1 and 2 (*RAG-1 and RAG-2*). These enzymes make nicks between coding regions and heptamers in each DNA strand, and the released 3′ OH of the coding end makes a covalent bridge to the phosphodiester bond of the other DNA strand, creating a hairpin
- *Hairpin opening and reprocessing*: the hairpins are opened up by an endonuclease called "Artemis." Mutations of Artemis in mice are

causes of disrupted maturation of B and T cells leading to the generation of mice with severe combined immunodeficiency (SCID). After opening the hairpins, an enzyme called terminal deoxynucleotidyl transferase (TdT) adds bases to broken DNA ends and contributes substantially to a rather extent antibody diversity

- *Joining* is the process of ligation of the open ends of hairpins after TdT-induced processing. This process is called "nonhomologous end joining." Several proteins contribute to this process, such as the proteins Ku70 and Ku80 which recruit to the open DNA ends the catalytic subunit of the enzyme DNA-dependent protein kinase (DNA-PK) which catalyzes a repair process. Mice deficient to DNA-PK are presented with the phenotype of SCID mice

(b) The diversity of B-cell antigen receptors is attributed to two distinct processes: (a) combinatorial diversity which is attributed to the VDJ rearrangements and (b) junctional diversity which is operated by removal or addition of nucleotides at the junctions of the V and D, D and J, and V and J segments, catalyzed by the enzyme TdT as previously described

31. What are immunoglobulin idiotype, idiotope, paratope, and isotype? (Fig. 1.5)

Idiotope is the unique set of antigenic determinants (epitopes) of the variable portion of an antibody.

Paratope is a part of five to ten amino acids of an antibody's variable region which recognizes and binds to an antigen. It contains parts of the antibody's heavy and light chains.

Idiotypes are unique genetically controlled determinants which represent the antigenic specificity of the antibody. The idiotypic determinants are located into the immunoglobulin variable region of both immunoglobulin polypeptide chains.

Isotype defines the class of immunoglobulin, as it is determined by the type of its heavy chain. Immunoglobulin isotypes are IgG1, IgG2, IgG3, IgG4, IgA1, IgA2, IgM, IgE, and IgD. Some authors use also the term "isotype" to differentiate the types of κ- and λ-light chains.

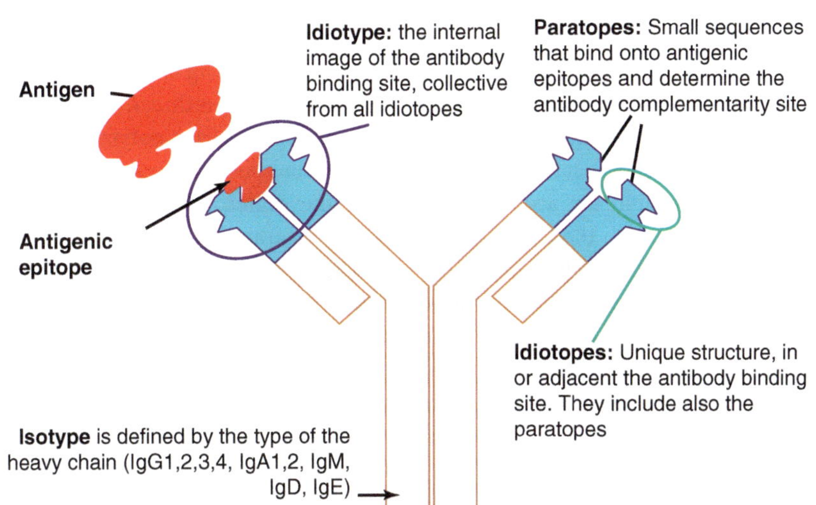

Fig. 1.5 Immunoglobulin idiotype, idiotope, paratope, and isotype: Idiotopes are unique structures in the antibody-binding site or adjacent to this site. The collection of the entire number of idiotopes in a particular site of antibody-binding structure forms the idiotype; therefore, idiotype represents the internal image of the antibody-binding site. Paratopes are small sequences that bind onto antigenic epitopes and determine the antibody complementarity site (*Figure created by Professor Panayiotis G. Vlachoyiannopoulos, MD*)

32. What is the function of the Fc portion of Immunoglobulin?

The Fc portion of immunoglobulins (Igs) contributes to the executive actions of antibodies; these actions are mainly dependent on the fact that many body cells possess receptors for the Ig Fc portion. The Fc functions can be classified as follows:

(a) Transportation of Igs:

- Polymeric IgA and IgM bind through their Fc portions to the polymeric immunoglobulin receptor (pIgR) secretory component, and they are transported across epithelial barriers
- The Fc portion of the maternal IgG binds to the neonatal Fc receptor in the placenta and facilitates IgG transport to the fetus

(b) Opsonization and phagocytosis of bacteria and immune complexes:

- Antibodies bind to bacterial cell wall polysaccharides and/or proteins and activate complement by interacting with the C1q, with the CH2 areas of the heavy Ig chains. Complement activation leads to the generation of C3b, which also binds to bacterial cell wall. This process is called opsonization. Opsonization is followed by bacterial phagocytosis which can be carried out by binding of the Fc portion of antibody and the C3b complement component to appropriate receptors on phagocytes
- Immune complexes enable the accumulation of many antibodies together; the CH2 areas of the heavy Ig chain of the antibodies upon binding to the C1q induce complement activation and generation of C3b; subsequently, the Fc portions of Igs alone with the C3b complement component facilitate phagocytosis of immune complexes as previously described, and eventually immune complexes are destroyed

(c) The Fc portion of antibodies induces cellular signaling by binding to Fc receptors:

- Antibody-coated targets bind to Fc receptors on natural killer (NK) cells and activate these cells in order to destroy the target
- The Fc portion of IgE antibody binds with high affinity to IgE Fc receptors on mast cells and basophils and induces the release of enzymes and vasoactive amines from their granules
- Ig Fc portion through interaction with the appropriate Fc receptors on phagocytes, in addition to bacterial uptake, induces macrophage, neutrophil, and eosinophil signaling leading to activation of the respiratory burst and induction of foreign cell killing
- IgA and IgG which are specific for parasites are important for eosinophil binding via interaction with the eosinophil Fc receptors; then eosinophils then attack and kill parasites, by releasing toxic constituents from their granules. This process is known as "exocytosis"

33. What is the structure of secretory immunoglobulins?

Secreted polymeric immunoglobulins A and M (pIgA and pIgM, respectively) play vital roles in protecting the ~400 m^2 of human mucosa from invasion by pathogens. IgA and IgM contain 18-residue tailpiece extensions on their heavy chains that bestow polymer-forming capabilities. IgM can independently oligomerize to form hexamers, whereas IgA polymerization requires the 137-residue joining chain (JC). The predominant IgA oligomer is a dimer, though a smaller fraction of higher-order polymers up to pentamers have been described. Although less abundant than the dimer, higher-order polymers display better neutralizing capabilities, specifically for low-affinity antigens. The pIgA that is synthesized by mucosal plasma cells undergoes transcytosis, crossing the epithelium to reach the external secretions and perform its protective function. To initiate this process, pIgA binds the ectodomain of basolaterally expressed pIg receptor (pIgR), an interaction that requires the JC and is stabilized through a disulfide bond between the receptor and one Fc. Once bound, the receptor and pIgA undergo transcytosis through the epithelial cell to the mucosa. Upon transcytosis, proteolytic cleavage releases the secretory component (SC) of the receptor, which remains covalently attached to pIgA to form secretory

IgA (sIgA). In this mature form, sIgA performs its antimicrobial, neutralization, and protective functions.

34. In which fraction of proteins do immunoglobulins belong?

Several methods to perform serum or plasma protein fractionation exist. The most useful, easy, reliable, and clinically applicable in everyday medical practice is the serum protein electrophoresis, applied by Tiselius in 1937. Serum is applied to a trough (initiation point) on agarose gel or on a cellulose acetate membrane, and constant current is applied with a cathode to the site of the application of the serum. Serum proteins (which used to be called "globulins") are separated by their size and electrical charge through electrical forces and electroendoosmotic forces. Proteins with negative charges such as albumin migrate to the anode, while proteins with positive charges remain close to the cathode. Using this technique, serum proteins can be fractionated in the following fractions (which are depicted as separate zones in electrophoresis), from the anode to the cathode: albumin, α1 globulins, α2 globulins, β1 globulins, β2 globulins, and γ-globulins.

Immunoglobulins migrate to the area of γ-globulins and in fact constitute a large part of the γ-globulin fraction, which appears as a smooth "blush," or smear, close to the cathode. The majority of immunoglobulin molecules move to the cathode, but some of them move slightly toward the anode, so immunoglobulins occupy both sides of the initiation point. IgG moves toward the cathode and occupies the largest part of the γ-globulin fraction, together with IgM and IgD. However, IgA migrates to the anode and occupies the interzone between β- and γ-globulins as well as the β globulin zone.

35. Based on what markers can lymphocyte populations be characterized as monoclonal?

A monoclonal T- or B-cell population is defined as a collection of cells derived from a single precursor, and therefore, these cells share common characteristics to each other and also to the precursor cell. In addition, monoclonal B or T cells derive from a pull of immature cells, and thus they may express surface molecules known as "clusters of differentiation" (CDs) which are unusual for healthy, mature cells. Light microscopy may also detect monoclonal B and T cells in case these cells possess morphological changes indicating an aggressive, non-regular phenotype. However, all these changes are suggestive of monoclonality, but they are nonconclusive. The following changes or markers—detected by various methods—indicate monoclonality:

Immunopathological methods:

B cells: a monoclonal B-cell population is defined by a monoclonal immunoglobulin on the surface of B cells. This monoclonal immunoglobulin should include only κ- or λ-light chains. Therefore, monoclonal antibodies to κ- or λ-light chains can differentiate a monoclonal B-cell population, defining B cells baring only immunoglobulins which contain exclusively κ- or λ-chains.

T cells: there is not any immunopathological method to detect monoclonal T cells. T cell clonality is routinely evaluated with a PCR-based method using genomic DNA.

Southern blot to detect B and T cell gene rearrangement: the Southern blot is a sensitive and specific technique to detect monoclonal B- and T-cell populations by detecting precisely the same B- or T-cell receptor gene rearrangement in a collection of B or T cells, respectively. This technique can identify even small monoclonal cell populations compared to the total number of cells under study. Samples appropriate for analysis include fresh cell supernatants, fresh body fluids, or well-preserved frozen tissue sections.

36. Which are the T and B lymphocyte receptors?

T-cell antigen receptors are constituted of eight transmembrane polypeptide chains termed α, β, γ, δ, ε, and ζ. Each receptor possesses one α-, one β-, one γ-, one δ-chain, as well as two ε- and two ζ-chains. Chains α and β are covalently linked to each other by a disulfide bridge between cysteine residues, close to the area of their emersion from the cell surface. Each of α- and β-chains contains one variable (V) and one constant (C) domain. Within the V domains, there are regions which differ significantly between individual T cells, and these are called "hypervariable (HV) regions" which come close to each other as the V regions of α- and β-chains are folded; eventually, the HV regions form an area which is complementary to structures constituted of complexes of antigenic peptides with major histocompatibility complex (MHC) antigens; thus, the HV regions are called "complementarity-determining regions" (CDRs). The remaining transmembrane polypeptide chains are not involved in antigen recognition, but in intracellular signaling. They are joined to each other by charged residues as follows: one ε is joined to γ, and one ε is joined to δ-chain, constituting the so-called CD3 complex, while ζ-chains are mutually joined. The CD3 complexes, as well as the ζ-chains, contain in their intracellular parts conserved sequences of four amino acids of which one is tyrosine; these motifs are called "immunoreceptor tyrosine-based activation motifs" (ITAMs) and facilitate signaling after interaction of the receptor with the MHC-antigenic peptide complex.

B-cell antigen receptor is constituted of membrane IgM or IgD immunoglobulins associated with two transmembrane invariant chains called Igα and Igβ, which are joined to each other by a disulfide bridge just after their emersion from the cell surface. Thus, the B-cell antigen receptor is the surface immunoglobulin, while Igα and Igβ contain ITAMs in their intracellular domains and facilitate signaling. After class switching, B cells as well as memory B cells express IgG, IgA, and IgE class surface immunoglobulins as antigen receptors.

37. How can B- and T-cell antigen receptors recognize millions of different antigens?

In each individual B or T cell, a unique rearrangement of VDJ gene segments occurs and a unique antigen receptor emerges on their surface. Therefore, millions of different B or T cells exist, each expressing an antigen receptor of unique specificity. Thus, by taking B and T cells as a whole, they carry a huge diversity of antigenic receptors. As soon as a B or T cell encounters an antigen, the cell proliferates to make daughter cells identical to the precursor cell. This phenomenon is called "clonal expansion." The B cells differentiate to plasma cells and produce huge amounts of antibodies against the antigen they encountered, while T cells are transformed into "armed effectors T cells" (or simply "effector T cells"). Then T cells express their executive actions as helper, inflammatory, or cytotoxic cells in the injured tissues. The first encounter of antigen by T and/or B cells in order to successfully activate the cells for proliferation and differentiation should take place in the lymph nodes and other lymphoid tissues because these tissues provide the appropriate "environment" for T- and B-cell activation. Indeed, the lymphoid tissues contain soluble antigens drained by infected tissues, reaching the lymph nodes through the lymphatic vessels; in addition, antigen-presenting cells, such as dendritic cells coming from peripheral tissues and resident macrophages, present antigen "appropriately" to B or T cells; this means that antigen-presenting cells, in addition to antigen presentation, express co-stimulatory molecules and cytokines and provide T or B cells with additional signals for survival, proliferation, and differentiation.

38. Which are the main co-stimulatory molecules on the cell surface of lymphocytes and antigen-presenting cells?

CD28 is expressed on T cells and interacts with CD80 (B7.1) and CD86 (B7.2) on antigen-presenting cells. The inducible T cell co-stimulator (ICOS, CD278) is expressed also on T cells is interacts with ICOS-Ligand.

Co-stimulation for B cells is provided alternatively by complement receptors (CR2). CR2 (CD21) on mature B cells formulates a complex with CD19 and CD81, which is often called B cell co-receptor complex because CR2 binds to opsonized antigens through attached C3d when the B-cell receptor binds the antigen.

CD40 is expressed on B cells and antigen-presenting cells which acts as a co-stimulatory molecule necessary for their activation. This is accomplished when it binds on its ligand CD154 (CD40L) on activated T helper cells. CD40 engagement on the surface of dendritic cells (DCs) promotes their cytokine production, the induction of co-stimulatory molecules on their surface, and facil-

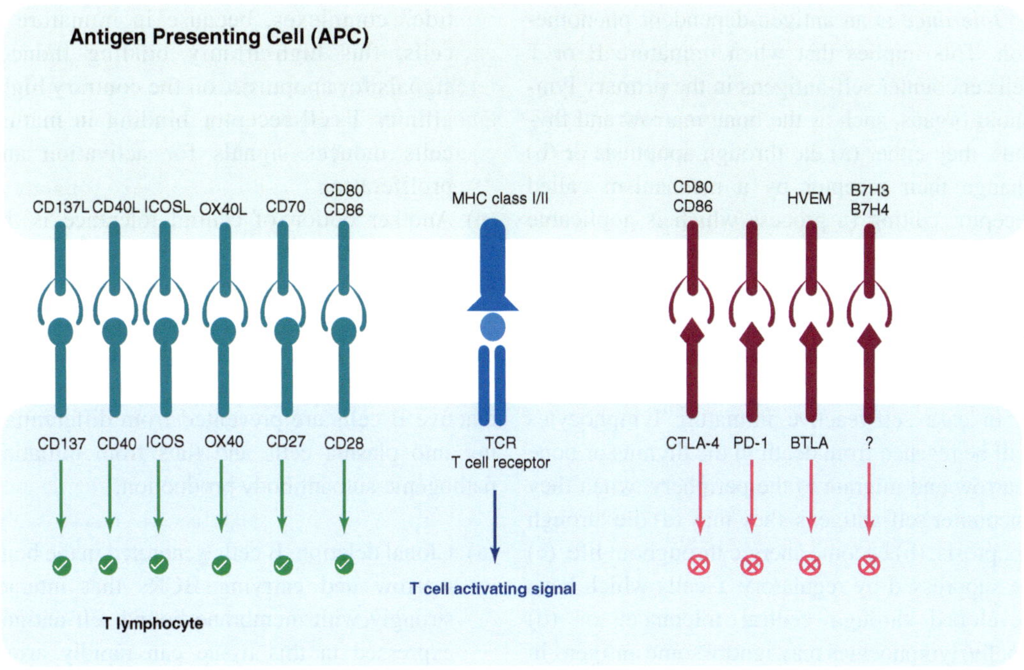

Fig. 1.6 Co-stimulatory and co-inhibitory molecules expressed by lymphocytes and antigen-presenting cells. Co-stimulatory molecules deliver positive signals to T cells (green) following their binding to ligands and receptors on APCs. Co-inhibitory molecules deliver negative signals (pink) to T cells upon interaction with their counterparts on the APCs. The balance between co-stimulatory and co-inhibitory signals (red) alters the net stimulating effect of TCR signaling mediated through antigen presentation on MHC (blue) (*Figure created by Evangelia Zampeli, MD*)

itates the cross-presentation of antigen (Fig. 1.6). CD40 signaling of B cells promotes germinal center (GC) formation, immunoglobulin (Ig) isotype switching, somatic hypermutation (SHM) of the Ig to enhance affinity for antigen, and finally the formation of long-lived plasma cells and memory B cells.

39. What are immune checkpoints?

Immune checkpoints (ICPs) are co-stimulatory and inhibitory signals transmitted by an assortment of receptors and their respective ligands (Fig. 1.6) in order to maintain immune homeostasis and self-tolerance. Under normal physiological conditions, ICPs are implicated in the initiation and in the determination of the intensity/duration of the immune response. They operate to limit collateral tissue damage during immune responses and therefore are critical for preventing autoimmune diseases.

Co-stimulatory checkpoint molecules (CD28, ICOS, CD27, CD40, OX40, and CD137) are necessary to provide the "second signal," after the interaction between the T-cell receptor (TCR) on the surface of T-cells and a major histocompatibility complex (MHC) molecule, in order to promote T cell activation. Absence of the co-stimulatory signal may lead to T cell anergy or apoptosis and decrease the strength of the immune response.

Co-inhibitory checkpoint molecules (CTLA-4, PD-1, BTLA, B7-H3, B7-H4, and VISTA) prevent T-cell activation. These checkpoints normally function to prevent exaggerated immune responses and subsequent autoimmune disease. Cancer cells can "hijack" immune checkpoints and escape immune destruction by acquiring abilities to inhibit immune checkpoint pathways and suppress anti-cancer T cell responses (Fig. 1.6).

40. Which are the mechanisms leading to the development of self-tolerance?

An outline of self-tolerance is as follows:

Tolerance is an antigen-dependent phenomenon. This implies that when immature B or T cells encounter self-antigens in the primary lymphoid organs, such as the bone marrow and thymus, they either (a) die through apoptosis or (b) change their receptor by a mechanism called receptor editing (a process which is applicable for B cells) or (c) become regulatory; that means the cell does not further react to self-antigens (a process which is applicable for $CD4^+$ T cells). The above processes constitute the so-called central tolerance.

In case self-reactive immature lymphocytes will be rescued from death in the thymus or bone marrow and migrate to the periphery, when they encounter self-antigens, they may (a) die through apoptosis, (b) become anergic throughout life, (c) be suppressed by regulatory T cells which have developed through central tolerance; or (d) finally, lymphocytes may ignore some antigens in the periphery, such as antigens of the testes or the eyes, which lie in immune-privileged sites. These processes constitute the so-called "peripheral tolerance."

Mechanisms in detail, inducing tolerance, are as follows:

Central T-cell tolerance:

(a) Thymic medullary epithelial cells express many antigens exposed in the peripheral tissues under the influence of a protein which acts as a transcriptional regulator and promotes the expression of many antigens of peripheral tissues to thymus. This protein is called AIRE (autoimmune regulator); in the absence of AIRE, an autoimmune polyendocrinopathy syndrome is developed, because antigen-specific T cells for endocrine gland tissues escape central tolerance. AIRE does not explain the expression of so many antigens of the peripheral tissues in thymus, but it is a paradigm of how the system works. Central T-cell tolerance takes place in the thymus through the process of negative selection. This process affects both $CD8^+$ and $CD4^+$ T cells when their T-cell receptors bind with high affinity to "MHC/antigenic peptide" complexes, because in immature T cells, this high-affinity binding induces signals for apoptosis; on the contrary high-affinity T-cell receptor binding in mature cells induces signals for activation and proliferation
(b) Another option of central tolerance is the transformation of immature $CD4^+$ T cells in the thymus to regulatory T cells

Central B-cell tolerance: A range of mechanisms exist that collectively ensure that most self-reactive B cells are prevented from differentiating into plasma cells and thus from initiating pathogenic autoantibody production.

(a) Clonal deletion. B cells generated in the bone marrow and carrying BCRs that interact strongly with membrane-bound self-antigen expressed in this tissue can rapidly arrest maturation and die
(b) Receptor editing. Instead of directly triggering apoptosis, strongly self-reactive BCR specificities can be purged from the repertoire by the process of receptor editing. Strong cross-linking of BCRs on immature bone marrow B cells by self-antigen reactivates expression of their combinase-activating gene (RAG) proteins, thus triggering further VJ rearrangements within the immunoglobulin light chain genes. A new immunoglobulin light chain is expressed which offers a new (probably non-autoreactive specificity) to B-cell surface immunoglobulin (B-cell receptor)
(c) Clonal anergy. While both clonal deletion and receptor editing effectively remove self-reactive specificities from the primary B cell repertoire, many self-reactive B cells instead survive in the periphery in a functionally compromised state of anergy, characterized by desensitized BCR signaling and a suppressed ability to undergo plasma cell differentiation
(d) Clonal ignorance. Although not a tolerance mechanism per se, clonal ignorance describes the fate of self-reactive B cells that fail to encounter their self-antigen target, due to

either its scarcity or its sequestration inside cells or other inaccessible physiological structures

41. How does peripheral T- and B-lymphocyte self-tolerance develop?

Peripheral T cell tolerance:

(a) When autoreactive $CD4^+$ T cells encounter antigen in the periphery in the absence of co-stimulatory molecules, they become anergic; that is, they are not activated. There is some evidence that intracellular molecules important for T-cell receptor signaling are ubiquitinated, and the signal for T-cell activation is terminated. Another mechanism for autoreactive T-cell inactivation is the overexpression of CTLA4 surface molecule which belongs to the CD28 family, but when it binds to B7 molecules at the surface of antigen-presenting cells, it prevents B7:CD28 interaction and the T cell fails to be activated. Another molecule that belongs to the CD28 family and like CTLA4 inactivates autoreactive T cells is the PD-1. Ligands for PD-1 are expressed in antigen-presenting cells and other cells
(b) Suppression of autoreactive T cells by T_{regs}. The suppressive action of T_{regs} is mediated by three mechanisms: (a) production of immunosuppressive cytokines IL-10 and TGF-β, (b) overexpression of CTLA4, and (c) consumption of IL-2, a phenomenon which results in deprivation of effector T cells which also need IL-2 for survival, proliferation, and activation
(c) Issues regarding $CD8^+$ T-cell tolerance are not very well substantiated

Peripheral B cell tolerance is attributed to the following mechanisms:

(a) Anergy and deletion which occurs when autoreactive B cells are repeatedly stimulated by autoantigen in lymphoid follicles. They need high levels of the growth factor BAFF/Blys; therefore they are unable to compete normal naive B cells which can differentiate with much less amounts of BAFF/Blys, and eventually autoreactive B cells become anergic or die
(b) Inhibition of autoreactive B cells by inhibitory molecules as depicted in mice but it is not substantiated in humans. Such molecules are CD22, Lyn, and SHP-1. The ligand for CD22 is not known

42. What are the different cells interacting in a germinal center and their functions?

Different cell types collaborate to ensure positive selection of high-affinity germinal center (GC) B cells and differentiation into effector plasma cells and memory B cells.

(a) Light zone and dark zone B cells. Light zone (LZ) and dark zone (DZ) domains within GC contain morphologically distinct populations of lymphocytes termed centrocytes (LZ, small, $CD86^{hi}CXCR4^{lo}$) and centroblasts (DZ, large, $CD86^{lo}CXCR4^{hi}$). Centroblasts and centrocytes are not separate B cell lineages but represent alternating phenotypes adopted by GC B cells as they move through the cyclic processes that underpin positive selection in the GC
(b) Follicular dendritic cells. FDCs are specialized, nonhematopoietic cells that derive from perivascular precursors, form the nucleation site for nascent GCs, and are essential for both initiation and maintenance of GCs. As B cell proliferation continues and the GC matures to form LZ and DZ compartments, FDCs localize exclusively to the LZ. Their primary role is to act as a depot for intact antigen, which they maintain for extended periods (weeks to months) on their plasma membrane in the form of immune complexes or opsonized macromolecules
(c) T follicular helper cells. As with GC B cells, T follicular helper (T_{fh}) cells derived from the original antigen-specific lymphocyte clones responsible for initiating the T-dependent B cell responses that ultimately result in GC formation. Like FDCs, T_{fh} cells

are found almost exclusively within the LZ of the GC, where they act as the source of T cell help that sustains the ongoing proliferation and selection of GC B cells. In addition to T_{fh} cells, a related population of Foxp3$^+$ T cells designated T follicular regulatory (T_{fr}) cells has also been identified within GCs and seems to suppress GC responses at least under some circumstances
(d) Tingible body macrophages. Tingible body macrophages (TBMφs) are phagocytic cells unique to the GC that, although relatively rare, have a prominent phenotype characterized by internal tingible bodies corresponding to lymphocytes in various states of degradation. TBMφs are typically found in close proximity to the border between the LZ and DZ and act as the GC's garbage disposal system, removing there mains of the large numbers of B cells that undergo apoptosis in the GC

43. What are tertiary lymphoid structures?

Tertiary lymphoid structures (TLS) or ectopic lymphoid structures often occur at sites of autoimmune inflammation, organ transplantation, and cancer. Unlike secondary lymphoid organs, TLS lack a capsule and afferent lymphatic vessels and they are transient structures, which resolve after antigen clearance. TLS are characterized by B- and T-cell segregation, ectopic expression of lymphoid chemokines CXCL13, CCL19, and CCL21 that regulate T and B lymphocyte compartmentalization, high endothelial venules, and often by the presence of CD21$^+$ follicular dendritic cell (FDC) network which sustains the local humoral B-cell response. TLS can display features of active germinal centers (GCs), including the expression of the enzyme activation-induced cytidine deaminase (AID) which regulates immunoglobulin gene affinity maturation via the process of somatic hypermutation, and they support a local antigen-driven B-cell proliferation and differentiation into antibody-producing plasma cells. TLS support the local proliferation and differentiation of autoreactive B cells in a disease-specific manner suggesting that the maintenance of TLS is also sustained, at least in part, by an autoantigen-dependent process with the differentiation of autoreactive plasma cells toward disease-specific autoantigens. Recently, TLS have been associated with a favorable response to immunotherapy.

44. Which are some examples of pro-inflammatory cytokines and the cells that produce them?

Tumor necrosis factor-α: produced by macrophages, T cells, mast cells, and NK cells. Its main functions are increase of adhesion molecules, stimulation of the production of interleukin (IL)-1 and IL-6, activation of neutrophils, and initiation of acute inflammatory response.

IL-1: produced by macrophages, dendritic cells, neutrophils, and endothelial cells. Its main functions are increase of adhesion molecules and stimulation of hepatocytes to produce acute-phase reactants.

IL-12: produced by dendritic cells and macrophages. Its main functions are to increase IFN-γ production, transform CD4$^+$ T cells to Th1 phenotype, and increase cytotoxic activity of NK cells and CD8$^+$ T cells.

IL-6: produced by macrophages, endothelial cells, and fibroblasts. Its main functions are maturation of B cells and antibody production, differentiation of neural cells, and stimulation of hepatocytes to produce acute-phase reactants.

45. What is the cytokine release syndrome?

Cytokine release syndrome (CRS) or cytokine storm syndrome is a systemic inflammatory response, which can be caused by infections, some drugs, and other factors, characterized by a sharp increase in the level of a large number of pro-inflammatory cytokines. CRS is more common in immune system-related diseases or immune-related therapy, such as Chimeric antigen receptor (CAR)-T cell therapy, organ transplantation sepsis, and virus infection (i.e., SARS-CoV2). CRS can be induced by direct target cell lysis with consecutive release of cytokines like interferon-gamma (IFN-γ) or tumor necrosis factor-alpha (TNF-α) or by activation of T cells due to therapeutic stimuli with subsequent cytokine release. These cytokines trigger a chain reaction due to the activation of innate immune cells like macrophages and endothelial cells with further cytokine release. IL-6 contributes to many of the key symptoms of CRS.

46. Which are some examples for the function of Th1, Th2, and Th17 cells and cytokines?

Th1 cytokines: IFN-γ, IL-2, and TNF. They are produced by $CD4^+$ Th1 cells. Their main functions are cell-mediated immunity and phagocyte-dependent inflammation.

Th2 cytokines: IL-4, IL-5, IL-6, IL-10, and IL-13. They are produced by $CD4^+$ Th2 cells and innate lymphoid cells-2 (ILC-2). Their main functions are to evoke strong antibody responses (including IgE) and eosinophil accumulation (phagocyte-independent defense) and inhibition of Th1-mediated macrophage activation.

Th17 cytokines: IL-17, IL-22, and IL-21. They are produced by Th17 cells. Their main functions are recruitment of neutrophils, induction of antimicrobial peptides in epithelial tissues, and stimulation of inflammation.

47. What is the interferon (IFN) signature?

Multiple type I interferons (consist of 13 IFN-α subtypes, IFN-β, IFN-ω, IFN-κ, and IFN-ε), interferon-γ (IFN-γ) and type III IFNs (IFN-λ1 (IL-29), IFN-λ2 (IL-28A), IFN-λ3 (IL-28B), and IFN-λ4) are expressed under physiological conditions and are increased by stress and infections, and in autoinflammatory and autoimmune diseases. Interferons activate the Jak–STAT signaling pathway and induce overlapping patterns of expression, called "interferon signatures," of canonical interferon-stimulated genes (ISGs) encoding molecules important for antiviral responses, antigen presentation, autoimmunity, and inflammation. Although the three IFN types signal via distinct receptors, the genes or signatures controlled by these IFNs overlap substantially. Although the potential pathogenic roles of IFN signatures in autoimmune diseases has been highlighted, both type I and II IFNs induce negative feedback and inhibitory pathways and have been implicated in suppressive effects, such as immune cell exhaustion. Thus, IFNs are likely to mediate both pathogenic and protective mechanisms in autoimmune diseases.

48. Which cells produce chemokines and what is their function?

Chemokines are produced by leukocytes and by several types of tissue cells such as endothelial cells, epithelial cells, tissue macrophages, fibroblasts, and other cells of the stroma, under the stimulation of cytokines like TNF and IL-1β or under the recognition of pathogen-associated molecular patterns.

Chemokines are divided into two major subfamilies defined as CXC (when two cysteine residues are separated by every other amino acid), which are called α chemokines, and the CC (when two cysteine residues are adjacent), which are called β chemokines. A subgroup of CXC chemokines (for instance, CXCL8, also termed IL-8) with the sequence "glutamic acid-leucine-arginine" (ELR) motif just before the CXC motif support neutrophil migration to infected or damaged tissues. The remaining CC (for instance, CCL2, also termed MCP-1) and CXC (for instance, CXCL10, also termed IP-10) chemokines support the migration of monocytes, lymphocytes, and other immune cells.

Suggested Reading

1. Abbas AK, Lichtman AHH, Pillai S. Cellular and molecular immunology. 9th ed. Philadelphia: Elsevier; 2018.
2. Coleman WB, Tsongalis GJ, editors. Molecular diagnostics: for the clinical laboratorian. 2nd ed. Totowa, NJ: Humana Press; 2006. ISBN 1-58829-356-4 (alk. paper) eISBN 1-59259-928-1.
3. Murphy K, Weaver C, with contributions by Mowat A, Berg L, Chaplin D. Janeway's immunobiology. 9th ed. New York: Garland Science/Taylor and Francis Group; 2016. ISBN 978-0-8153-4505-3 978-0-8153-4551-0 (International Paperback).
4. Delves PJ, Martin SJ, Burton DR, Roitt IM. Roitt's essential immunology. 13th ed: Wiley-Blackwell; January 2017. ISBN: 978-1-118-41577-1.
5. Punt J, Stranford S, Jones P, Judith A. Kuby immunology. 8th ed: Owen Published; 13th June 2018. ISBN: 9781319114701.

6. Shikhagaie MM, Germar K, Bal SM, Ros XR, Spits H. Innate lymphoid cells in autoimmunity: emerging regulators in rheumatic diseases. Nat Rev Rheumatol. 2017;13:164–73.
7. Xu D, Matsumoto ML, McKenzie BS. TPL2 kinase action and control of inflammation. Pharmacol Res. 2018;129:188–93.
8. Bal SM, Golebski K, Spits H. Plasticity of innate lymphoid cell subsets. Nat Rev Immunol. 2020;20: 552–65.
9. Brink R, Phan TG. Self-reactive B cells in the germinal center reaction. Annu Rev Immunol. 2018;36:339–57.
10. Kumar N, Arthur CP, Ciferri C, Matsumoto ML. Structure of the secretory immunoglobulin A core. Science. 2020;367:1008–14.
11. Barrat FJ, Crow MK, Ivashkiv LB. Interferon target-gene expression and epigenomic signatures in health and disease. Nat Immunol. 2019;20:1574–83.
12. Corsiero E, Delvecchio FR, Bombardieri M, Pitzalis C. B cells in the formation of tertiary lymphoid organs in autoimmunity, transplantation and tumorigenesis. Curr Opin Immunol. 2019;57:46–52.
13. Pardoll DM. The blockade of immune checkpoints in cancer immunotherapy. Nat Rev Cancer. 2012;12:252–64.
14. Provine NM, Klenerman P. MAIT Cells in Health and Disease. Annu Rev Immunol. 2020;38:203–28. .
15. Macpherson AJ, Yilmaz B, Limenitakis JP, Ganal-Vonarburg SC. IgA function in relation to the intestinal microbiota. Annu Rev Immunol. 2018;36:359–81.
16. Narasimhan PB, Marcovecchio P, Hamers AAJ, Hedrick CC. Nonclassical monocytes in health and disease. Annu Rev Immunol. 2019;37:439–56.
17. Fousert E, Toes R, Desai J. Neutrophil extracellular traps (NETs) take the central stage in driving autoimmune responses. Cell. 2020;9:E915.

Autoimmune Rheumatic Disorders: Pathogenetic and Laboratory Aspects

2

Jacques-Olivier Pers,
Panayiotis G. Vlachoyiannopoulos,
Evangelia Zampeli,
and Haralampos M. Moutsopoulos

Abstract

Autoimmune disorders result from the attack of the immune system against self, since patients with these diseases have lost a major characteristic of the immune system, the *immune tolerance* (ability not to react against self). They can affect one organ (*organ-specific*) or many organs (*systemic*). The majority of autoimmune rheumatic diseases are systemic. The disorders occur in genetically predisposed individuals (associated with major histocompatibility antigens and other immunoreactive molecules) when they come across with chemical, physical, or microbial agents in the context of a particular hormonal background (majority are females) and under circumstances that create incompetence to cope with life stressful events. The autoimmune attack can be mediated by autoantibodies, immune complexes, B or T lymphocytes and can result in organ hyperfunction (e.g., hyperthyroidism), hypofunction (e.g., myasthenia gravis), or destruction of the affected organ (e.g., synovium in rheumatoid arthritis). The presence of leukocytosis and acute-phase proteins (C-reactive protein) characterizes the autoimmune disorders as inflammatory (e.g., vasculitis), while their absence as not inflammatory (e.g., systemic lupus erythematosus, SLE). B-lymphocyte hyperactivity, as attested by hyperglobulinemia and a plethora of circulating or tissue-deposited autoantibodies, is a common manifestation in the majority of autoimmune diseases, while different types of T-helper lymphocytes (Th1, Th2, and Th17) operate in different autoimmune diseases. The autoantibodies can be diagnostic (high specificity for disease, e.g., anti-Sm for SLE), pathogenetic (e.g., DNA-anti-DNA immune complexes activate the complement cascade and induce tissue injury), or predictive for disease development (e.g., rheumatoid factors and anti-cyclic citrullinated autoantibodies).

J.-O. Pers
UMR1227, Lymphocytes B et Autoimmunité, Université de Brest, Inserm, Brest, France
e-mail: pers@univ-brest.fr

P. G. Vlachoyiannopoulos
Department of Pathophysiology, School of Medicine, National University of Athens, Athens, Greece
e-mail: pvlah@med.uoa.gr

E. Zampeli
Bioclinic General Hospital of Athens and Institute for Autoimmune Systemic and Neurological Disorders, Athens, Greece
e-mail: ezampeli@bioclinic.gr

H. M. Moutsopoulos (✉)
Academy of Athens, Athens, Greece
e-mail: hmoutsop@med.uoa.gr

H. M. Moutsopoulos, E. Zampeli (eds.), *Immunology and Rheumatology in Questions*, https://doi.org/10.1007/978-3-030-56670-8_2

1. **On the basis of what facts a disorder can be characterized as autoimmune disease?**

A disease is termed as autoimmune when (a) antibodies or immune cells recognize self-antigens, (b) these autoreactive antibodies (autoantibodies) and immunocytes result either in hypo- or hyperfunction or tissue injury of the affected organ(s), and (c) transfer of the autoantibodies or autoreactive immunocytes to another human (e.g., maternal autoantibodies to Ro/SSA and La/SSB autoantigens transferred to embryo induce neonatal lupus) or to an experimental animal (e.g., transfer of autoantibodies to acetylcholine receptor from a patient to a rabbit induces myasthenia gravis) can produce a similar clinical syndrome.

2. **Which is the proposed mechanism for autoantibodies development?**

Autoantibodies are detected in the sera of patients many years before the diagnosis of an autoimmune disease is set. It has been proposed that their development is due to defective cellular apoptosis which results in redistribution of nuclear and cytoplasmic cellular antigens to cell surface. Subsequently, autoreactive natural immunocyte clones target the physiologically protected intracellular antigens leading to increased autoantibody generation. The defective clearance of the apoptotic cell autoantigens leads to increased amounts of circulating autoantigens which together with the circulating autoantibodies form immune complexes. In the presence of large amounts of autoantigens, the formed immune complexes deposit to different tissues and activation of complement system begins which fuels the tissue inflammatory process [1].

3. **How are autoimmune diseases classified?**

The autoimmune diseases can affect one organ of the human body (e.g., autoimmune diseases of the thyroid gland) and are called *organ-specific autoimmune diseases*. Others affect simultaneously or sequentially many organs and are termed *systemic autoimmune diseases*. The majority of autoimmune rheumatic (connective tissue) diseases are systemic autoimmune disorders.

4. **Which are the pathologic results of an autoimmune attack?**

- Loss of organ function of the affected target tissue: e.g., in diabetes mellitus type I, the β-Langerhans pancreatic cells are destroyed by autoreactive cytotoxic T cells
- Suppression of the affected organ function: e.g., in myasthenia gravis, autoantibodies directed against the acetylcholine receptor (AChR) prohibit the transfer of message from the nerves to the muscles, mainly by internalizing the AChR which is destroyed in the phagosome
- Hyperstimulation of the affected organ function: e.g., in Graves' disease (hyperthyroidism), autoantibodies directed against the thyroid-stimulating hormone (TSH) receptor mimic the function of TSH, thus providing a constant stimulation of the thyroid gland to produce thyroid hormones, ultimately resulting in the clinical picture of hyperthyroidism
- In systemic autoimmune diseases, the immune-mediated events are multiple and complex and can lead to the impairment or destruction of many organs, as is seen in patients with systemic lupus erythematosus

5. **What is termed hypersensitivity reaction?**

Hypersensitivity refers to a pathologic immune reaction that is brought about from an immune response after repeated exposure to an antigen. Hypersensitivity diseases include autoimmune diseases, in which immune responses are directed against self-antigens and diseases that result from uncontrolled or excessive responses to foreign antigens. Primary mediators are the adaptive immune system components such as B cells, T cells, and their products, namely, antibodies and cytokines. The term "hypersensitivity" historically defines what we call today "immunity" and was based on the observation that individuals exposed to an antigen are sensitive to respond more aggressively to subsequent exposures to the same antigen. Damage is mediated by the same attack mechanisms that mediate normal immune responses to pathogens. There are four types of hypersensitivity reactions: type I, immediate type; type II, antibody-dependent, cytotoxic; type III, immune complex mediated; and type IV, delayed type.

6. How do the different types of hypersensitivity reactions occur?

Type I hypersensitivity reaction: When genetically predisposed individuals are exposed to an allergen, their dendritic cells, as well as their B cells, recognize the allergen and present antigenic peptides to naive T cells which become T-helper (Th)-2 cells in the periphery and T follicular helper (T_{fh}) cells in the lymph nodes, both of which secrete the cytokine interleukin-4 (IL-4). Upon activation with IL-4, B cells that have also been exposed to the allergen undergo immunoglobulin (Ig) E class switching and secrete allergen-specific IgE, which binds to the FcεRI receptors on mast cells. Repeated exposure to the allergen leads to allergen-IgE interaction on the surface of mast cells resulting in mast cell activation, with two major consequences: (a) immediate hypersensitivity reaction (minutes after allergen exposure) due to vasoactive amines (histamine, heparin), and lipid mediators, which cause increased vascular permeability and leakage, bronchospasm, and intestinal hypermotility, and (b) late-phase reaction (2–4 h after allergen exposure) due to cytokine secretion, characterized by inflammation due to accumulation of eosinophils and Th2 cells.

Type II hypersensitivity reaction: it takes one of the following patterns: (a) autoantibodies directed against self-antigens lead to opsonization, activation of complement cascade, as well as recruitment of polymorphonuclear leukocytes, macrophages, and natural killer cells, which results in phagocytosis and killing of the target cell; (b) Fc receptor binds antibodies which have recognized either soluble or fixed antigens in various tissues and activates immunocytes bearing Fc receptor; and (c) abnormal functions without inflammation, such as antibody binding and hyperactivation of the thyroid-stimulating hormone (TSH) receptor inducing hyperthyroidism (Graves' disease) or antibody binding to acetylcholine receptor internalizing it into phagosomes where the receptor is degraded and eventually the muscle endplate is deficient of acetylcholine receptors.

Type III hypersensitivity reaction: is induced by autoantibodies that bind to self-antigens and form antigen–antibody complexes (immune complexes). Immune complexes, formed in excess of antigen, are soluble and circulate in the blood, but finally they get entrapped in the capillaries, where they lead to complement system activation and tissue damage. Tissue damage extended in many tissues at the microcirculation level results in disease.

Type IV hypersensitivity reaction: is a cell-mediated immune response, which can be implemented either by $CD4^+$ T cells or by $CD8^+$ T cells. $CD4^+$ T cells are activated when they recognize antigenic peptides bound to type II major histocompatibility complex antigens (MHC-II) on the surface of antigen-presenting cells such as dendritic cells or macrophages. Macrophages secrete the cytokine interleukin (IL)-12 which induces maturation and activation of naive $CD4^+$ T cells to become Th1 cells that secrete interferon-γ (IFN-γ) which in turn activates macrophages to secrete the cytokines tumor necrosis factor α (TNF-α), IL-1, and IL-6. These cytokines induce capillary leaking, edema, and fever. In addition, macrophages secrete lysosomal enzymes and reactive oxygen species that induce tissue damage. $CD8^+$ T cells recognize antigenic peptides derived from viral antigens; these peptides are bound to MHC-I molecules on the surface of any nucleated somatic cell which has been infected by viruses. Thus, $CD8^+$ (cytotoxic) T cells kill the virus-infected cells without any additional help and eliminate the reservoir of the virus. To accomplish cell killing, $CD8^+$ T cells secrete perforins and granzymes; the former penetrate the membrane of the target cell and after polymerization form a hole in the cellular membrane; the latter enter the cell through this hole and destroy DNA and intracellular proteins leading to apoptotic cell death.

7. In which disorders hypersensitivity reactions types I, II, III, and IV predominate?

It should be emphasized that in inflammatory/autoimmune/allergic diseases, different types of hypersensitivity reactions may operate synchronously. However, in some diseases, a particular type prevails, as, for example:

- Type I: Asthma, hay fever, eczema, food allergies, anaphylaxis, and urticaria
- Type II: Autoimmune hemolytic anemia/thrombocytopenia, pernicious anemia, Goodpasture syndrome, and pemphigus
- Type III: Systemic lupus erythematosus/lupus nephritis, post-streptococcal glomerulonephritis, serum sickness, and Arthus phenomenon
- Type IV: Chronic delayed-type hypersensitivity reactions to persistent pathogens (tuberculosis, leprosy, leishmaniasis), to chemical agents (silicosis), contact dermatitis, and rheumatoid arthritis

8. What is the major pathophysiologic phenomenon observed in patients developing autoimmune diseases?

The immune system has the ability not to respond to self-antigens. This physiologic phenomenon is called immune tolerance. It is accomplished through central and peripheral mechanisms. In patients with autoimmune diseases, immune tolerance, in other words discrimination of self- and non-self-antigens, is lost.

9. How can self-tolerance be broken?

Taking into account that genetic predisposition is a prerequisite for this phenomenon, the following mechanisms/agents have been implicated in breaking self-tolerance:

(a) Disruption of tissue barriers by trauma or infection and release of autoantigens previously hidden from the immune system. A clinical paradigm of this mechanism is the sympathetic ophthalmia. An injury to one eye releases hidden endophthalmic antigens that are recognized from the immune system as foreign and immune response against them is elicited. These autoreactive immune cells then attack not only the injured eye but also the healthy one

(b) Molecular mimicry. Some pathogens contain epitopes on antigens, which resemble epitopes on self-antigens. When an individual is offended by those pathogens, the immune system elicits response not only against the foreign molecules but also against self-antigens. This leads to tissue injury and can induce autoimmune disease. MHC class II polymorphisms are associated with the development of autoimmune disease, implicating this antigen presentation pathway in breaking tolerance. A characteristic example of this mechanism is the one operating in the development of rheumatic fever. Genetically prone individuals after an infection with group A β-hemolytic streptococci develop immune reactivity which recognizes not only the M protein of streptococci but also the autoantigens (myosin/glycogen of the patient's heart muscle and smooth muscle cells of the patient's heart vessels), thereby initiating a type II hypersensitivity reaction against heart structures resulting in their injury

(c) Activation of the innate immune response through recognition of viral proteins and tissue components released from apoptotic and/or necrotic cells results in induction of autoimmune reactivity (Fig. 2.1a, b)

(d) UV irradiation (induction of apoptosis and release of autoantigens), drugs (acting as haptens), hormones (augmenting immune response), and smoking (induces citrullination of self-proteins stimulating autoimmune responses); all can break self-tolerance and can induce autoimmune disease

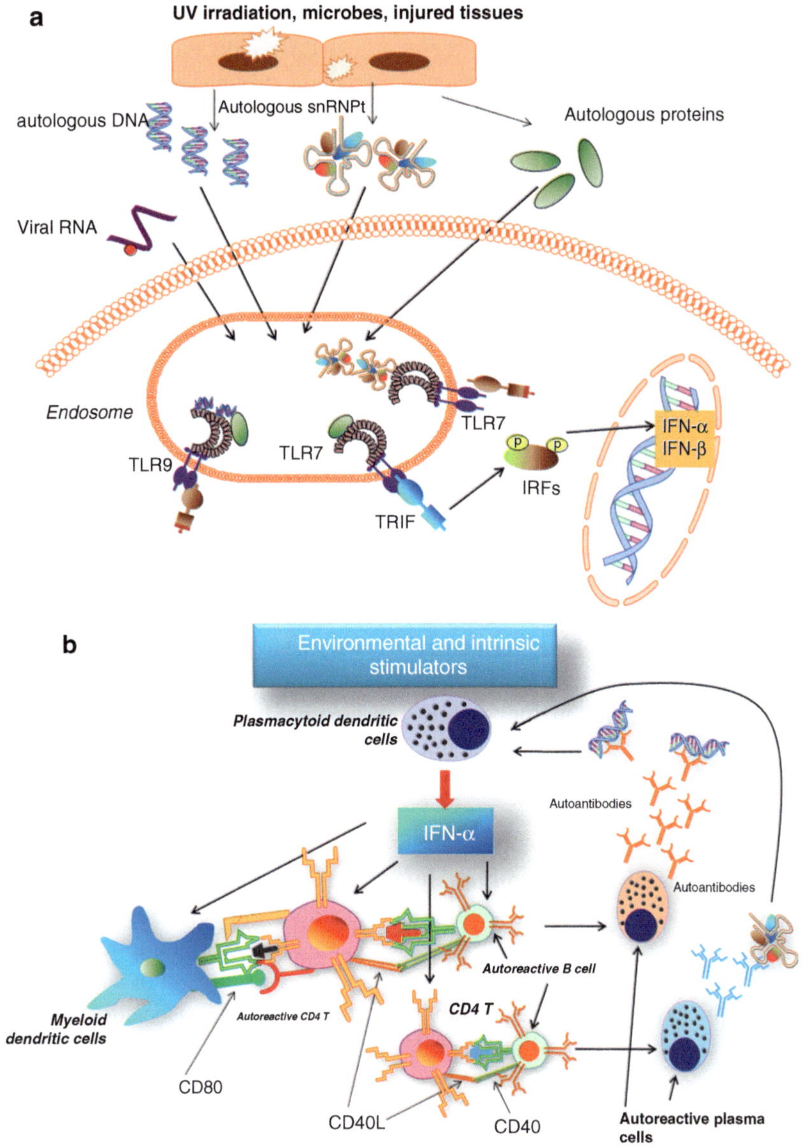

Fig. 2.1 Activation of the innate immune response. (**a**) Several environmental insults, such as UV irradiation, tissue injuries, and viral or bacterial infections, release substances such as autologous DNA, autologous small nuclear ribonucleoprotein particles, and autologous proteins. These substances enter the early endosomes of plasmacytoid dendritic cells and activate the Toll-like receptors (TLRs) which through signaling via transcription factors such as MyD88 (myeloid differentiation primary response protein 88) and TRIF (Toll/interleukin-1 receptor domain-containing adapter inducing interferon-β) activate interferon regulatory factor (IRF) which enters the nucleus and stimulates the transcription of genes producing interferon-α and interferon-β (IFN type I). Viral RNAs and C-p-G DNA fragments may also activate plasmacytoid dendritic cells in the same manner. (**b**) IFN I (α and β) stimulate dendritic cells, B cells, and macrophages to express co-stimulatory molecules and activate autoreactive T cells which have been in a stage of immunological ignorance, that is, they did not recognize autoantigens in the absence of co-stimulation. These processes lead eventually to the activation of autoreactive B cells to become plasma cells and produce autoantibodies (*Figures created by Professor Panayiotis G. Vlachoyiannopoulos, MD*)

(e) A defect in regulatory T cell and B cell numbers and/or function is found to be associated with the development of autoimmune disease in several experimental models and human autoimmune diseases. Regulatory T and B cells play an essential role in suppressing autoimmune response directed against self-antigens and thereby regulate self-tolerance

10. What is the biologic phenomenon of citrullination and in which diseases autoantibodies to citrullinated antigens can be detected?

Citrullination or deimination is a post-translational modification of the positively charged amino acid arginine in a protein into the neutral amino acid citrulline. Autoantibodies against citrullinated antigens are primarily detected in the sera of patients with rheumatoid arthritis and infrequently (5%) in the sera of patients with Sjögren's syndrome or systemic lupus erythematosus with arthritis.

11. What is hapten phenomenon? Provide examples of therapeutic agents commonly inducing it

Haptens are chemical moieties too small to elicit immune responses in their free soluble form, because they cannot cross-link B-cell receptors and cannot recruit T-cell help. However, when they are coupled to a carrier protein, they can become immunogenic. An example of a therapeutic agent inducing immune reactions through hapten-carrier phenomenon is heparin causing heparin-induced thrombocytopenia and thrombosis (HITT). In HITT, the immune system develops antibodies against heparin when it is bound to a protein called platelet factor 4 (PF4). Of note, unfractionated heparin forms more easily complexes with PF4 than the low-molecular-weight heparin. Thus, HITT develops more commonly in patients who are treated with unfractionated heparin. Other examples of medications that can act as haptens are the penicillins which may cause autoimmune hemolytic anemia/thrombocytopenia and hydralazine which in certain individuals can cause drug-induced lupus erythematosus. There are many proteins able to bind haptens. Studies have shown that penicillins make covalent bonds with lysine residues in multiple sites of many proteins. These proteins undergo degradation in the phagolysosomes and then are presented as peptides covalently linked to penicillins on several major histocompatibility complex (MHC) molecules on the surface of antigen-presenting cells.

12. What is autophagy? How does it interfere with the pathogenesis of autoimmune diseases?

Autophagy is a protective and life-sustaining process by which cellular "debris" are packaged into double-membrane vesicles and degraded by lysosomes. This process of cellular self-digestion is an essential stress response and is cytoprotective by removal or recycling of damaged organelles and proteins that threaten the cell's survival. In the immune system, autophagy regulates processes such as antigen uptake and presentation, removal of pathogens, survival of short- and long-lived immune cells, cytokine-dependent inflammation, and therefore should be considered as an important node in the activation and expansion of autoreactive clones.

Genome-wide association studies have linked polymorphisms in autophagy-related genes with a predisposition to tissue-destructive inflammatory diseases, such as inflammatory bowel disease and systemic lupus erythematosus. Autophagy activation has recently been involved in the pathogenesis of rheumatoid arthritis by contributing to the survival of synoviocytes and lymphocytes, and is implicated in protein citrullination and osteoclastogenesis.

13. Which factors may play a role for the development of autoimmune diseases?

The effect of environmental factors (microbial, chemical, and physical stressors) which break self-tolerance of individuals carrying a genetic predisposition results in autoimmune reactivity. Family and monozygotic twin studies, as well as association of autoimmune diseases with certain genes (HLA class I/II and others), have attested to the genetic predisposition of these diseases. Additionally, life stressful events and inability to cope with them, as well as hormones (female predilection), also strongly influence autoimmune disease development.

14. What is the probability for a monozygotic twin to develop an autoimmune disease if its identical sibling suffers from one?

Different studies of monozygotic twins have demonstrated that genetics account for about 15–60% of the disease occurrence, while environmental factors, such as exposure to infectious, chemical, or physical agents, are responsible for the remaining.

15. What is the major histocompatibility complex (MHC) and what is its role?

The MHC is a group of genes (to date more than 200 genes) located on chromosome 6 in humans encoding the human leukocyte antigen (HLA). The most important known function of the gene products of the MHC is the processing and presentation of antigens to T cells. Within the MHC region, there are three different subregions encoding for HLA class I (HLA-A, HLA-B, and HLA-C), class II (HLA-DR, HLA-DP, and HLA-DQ), and class III (C2, C4A, C4B, and factor B of complement system; some heat shock proteins, tumor necrosis factor-α [TNF-α], and lymphotoxin) proteins. This means that within each locus (for instance, HLA-DR), there are different gene alleles such as HLA-DR1, HLA-DR2, and HLA-DR3. Each individual inherits one HLA gene for each locus, one from the mother and one from the father.

16. Which are the HLA class II allele associations with different autoimmune diseases?

- HLA-DR2: Systemic lupus erythematosus, multiple sclerosis, and negatively correlated with diabetes mellitus type I
- HLA-DR3: Sjögren's syndrome, myasthenia gravis, systemic lupus erythematosus, and diabetes mellitus type I
- HLA-DR4: Rheumatoid arthritis, diabetes mellitus type I, and pemphigus vulgaris
- HLA-DRB1-DQA1-DQB1: Rheumatoid arthritis, diabetes mellitus type I, and Graves' disease
- HLA-DR15: Systemic lupus erythematosus
- HLADQA1*0501: Sjögren's syndrome
- HLA-DQ2 and HLA-DQ8: Celiac disease
- HLA-DR15: Systemic sclerosis

17. Which other associations besides the HLA have been detected with genomic analysis in autoimmune diseases?

- Rheumatoid arthritis:
  - PTPN22 (protein tyrosine phosphatase, non-receptor type 22)
  - IL-23R (interleukin-23 receptor)
  - TRAF1 (TNF receptor-associated factor 1)
  - CTLA4 (cytotoxic T-lymphocyte-associated antigen 4)
  - IRF5 (interferon regulatory factor 5)
  - STAT4 (signal transducer and activator of transcription 4)
  - CCR6 (chemokine receptor 6)
  - PADI4 (peptidyl-arginine deiminase 4)
- Ankylosing spondyloarthritis:
  - IL-23R
  - TYK2 (tyrosine kinase 2)
  - IL-6R (interleukin-6 receptor)
- Systemic lupus erythematosus:
  - FcGR3A and FcGR2A (Fc fragment of IgG receptor IIIa, Fc fragment of IgG receptor IIa)
  - IRF5 (interferon regulatory factor 5)
  - TYK2 (tyrosine kinase 2)
  - TLR7 and TLR9 (Toll-like receptor 7, Toll-like receptor 9)
  - PTPN22
  - CTLA4
  - PDC D1 (programmed cell death 1)
- Scleroderma:
  - IRF5
  - STAT4
  - BANK1 (B-cell scaffold protein with ankyrin repeats 1)
  - BLK (B-lymphocyte kinase)
  - TNFSF4 (tumor necrosis family superfamily member 4)

- Sjögren's syndrome:
  - IRF5 (interferon regulatory factor 5)
  - STAT4 (signal transducer and activator of transcription 4)
  - BAFF (B-cell activating factor)
  - EBF1 (Early B-Cell Factor)
  - BLK (B-cell lymphocyte kinase)
  - TRAF3IP2 (TRAF3-interacting protein 2)
  - IL-10 (interleukin-10)

18. In which autoimmune disorders T-helper (Th)1, Th2, or Th17 immune response prevails?

Approximately 48–72 h after antigenic stimulation, naive T cells (Th0) begin to differentiate into either Th1 or Th2 cells. Which subset emerges depends on the cytokines in the local microenvironment, which are in turn determined by the type of innate response cells that have been activated by the invading entity. Intracellular bacteria and viruses trigger macrophages and dendritic cells to produce interleukin-12 (IL-12). A Th0 that encounters IL-12 becomes irreversibly committed to the Th1 subset.

Th1-related autoimmune diseases are diabetes mellitus type I, rheumatoid arthritis, Sjögren's syndrome, multiple sclerosis, autoimmune thyroiditis, psoriasis, celiac disease, Crohn's disease, and chronic viral infections.

On the other hand, extracellular pathogens such as certain bacteria and parasites induce IL-4 production. In the absence of IL-12 but in the presence of IL-4, a Th0 cell generates Th2 effectors.

Th2-related autoimmune diseases are systemic lupus erythematosus, scleroderma, allergy/atopy/asthma, and ulcerative colitis.

Th17 development is distinct from that of Th1 and Th2. It is hypothesized that transforming growth factor-beta (TGF-β) inhibits the production of IL-12 and IL-4 needed for Th1 and Th2 differentiation, respectively, and together with IL-6 promotes the Th17 differentiation. Once differentiated, Th17 cells require IL-23 and IL-1 to support their survival and proliferation.

Th17-related autoimmune diseases are systemic lupus erythematosus, rheumatoid arthritis, psoriasis, ankylosing spondylitis, inflammatory bowel disease, autoimmune thyroiditis, and scleroderma.

19. On what basis systemic autoimmune disorders are classified as inflammatory and non-inflammatory?

Inflammatory systemic autoimmune disorders are characterized by leukocytosis, thrombocytosis, elevated acute-phase proteins (e.g., C-reactive protein), and pro-inflammatory cytokines. This group of diseases encompasses vasculitic syndromes, rheumatoid arthritis, seronegative spondyloarthritis, and juvenile idiopathic arthritis. In non-inflammatory systemic autoimmune disorders, leukopenia, thrombocytopenia, and normal acute-phase proteins prevail. Systemic lupus erythematosus, Sjögren's syndrome, scleroderma, and allied conditions belong to this group of disorders.

20. What is Arthus reaction?

Arthus reaction is reported after vaccinations containing diphtheria and tetanus toxoid. It is a local type III hypersensitivity reaction. It involves the in situ formation of antigen/antibody complexes after the intradermal injection of an antigen. If the individual has been previously sensitized (has circulating antibodies), an Arthus reaction occurs. Arthus reaction manifests as local vasculitis expressed as a raised erythematous painful nodule due to the deposition of immunoglobulin (Ig) G-based immune complexes in dermal blood vessels and activation of the complement cascade.

21. What is the biologic phenomenon of autoantibody epitope spreading?

Autoantibody epitope (determinant) spreading is an acquired biologic phenomenon seen in autoimmunity that involves a continuous acquisition of new self-recognition antigens. Early in the course of an autoimmune disease, patients make antibodies against one epitope, but during the chronic progression of the autoimmune response, they make additional antibodies against moieties in the same molecule (intramolecular epitope spreading) or even against a different molecule (intermolecular epitope spreading), which are closely associated in a tissue (e.g., nucleosome, spliceosome, and ribosome). Autoantibody epitope spreading shifts T-cell autoreactivity from primary initiating self-determinants to secondary determinants.

Examples of autoantibody epitope spreading are the anti-Ro/SSA, anti-La/SSB responses, and the autoantibody spreading in spliceosome from the U1RNP (ribonuclear protein) peptides to Sm (Smith) antigenic molecules.

22. In which immunoglobulin class rheumatoid factors belong? In the routine test, which autoantibody having rheumatoid factor activity is detected? In which diseases or situations rheumatoid factors can be found in the patient's serum?

Rheumatoid factors (RFs) are autoantibodies against the Fc portion of immunoglobulin (Ig) (immunoglobulins against immunoglobulins IgM, IgA, and IgG). IgM rheumatoid factor is detected during routine latex agglutination test. IgM is a large pentameric molecule which binds at least ten other Ig molecules and thus demonstrates a strong agglutinability. RFs are found in the sera of two-thirds of rheumatoid arthritis, Sjögren's syndrome, mixed connective tissue disease, and idiopathic mixed cryoglobulinemia patients. In the other autoimmune diseases like systemic lupus erythematosus and scleroderma, RFs are found in around one-fourth of the patients. It should be noted, however, that RFs can also be present in the sera of patients with chronic infections (bacterial endocarditis, syphilis, tuberculosis) as well as in the sera of elderly individuals.

23. What is the prozone phenomenon?

Prozone phenomenon is a false-negative laboratory result. It is observed when high antibody titer in the sera under examination interferes with the formation of antigen–antibody lattice, necessary to visualize a positive flocculation test.

24. What are natural autoantibodies, in which immunoglobulin class do they belong, and what is their physiologic and pathophysiologic role?

Natural autoantibodies are found in the circulation of all normal individuals. They belong to all immunoglobulin classes (IgM, IgG, and IgA) and are multireactive in the sense that they react with a variety of human components (proteins, cell surface, and intracellular structures). Compelling evidence indicates that not all human autoantibodies are pathogenic. Based on the context in which natural autoantibodies encounter antigenic targets, these immunoglobulins have the specific ability to exert either physiological or pathological effector functions. Self-reactive IgM antibodies are common in healthy individuals and are already present in the cord blood of human newborns. These low-affinity natural IgM autoantibodies usually lack N-region additions and are germline-encoded or exhibit minimal somatic hypermutation. In contrast, pathogenic natural autoantibodies found in adults are predominantly high-affinity, somatically mutated IgGs that may result from failure of counterselection processes against specific autoantigens.

B lymphocytes, termed B1 cells, are produced initially in the fetus, express particularly IgM antibodies, and have the ability to polyreact with many antigens. B-1a cells that express CD5 have long been considered the major source of natural IgM, which is possibly driven by microorganisms residing in the host, such as bacteria living in the intestine. Natural autoantibodies do not undergo affinity maturation in healthy individuals. They may participate in a variety of physiological activities, such as regulation of B-cell responses, control of B-cell development, selection of the B-cell repertoire, suppression of allergic responses, protection against cancer, and first-line defense against various bacterial cell wall components or parasites. In autoimmune diseases, expansion of natural autoantibody clones may occur, giving rise to development of pathogenic autoantibodies [1, 2].

25. Which are the characteristics of pathogenic autoantibodies?

- Serum titers are high
- Immunoglobulin G isotype predominates
- Autoantigen specificity is high
- Somatic mutations occur

26. Which antigen(s) recognize the autoantibodies that in the immunofluorescence antinuclear antibody (ANA) test in Hep2 cells give a homogeneous pattern?

The homogeneous pattern is characterized by diffuse fluorescence of the entire nucleus of cells in interphase and pronounced fluorescence in the condensed chromatin of cells in the mitotic phase (Fig. 2.2a). The target antigens can be double-stranded (ds) DNA, single-stranded (ss) DNA, nucleosome, chromatin, and histones. Intense fine speckled patterns may appear homogeneous as, for example, in case of high titers of anti-Scl70 (topoisomerase I) autoantibodies. Anti-Ku autoantibodies may produce homogeneous immunofluorescence pattern but do not stain the condensed chromatin of cells in metaphase.

27. Which ANA immunofluorescence patterns are diagnostic?

- Anti-centromere antibodies: Immunofluorescence of the centromere is characterized by staining of 40–60 discrete

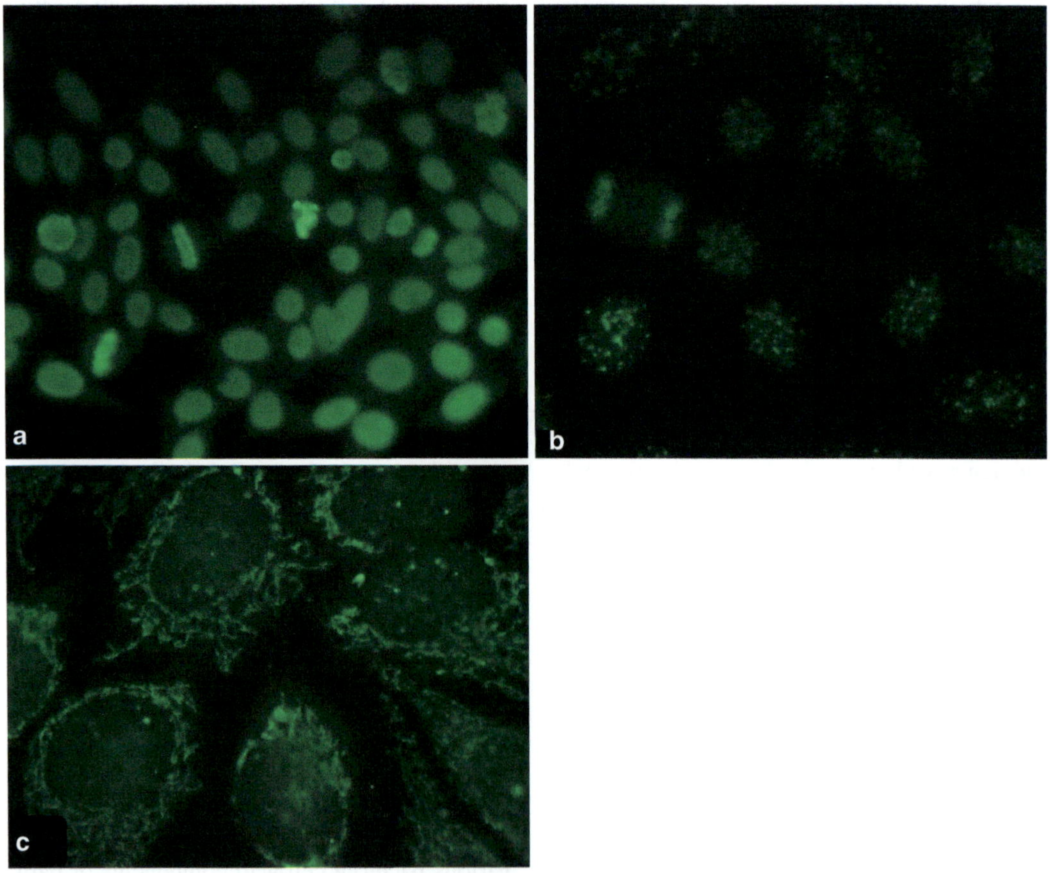

Fig. 2.2 Antinuclear antibody (ANA) immunofluorescence patterns: (**a**) homogeneous pattern, (**b**) autoantibodies to centromere, and (**c**) autoantibodies to mitochondria (*Figure courtesy of Professor Fotini N. Skopouli, MD*)

speckles distributed in the nuclei of cells in interphase, which are localized in the condensed nuclear chromatin in mitotic cells and appear as bars of closely associated speckles (Fig. 2.2b). These autoantibodies are found primarily in patients with limited scleroderma (CREST syndrome: calcinosis, Raynaud's phenomenon, esophageal dysmotility, and telangiectasia). However infrequently (<5%), these autoantibodies can be found in the sera of patients with Sjögren's syndrome and autoimmune cholangitis (primary biliary cholangitis, PBC)

- Anti-mitochondrial antibodies: They produce a granular filamentous staining extending throughout the cytoplasm and around the nucleus (Fig. 2.2c). These autoantibodies are found primarily in the sera of patients with PBC and infrequently (around 5%) in the sera of patients with limited scleroderma (CREST), Sjögren's syndrome, and overlap syndromes (systemic lupus erythematosus, scleroderma, and Sjögren's syndrome)

28. Which mitochondrial antigens (M) patients with primary biliary cholangitis (PBC) recognize?

Anti-mitochondrial antibodies recognize nine autoantigens (M1–M9) with different physical and chemical properties. Reactivity against M2 autoantigen is a specific autoantibody marker in the majority of PBC patients whereas M4, M8, and M9 classes are also well-described. In contrast autoantibodies against other M-autoantigens can be found in the sera of patients with infectious diseases (secondary syphilis, anti-M1) and undefined collagen diseases (anti-M5) as well as in patients with drug-induced hepatitis (anti-M6).

29. Which antigen(s) recognize the autoantibodies that in the immunofluorescence ANA test in Hep2 cells give nucleolar pattern?

Firstly two main types of nucleolar immunofluorescence staining can be observed using sera of patients with systemic rheumatic disorders, the homogeneous and the speckled. Autoantibodies that recognize the PM/Scl complex (main antigenic components 75 and 100 kDa) and Th/To (40 kDa ribonucleoprotein) can produce homogeneous nucleolar staining (Fig. 2.3a). Autoantibodies to PM/Scl are found in sera of patients with myositis/scleroderma overlap, while autoantibodies to Th/To can be found infrequently in sera of patients with limited cutaneous scleroderma. Speckled nucleolar pattern is produced from antibodies to RNA polymerases and is found primarily in the sera of patients with systemic sclerosis. Infrequently they can be detected in the sera of patients with mixed connective tissue disease (MCTD). Autoantibodies to Scl70 (topoisomerase I) can produce both staining patterns of the nucleoli and are found primarily in the sera of patients with systemic sclerosis.

30. Which autoantibodies give in the immunofluorescence ANA test in Hep2 cells a rim pattern?

Autoantibodies against nuclear membrane show, in immunofluorescence, a fine, linear fluorescence pattern of the nuclear membrane with less intense homogeneous staining of the entire nucleus. The target antigens are a family of intermediate filaments comprising lamins and lamin-associated proteins (GP210, lamin A, lamin B, lamin C, Lap 1A, and Lap 2).

This rare ANA pattern can be detected infrequently in the sera of overlapping autoimmune disorders such as hepatitis and cholangitis and is variably associated with vasculitis, thrombocytopenia, as well as systemic lupus erythematosus. Low-titer antibodies have been also observed in patients (50%) with chronic fatigue syndrome.

31. Which autoantibodies give in the immunofluorescence ANA test in Hep2 cells a speckled pattern?

Two main immunofluorescence speckled patterns can be seen: coarse and fine speckled. Coarse speckled pattern consists of dense intermediate-sized particles in interphase nucleus together with large speckles. Fine speckled pattern presents fine discrete speckled staining of interphase nuclei. Mitotic cells are not stained (Fig. 2.3b). Coarse speckled pattern is produced

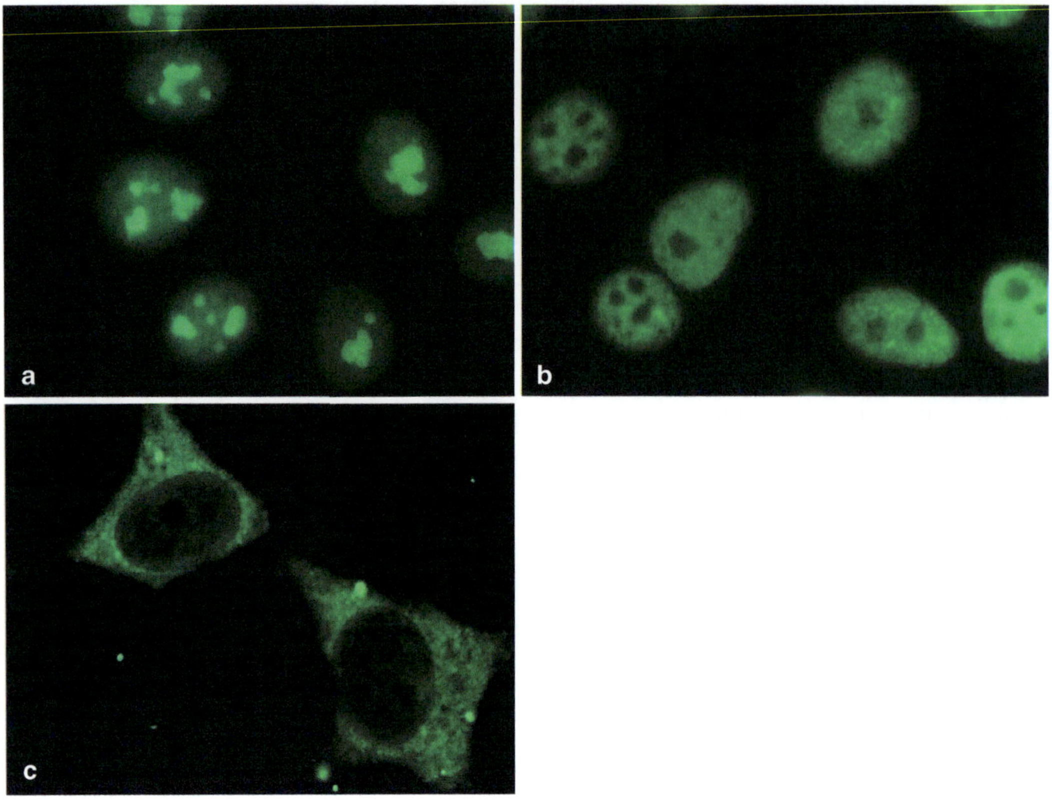

Fig. 2.3 Antinuclear antibody (ANA) immunofluorescence patterns: (**a**) autoantibodies to nucleolar antigens, (**b**) nuclear fine speckled pattern, and (**c**) cytoplasmic pattern (the figure has been developed from the sera of a patient with anti-ribosomal P protein antibodies) *(Figure courtesy of Professor Fotini N. Skopouli, MD)*

from autoantibodies to U1RNP and Sm autoantigens, while fine speckled from autoantibodies to Ro/SSA, La/SSB, RNA polymerases, Ku, and Mi-2 autoantigens.

32. Which autoantibodies give in the immunofluorescence ANA test in Hep2 cells a cytoplasmic pattern?

The cellular cytoplasm contains organelles (e.g., mitochondria, Golgi apparatus, endoplasmic reticulum, and others), different proteins, as well as RNA–protein complexes against which autoantibodies can develop. Anti-mitochondrial autoantibodies, which transfer RNAs, as is the anti-histidyl-tRNA synthetase (anti-Jo-1), anti-ribosomal P protein (Fig. 2.3c), and anti-signal recognition particle (anti-SRP), are some of the commonest autoantibodies which produce cytoplasmic immunofluorescence pattern.

33. Which antigens are detected with direct and indirect Coombs test?

The direct Coombs test is used to detect immunoglobulins or complement proteins that are bound to the surface of red blood cells (RBCs). The indirect Coombs test detects immunoglobulins against RBCs that are found in the patient's serum and are not bound to RBCs.

34. In which autoimmune conditions autoantibodies to histones are found?

Anti-histone antibodies are found in drug-induced lupus patients. Most symptomatic patients (95%) with drug-induced disease due to procainamide, hydralazine, and quinidine will have elevated immunoglobulin (Ig) G anti-histone levels, while most asymptomatic will have IgM anti-histone antibodies. Patients with drug-induced lupus due to minocycline, statins, or propylthiouracil will have less frequently positive anti-histone antibodies (40%). Antibodies to histones are also frequently (50–80%) found in systemic lupus erythematosus patients depending on disease activity status. The anti-histone antibodies are directed to different histones in drug-induced lupus and in systemic lupus erythematosus.

35. In which autoimmune diseases anti-nucleosome antibodies can be detected?

Anti-nucleosome antibodies were firstly indirectly described when the lupus phenomenon was observed in 1948. Today, with the use of specific assays, anti-nucleosome antibodies are found in systemic lupus erythematosus (SLE) patients with active disease, in patients with drug-induced systemic lupus erythematosus as well as in some scleroderma patients. In SLE patients, they correlate directly with renal disease, and in anti-dsDNA negative SLE patients, they inversely correlate with serum complement levels. In antiphospholipid syndrome patients, their presence predicts SLE development.

36. Toward which proteins and/or phospholipids the anti-phospholipid antibodies are directed?

Anti-phospholipid antibodies (aPL) comprise a group of antibodies that recognize *negatively charged* phospholipids including cardiolipin, phosphatidylserine, phosphatidylinositol, phosphatidylglycerol, and phosphatidic acid, as well as *neutrally charged* phospholipids including phosphatidylethanolamine, phosphatidylcholine, platelet-activating factor (PAF), sphingomyelin, a phospholipid-binding protein cofactor, called β2 glycoprotein I (β2GPI), and the protein prothrombin [3].

37. What is lupus anticoagulant and how does it affect prothrombin and activated partial thromboplastin time?

Lupus anticoagulant (LA) is an immunoglobulin binding to phospholipids and cell membrane proteins. The term is a misnomer as LA is, in fact, a prothrombotic agent. The term "anticoagulant" refers to its in vitro properties, since in laboratory tests, this immunoglobulin increases activated partial thromboplastin time (aPTT) which cannot be corrected by addition of normal plasma, whereas in vivo it interacts with platelet membrane phospholipids, increasing adhesion and aggregation of platelets. Prothrombin time (PT) is not affected by the presence of LA. If PT is prolonged, it might indicate a high level of LA, but it can also be due to prothrombin (factor II) deficiency, which is associated with bleeding tendency rather than hypercoagulability. Prolonged aPTT is seen in half of the patients with LA; however, a normal aPTT does not exclude LA presence.

38. Why is Venereal Disease Research Laboratory (VDRL) test positive in patients with antiphospholipid syndrome?

The VDRL test measures antibodies against negatively charged phospholipids, such as cardiolipin. Antibodies recognizing negatively charged phospholipids can cause agglutination, similar to what is seen in patients with syphilis. A false-positive VDRL test, in other words a positive test in patients without syphilis, can therefore be found in patients with antiphospholipid syndrome.

39. **Which autoantibody specificities can be found in the sera of patients with necrotizing autoimmune myositis?**

Anti-signal recognition particle (anti-SRP) and anti-3 hydroxy-3-methyl-glutaryl-coenzyme A reductase (HMGC) antibodies.

40. Which autoantibody specificities account for fetal loss?

Anti-β2GPI, lupus anticoagulant (LA), anti-cardiolipin, anti-Ro/SSA, anti-La/SSB, and anti-thyroglobulin antibodies.

41. Which are the constituents of Ro/SSA and La/SSB autoantigens?

Ro/SSA and La/SSB autoantigens are constituents of ribonucleoprotein complexes with small noncoding RNAs ("Y RNAs"). The antibodies to

Ro/SSA recognize two distinct proteins with different molecular weights (52 kDa and 60 kDa) and cellular locations. The 52-kDa protein is an interferon-inducible protein located in the cytoplasm. The 60-kDa protein binds to small noncoding RNAs ("Y RNAs") located in the nucleus. The Ro/SSA protein functions as an RNA chaperone that binds to defective cellular and viral RNAs to hasten their degradation, while the La/SSB protein functions as a termination factor for RNA polymerase III.

42. In which disease autoantibodies to Ro52 and/or Ro60 are found, what is their clinical relevance and with which other autoantibody reactivities can they associate?

Anti-Ro/SSA antibodies are among the most commonly detected autoantibodies in the routine screening for autoimmune diseases [4]. In a recent retrospective, observational study [5] comprising 272 autoimmune patients, the clinical relevance, the disease phenotype and other autoimmune reactivities' associations in patients with anti-Ro52 and/or anti-Ro60 autoantibodies were analyzed:

- Combined serum anti-Ro52/anti-Ro60 is the most frequently detected reactivity
- Sjögren's syndrome (SS) and systemic lupus erythematosus (SLE) patients have mostly combined anti-Ro52/anti-Ro60 autoantibodies in their sera
- In SS or SLE patients anti-Ro52/anti-Ro60 reactivity associates strongly with anti-La and/or anti-dsDNA autoantibodies
- SS patients with combined anti-Ro52/anti-Ro60 and anti-La reactivity present more frequently with clinical and/or laboratory risk factors for lymphoma development
- Solo anti-Ro52 reactivity is primarily found in idiopathic inflammatory myopathies (IIM), primary biliary cholangitis (PBC), rheumatoid arthritis (RA), and SS patients
- Solo anti-Ro52 associates with anti-Jo1 and anti-M2 autoantibodies and with interstitial lung disease (ILD) in a clinical context of IIM-related lung injury
- ILD patients with combined anti-Ro52/anti-Ro-60 reactivity are diagnosed mostly as RA and/or SS
- Solo anti-Ro60 reactivity often coexists with autoantibodies to Sm or U1RNP

As anti-Ro52 and anti-Ro60 reactivities, combined or isolated, can point to a certain spectrum of disease manifestations, guide diagnosis, and at times define prognosis of certain autoimmune diseases, it is important that they are tested and reported separately in everyday clinical practice [4, 5].

43. In which systemic lupus erythematosus patients anti-ribosomal P antibodies can be found?

Anti-ribosomal-P autoantibodies are found in the sera of systemic lupus erythematosus patients with neuropsychiatric manifestations, mainly psychosis and epilepsy.

44. Which is the clinical relevance of autoantibodies in the different forms of scleroderma?

Different autoantibodies are detected in the sera of scleroderma (systemic sclerosis, SSc) patients and can guide diagnosis and prognosis. Two autoantibody specificities, anti-centromere antibodies (ACA) and anti-Scl-70 can differentiate localized (ACA) from diffuse (anti-Scl-70) SSc. These autoantibodies are commonly found in SSc patients and infrequently in the sera of other autoimmune connective tissue diseases. Anti-RNA-polymerase III antibodies and anti-fibrillarin autoantibodies (which share significant serologic overlap with anti-U3-ribonucleoprotein antibodies) are found less frequently (11% and 4%, respectively) in the sera of systemic sclerosis patients. Additionally, autoantibodies to PM/Scl are seen in the sera of patients with limited skin disease and in patients with overlapping features of scleroderma and myositis. The clinical significance of anti-Ku autoantibodies is not well characterized [6].

45. What is the clinical significance of autoantibodies against CXCR3/4 in patients with diffuse cutaneous scleroderma (dcSSc)?

Previous studies have shown C-X-C motif chemokine receptor (CXCR)3 and CXCR4, through activation and accumulation of T cells, neutrophils, and monocytes in the lungs of dcSSc patients, play a significant pathogenetic role in interstitial pulmonary inflammation. In a recent study, it was shown that serum autoantibodies directed against the chemokine receptors CXCR3 and CXCR4 were mainly linked to the presence of interstitial lung disease (ILD) in dcSSc-patients. Higher anti-CXCR3 and anti-CXCR4 autoantibody levels were observed in patients with dSSc with lung fibrosis compared with those with limited cutaneous systemic sclerosis (lcSSc) and in those dcSSc patients without ILD. The autoantibody levels weakly and negatively correlated with lung function parameters. In addition, it was found that the expression of CXCR3 and CXCR4 in peripheral blood mononuclear cells correlated with the extent of lung and skin fibrosis. The deterioration of lung function parameters was associated with low anti-CXCR3 and anti-CXCR4 autoantibody levels. In addition, low anti-CXCR3 and anti-CXCR4 autoantibody levels predicted the progressive impairment of lung function parameters. In conclusion, it appears that anti-CXCR3/4 autoantibodies and their receptors are linked with the severity of dcSSc-ILD. The levels of these autoantibodies discriminate patients with stable or decreasing lung function. These findings should be re-evaluated in multicenter studies before these autoantibodies will be used in clinical practice for risk stratification of dcSSc patients [7].

46. In which autoimmune diseases anti-alpha enolase autoantibodies can be detected and with which clinical manifestations do they associate?

Human alpha-enolase is a ubiquitous glycolytic enzyme, highly expressed in the kidney and on the surface of endothelial cells. In recent years, citrullinated alpha enolase (CEP-1) has been recognized as a major antigenic target of antibodies against citrullinated proteins in several systemic autoimmune diseases. Anti-CEP-1 antibody reactivity has been reported in the serum of rheumatoid arthritis (RA), systemic lupus erythematosus (SLE), primary Sjögren's syndrome (pSS), and scleroderma (SSc) patients [8]. In RA the presence of anti-CEP-1 antibody seems to define a subset of RA patients with erosive arthritis and RA-associated interstitial lung disease (ILD) [9]. In SLE patients, alpha-enolase seems to play a role in the formation of circulating antibodies during disease flare and anti-CEP-1 antibody has been identified in both, kidney and serum samples of patients with lupus nephritis, and highest levels were associated with proteinuria [8]. In pSS patients anti-CEP-1 antibody presence associates with the occurrence of arthritis and possibly renal tubular dysfunction [10]. In SSc patients detection of anti-CEP-1 antibody seems to associate with ILD and anti-topoisomerase antibodies [8].

47. In which autoimmune disorders antibodies to Hsp-65 can be found?

Heat shock protein 65 (Hsp-65) is a mycobacterial protein that has common structural elements with several human host proteins. Through molecular mimicry, antibody production to mycobacterial HSP-65 has been associated with diabetes mellitus type I, autoimmune thyroiditis, Crohn's disease, rheumatoid arthritis, autoimmune hepatitis, primary biliary cholangitis (previously known as primary biliary cirrhosis), and scleroderma. Hsp-65 is also implicated in multiple vasculitis-associated systemic autoimmune diseases such as Kawasaki disease, Behçet's disease, and Takayasu arteritis.

48. Perinuclear immunofluorescence pattern of neutrophils develops from antibodies directed against myeloperoxidase, the so-called pANCA. Which other autoantibodies may give the same pattern and in which patient's sera can they be detected?

- α-Lactoferrin
- α-Elastase
- α-Cathepsin G
- They can be found in the sera of patients with ulcerative colitis, sclerosing cholangitis, and rheumatoid arthritis

49. What is the role of complement activation in systemic autoimmune diseases?

Complement proteins belong to the innate immune system. They recognize and eliminate foreign invaders either by killing them or by stimulating phagocytosis by opsonization. Activation of the complement plays a significant role in the pathogenesis of systemic autoimmune diseases. Activation of the classical pathway is the cornerstone in immune complex-mediated diseases such as systemic lupus erythematosus, cryoglobulinemic vasculitis, and post-streptococcal glomerulonephritis. In the recent decade, increasing evidence suggests that the alternative complement pathway is involved in several systemic autoimmune diseases such as ANCA-associated vasculitis, leading to new therapeutic options (monoclonal antibodies against C5 or C5a have shown to be effective in experimental models of ANCA-associated vasculitis and antiphospholipid syndrome). In the IgA-dominant Henoch-Schönlein purpura, activation of the lectin pathway has been shown to contribute to more severe disease.

50. Which autoimmune conditions can develop in patients with C4 null allele?

C4 has two allotypes, A and B. Deficiency in the C4A allotype is associated with systemic lupus erythematosus, diffuse systemic sclerosis (negative for anti-topoisomerase I antibody), and limited systemic sclerosis. A deficiency in the C4B allotype is associated with diffuse systemic sclerosis (positive for anti-topoisomerase I antibody), diabetes mellitus type I, and rheumatoid arthritis.

51. Which autoimmune conditions are characterized by low complement C3 and C4 levels?

Systemic lupus erythematosus, post-streptococcal glomerulonephritis, subacute bacterial endocarditis, cryoglobulinemia (types II and III), bacterial sepsis (pneumococcal, Gram negative), viremia (especially hepatitis B), and hypocomplementemic urticarial vasculitis.

52. What does CH50 test evaluate?

The hemolytic complement assay (CH50) assesses the integrity and function of the classical pathway of complement activation. Patient serum is added to standardized suspension of sheep red blood cells coated with rabbit anti-red blood cell antibodies, resulting in immune complex formation which in turn activates the classical pathway, resulting in lysis of the sheep red blood cells. CH50 is the reciprocal of the serum dilution that lyses 50% of the sheep red blood cells.

53. Why complement inhibitors could be used in autoimmune diseases?

Given the prevalence of autoantibodies in the various autoimmune and rheumatic diseases, complement inhibition holds promise as an effective strategy for blocking multiple pathways of injury common to these diseases. Therapeutic complement inhibitors may be effective at blocking direct tissue injury by the complement cascade. Complement inhibitors may also reduce the adaptive immune response by decreasing stimulation of dendritic cells, T cells, and B cells via the complement receptors. This class of drugs could, therefore, be effective in patients with acute disease flares, but also for chronic treatment of these diseases. In some autoimmune diseases, such as membranous neuropathy, activation may occur through the alternative or lectin pathways. Furthermore, the classical pathway may help to eliminate nuclear antigens in diseases such as systemic lupus erythematosus. Thus, there is a rationale to develop and test inhibitors that can specifically block these other pathways or specific downstream complement activation fragments, such as C5a [11].

54. Which are the physicochemical characteristics of C-reactive protein?

C-reactive protein (CRP) is localized in the serum protein electrophoresis between the beta and gamma zones producing beta/gamma zone fusion (Fig. 2.4). It is a pentameric protein composed of five individual subunits non-covalently linked, in cyclic symmetry in a single plane and

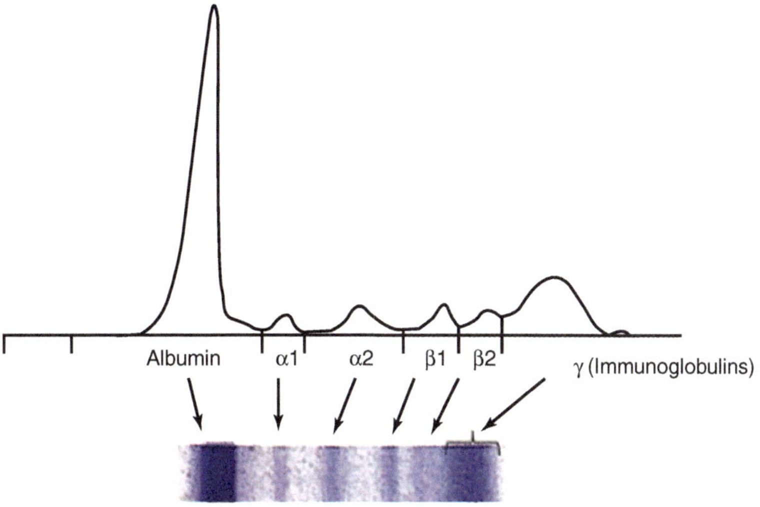

Fig. 2.4 Serum protein electrophoresis: the serum proteins are separated on an agarose gel or cellulose acetate membrane with the application of electric current. Negatively charged proteins (albumin) move faster toward the anode, while γ-globulins possessing a weaker charge move backward from the application site, separated primarily by endo-osmotic forces

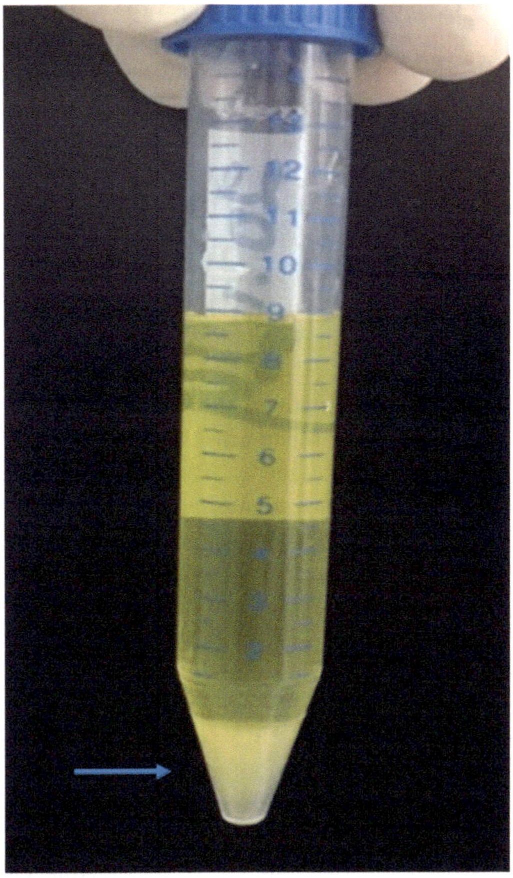

Fig. 2.5 Cryoglobulin precipitate (arrow) in a cryocrit tube

belongs to the family of pentraxins (together with serum amyloid P). CRP is produced by hepatocytes, when they receive message from IL-6 and other pro-inflammatory cytokines. CRP serum levels rise within 2–4 h after tissue injury, infection, or inflammation and peak within 24–72 h. In the absence of inflammatory stimuli, CRP levels fall rapidly with a half-life about 18 h. It can act as an opsonin by binding to phosphatidylcholine expressed on the surface of dead or dying cells and some bacteria and in that way activates the classical complement pathway (C1q), leading to their opsonization, by generating C3b complement component on cell surfaces.

55. Which are the characteristics of the three cryoglobulin types?

Cryoglobulins are immunoglobulins (Ig) or immunoglobulin-containing complexes that precipitate from serum and plasma at low temperatures (<37 °C), (Fig. 2.5) and become soluble again upon rewarming.

Type I cryoglobulins: are composed of a single monoclonal Ig, IgM being the most common Ig class. Their quantity is typically very high (cryocrit >5%) and precipitation occurs rapidly upon cooling (<24 h). This type of cryoglobulins is associated with underlying lymphoproliferative disorders (multiple myeloma, Waldeström's mac-

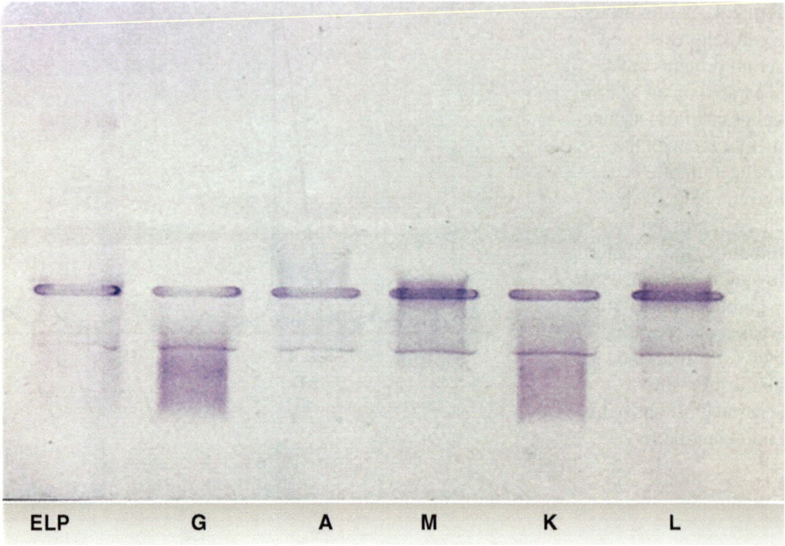

Fig. 2.6 Immunofixation of cryoprecipitate showing type III mixed polyclonal (IgG/IgM/IgA, κ, λ) cryoglobulins with rheumatoid factor activity

roglobulinemia, chronic lymphocytic leukemia, B-non-Hodgkin's lymphoma, and amyloidosis).

Type II cryoglobulins: are "mixed" cryoglobulins composed of a monoclonal Ig (usually IgM) that acts as an antibody (e.g., rheumatoid factor) against polyclonal Ig (typically IgG). Their quantity is usually intermediate (cryocrit 1–5%), and their precipitation may take a few days to occur. They are associated with hepatitis C infection (90%), Sjögren's syndrome, and lymphoproliferative processes.

Type III cryoglobulins: are "mixed" cryoglobulins similar to type II; the immunoglobulin with rheumatoid factor activity is polyclonal Ig directed against another polyclonal Ig (Fig. 2.6). Their quantity is usually small (cryocrit <1%) and their precipitation is slow (takes up to 7 days). They are associated with hepatitis C infection (90%), other infections (HIV, HBV, EBV, CMV, *Coxiella burnetii*, *Leishmania donovani,* parvovirus, and tuberculosis), autoimmune diseases (Sjögren's syndrome, systemic lupus erythematosus, rheumatoid arthritis), and lymphoproliferative processes.

56. Which proteins can become amylogenic?

In primary amyloidosis (AL), amyloid fibrils derive from the N-terminal region of the immunoglobulins' light chains (λ more often than κ) produced by a monoclonal population of plasma cells in the bone marrow. In chronic inflammatory conditions, serum amyloid A (SSA) protein precipitates in the tissues and induces the picture of secondary amyloidosis. Other amyloid proteins include calcitonin (ACal) which is associated with medullary carcinoma of the thyroid, atrial natriuretic factor (AANF) associated with senile amyloidosis of heart atria, prolactin (APro) associated with prolactinoma, β-amyloid (Aβ) associated with Alzheimer's disease, and transthyretin which is responsible for familial amyloidosis.

57. What factors do not allow the fast precipitation of red blood cells (RBCs) in the test tube and provide a within normal limit erythrocyte sedimentation rate (ESR)?

Four factors affect ESR: Size, concentration and shape of RBCs, and plasma protein composition.

Size of RBCs: Microcytes sink slower—lower ESR.

Concentration of RBCs: If high numbers of RBCs, they sink slower—lower ESR.

Shape of RBCs: Sickle cells and spherocytes sink slower—lower ESR.

Plasma protein composition: Increased levels of albumin cause RBC to sink slower—lower ESR, while increased γ-globulins and fibrinogen cause RBCs to sink faster-higher ESR.

References

1. Avrameas S, Alexopoulos H, Moutsopoulos HM. Natural autoantibodies: an undersugn hero of the immune system and autoimmune disorders-a point of view. Front Immunol. 2018;9:1320.
2. Fereidan-Esfahani M, Nayfeh T, Warrington A, Howe CL, Rodriguez M. IgM natural autoantibodies in physiology and the treatment of disease. Methods Mol Biol. 2019;1904:53–81.
3. Cozzani E, Drosera M, Gasparini G, Parodi A. Serology of lupus erythematosus: correlation between immunopathological features and clinical aspects. Autoimmune Dis. 2014;2014:321359.
4. Robbins A, Hentzien M, Toquet S, Didier K, Servettaz A, Pham BN, et al. Diagnostic utility of separate antibody detection in autoimmune diseases. Front Immunol. 2019;10:444.
5. Zampeli E, Mavrommati M, Moutsopoulos HM, Skopouli FN. Anti-Ro52 and/or anti-Ro60 immune reactivity: autoantibody and disease associations. Clin Exp Rheumatol. February 2020;18. [Epub ahead of print].
6. Mecoli CA, Casciola-Rosen L. An update on autoantibodies in scleroderma. Curr Opin Rheumatol. 2018;30:548–53.
7. Weigold F, Günther J, Pfeiffenberger M, et al. Antibodies against chemokine receptors CXCR3 and CXCR4 predict progressive deterioration of lung function in patients with systemic sclerosis. Arthritis Res Ther. 2018;20:52.
8. Pratesi F, Moscato S, Sabbatini A, et al. Autoantibodies specific for alpha-enolase in systemic autoimmune disorders. J Rheumatol. 2000;27:109–15.
9. Alunno A, Bistoni O, Pratesi F, et al. Anti-citrullinated alpha enolase antibodies, interstitial lung disease and bone erosion in rheumatoid arthritis. Rheumatology (Oxford). 2018;57:850–5.
10. Nezos A, Cinoku I, Mavragani CP, Moutsopoulos HM. Antibodies against citrullinated alpha enolase peptides in primary Sjogren's syndrome. Clin Immunol. 2017;183:300–3.
11. Thurman JM, Yapa R. Complement therapeutics in autoimmune disease. Front Immunol. 3 April 2019;10:672.

Suggested Reading

12. Bradwell AR, Hughes RG, Harden EL, editors. Atlas of Hep-2 patterns and laboratory techniques. 2nd ed. Birmingham: Binding Site; 2003.
13. Lorenz R, Nahm M, editors. Quick guide to autoimmune disease serology kindle edition: AACC Press; 2015.
14. Mackay I, Rose NR, editors. The autoimmune diseases. 5th ed: Academic; 2013.

Part II

Autoimmune Rheumatic (Connective Tissue) Diseases

Inflammatory Arthritides

3

Haralampos M. Moutsopoulos
and Evangelia Zampeli

Abstract

Inflammatory arthritides are systemic diseases characterized by synovial inflammation as well as cartilage and bone destruction, accompanied by increased levels of acute-phase reactants. They can be seropositive or seronegative based on the presence or absence of rheumatoid factor and/or anti-citrullinated peptide antibodies, respectively. Rheumatoid arthritis (RA) is the prototype of seropositive arthritis. RA is characterized by extensive synovitis resulting in articular cartilage erosions and joint destruction and presents as symmetrical arthritis of small and large joints along with a wide spectrum of extra-articular manifestations.

Seronegative spondyloarthropathies include psoriatic arthritis (PsA), ankylosing spondylitis (AS), enteropathic arthritis, post-infectious (reactive) arthritis, adult-onset Still's disease, juvenile idiopathic arthritis, and juvenile spondyloarthropathy. Type and location of articular involvement, extra-articular and systemic manifestations, as well as findings from joint imaging are important in distinguishing different types of arthritis. Sacroiliac joint and spine involvement alone or accompanied by asymmetrical arthritis of large peripheral joints and enthesitis are seen more often in seronegative spondyloarthropathies. Psoriasis and psoriatic nail changes are frequently encountered in PsA patients. Keratoderma blennorrhagica, conjunctivitis, and uveitis are some of the extra-articular manifestations of reactive arthritis. Enteropathic arthritis, seen in patients with Crohn's disease or ulcerative colitis, can affect the spine, sacroiliac joints, and large peripheral joints. *Tropheryma whipplei*, parvovirus 19, chikungunya virus, hepatitis B and C virus infection, *Borrelia burgdorferi*, and disseminated gonococcal infection are associated with arthritis, which is sometimes difficult to distinguish from inflammatory arthritis. Rheumatic fever, a sequel of group A streptococcal pharyngitis, manifests with febrile migratory polyarthritis, myocarditis, valvular heart disease, erythema marginatum, and chorea.

1. What is rheumatoid arthritis?

Rheumatoid arthritis is a chronic, systemic, autoimmune disease. Its main site of pathology is the joint synovium. Inflammation of the synovium leads to cartilage erosion and joint deformities.

H. M. Moutsopoulos (✉)
Athens Academy, Athens, Greece
e-mail: hmoutsop@med.uoa.gr

E. Zampeli
Bioclinic General Hospital of Athens and Institute for Autoimmune Systemic and Neurological Disorders, Athens, Greece
e-mail: ezampeli@bioclinic.gr

H. M. Moutsopoulos, E. Zampeli (eds.), *Immunology and Rheumatology in Questions*,
https://doi.org/10.1007/978-3-030-56670-8_3

Extra-articular manifestations may accompany joint disease, yet arthritis is the major manifestation of rheumatoid arthritis.

2. What is the role of genetic factors in the pathogenesis of rheumatoid arthritis?

The precise pathogenic mechanisms underlying rheumatoid arthritis (RA) are not yet fully understood. However, an increasing number of studies show that the interaction between genetic and environmental factors and the continuous activation of innate and adaptive immune systems trigger an abnormal autoimmune response. Large-scale genome-wide association studies (GWAS) on patients with RA have linked more than 30 genomic risk loci and single nucleotide polymorphisms (SNPs) to RA susceptibility; however, the genetic risk loci identified to date only account for approximately 60% of the total heritability of RA.

Class II major histocompatibility antigens/human leukocyte antigens (HLA-DR), as well as non-HLA genes, have been implicated in the pathogenesis of RA. Apart from susceptibility to RA, some genes are implicated in disease outcome and prognosis. HLA-DRB1 gene plays an important role in antigen presentation to T cells and is a well-known genetic risk factor for RA. Valine and leucine amino acids at position 11 in the HLA-DRB1 locus are identified as additional susceptibility factors for a more severe RA course and radiographic progression. Of note, certain gene profiles have also been associated with response or non-response to therapy. Recently, it has been demonstrated that the HLA-E 01:01/01:01 genotype may be associated with decreased RA risk and superior response to anti-TNF agents. Contrariwise, the HLA-E 01:03 variant may account for a lower probability of achieving disease remission. Among the non-HLA genes associated with RA predisposition, IL23R and PTPN22 genes have likely the strongest associations. Protein tyrosine phosphatase non-receptor type 22 (PTPN22), right after HLA-DRB1, shows the second strongest association with RA risk. According to the new GWASs, TNF receptor-associated factor 1 (TRAF1) may have the third strongest association with RA. Furthermore, TRAF1-C5 region has also been linked with anti-citrullinated peptide antibodies (ACPA) seropositive-RA. Moreover, different gene variants seem to be associated with specific clinical aspects of RA, rather than with disease susceptibility. This is the case of RARB gene (rs1161199914) which is linked to the development of subclinical atherosclerosis in RA.

3. What is the role of epigenetics in the pathogenesis of rheumatoid arthritis?

In the last few years, growing interest has been shown in elucidating, besides genetic factors, epigenetic mechanisms that could be implicated in the final interpretation of the encoded genetic information. Epigenetic modifications are inheritable and potentially reversible changes in DNA and chromatin that regulate gene expression without altering the DNA sequence. The major epigenetic mechanisms include DNA methylation, histone proteins modifications and changes in gene expression by microRNA (miRNA), and other non-coding RNA. Some miRNA (miR-23a-3p, miR4634, and miR 361-5p) are overexpressed in early RA, while others (miR-613) that have a protective role seem to be downregulated [1, 2].

4. What is the role of environmental factors in the pathogenesis of rheumatoid arthritis?

Various environmental factors have been postulated to be implicated in the pathogenesis of rheumatoid arthritis (RA). Of those, tobacco smoking is the most widely studied and recognized environmental risk factor for RA development.

- Smoking and smoking intensity are associated with increased risk of seropositive RA (rheumatoid factors and/or anti-citrullinated protein antibodies (ACPA)-positive). The increased risk of seropositive RA in smokers is associated with the presence of rheumatoid epitope (HLA-DRB1), confirming the genetic–environmental interaction between the alleles of the rheumatoid epitopes and tobacco. Besides triggering disease in genetically susceptible individuals, smoking has also been shown to have a negative impact on RA course and severity as well as on response to treatment

- Female hormones have been controversially implicated in RA susceptibility. In a recent study, it has been shown that oral contraceptives, as opposed to smoking, decrease the risk of RA, especially of ACPA-positive RA
- Several infectious agents have been studied as possible environmental factors implicated in RA development. *Porphyromonas gingivalis* and *Aggregatibacter actinomycetemcomitans*, causative agents of periodontitis, which is twice more frequent in RA patients than in the general population, have aroused as a potential risk factor for the development of RA. They induce activation of citrullinating enzymes and produce chronic inflammation and erosive destruction of periodontal bone. Periodontal disease, like RA, has been associated with HLA-DRB1. Of note, recently peptidyl arginine deiminase 4 (PADI4) was identified as the first non-MHC RA risk locus which is expressed in rheumatoid arthritis synovial tissues, as well as in *Porphyromonas gingivalis* and *Aggregatibacter actinomycetemcomitans* in gingival tissue and it post-translationally converts peptide-bound arginine residues into citrulline, leading to citrullinated epitope generation, which is recognized by ACPAs
- Exposure to crystalline silica and silicone breast implants are well-defined risk factors for RA [3–6]

5. **Which are the main immunopathological mechanisms involved in the pathogenesis of rheumatoid arthritis?**

The inflamed synovium in rheumatoid arthritis is characterized by distinct features:

- Fibroblast-like synoviocytes (FLS, synovial fibroblasts or type B synoviocytes) physiologically inhabit the intimal lining of the synovium and control the composition of the synovial fluid and the extracellular matrix (ECM) of the joints' lining. In rheumatoid arthritis (RA), FLS proliferate, acquire a pathogenic phenotype, and mediate inflammation which leads to destruction of the joint. RA FLS secrete enzymes able to destroy the ECM (such as matrix metalloproteinases, MMPs), aggrecanases, and cathepsins, which favor resorption of ECM and promote cartilage destruction. RA FLS are also potentially important promoters of bone erosion, since they are able to secrete receptor activator of nuclear factor-κB ligand (RANKL), which promotes osteoclast differentiation. The invasiveness of RA FLS is stimulated by local pro-inflammatory factors (interleukin (IL)-1 and IL-6, tumor necrosis factor (TNF), reactive oxygen and nitrogen species) whose formation is triggered by local hypoxia, growth factors (platelet-derived growth factor, PDGF), and ECM proteins. Another pathologic feature of RA FLS is their enhanced, compared to FLS of healthy individuals, ability to secrete many cytokines, chemokines, and proangiogenic factors, thus exerting a potent immunoregulatory function through interaction with immune cells
- Neoangiogenesis with endothelial activation and a massive invasion of inflammatory cells (macrophages, dendritic cells, lymphocytes, and mast cells) in the synovial sublining. Lymphocytes—B and T cells—infiltrate the synovium in different patterns: diffusely, in the form of aggregates (small aggregates consist mainly of T lymphocytes; in large aggregates, B cells are the dominant cell population), forming germinal centers which contain follicular dendritic cells and high endothelial venules (formed early in the disease process), which are responsible for ectopic neoangiogenesis
- T helper (Th)17/T regulatory (Treg) cell imbalance. RA has been classically identified as a Th1-mediated disease, yet recently the role of Th17 and Treg is being extensively investigated. Th17 cells represent a distinct effector T-cell subset, which are found in the inflamed rheumatoid synovium and produce the IL-17 family members, IL-21, and IL-22. IL-17 has been shown to play a leading role in pannus growth, RANKL-independent osteoclastogenesis, and synovial neoangiogenesis. Treg cells are found in abundance in the hyperplastic rheumatoid synovium and that their number increases in parallel with the worsening of inflammation. On the other hand, circulating

Treg cells are reduced during inflammation which seems to be a compensatory mechanism to counteract local inflammation
- Immunohistochemical analysis of synovial tissue specimens has shown that the numbers of CD38+ plasma cells and CD22+ B cells in RA synovium are increased in early seropositive rheumatoid arthritis [1]

6. **Can serum lipids be considered a risk factor of rheumatoid arthritis development?**

Besides environmental factors, several studies have suggested that hyperlipoproteinemia can be another predisposing factor for rheumatoid arthritis (RA) development. In a previous report [7] it was shown that patients with arthralgias, positive for rheumatoid factor (RF) and/or anti-cyclic citrullinated peptide antibodies (anti-CCP, ACPA), are at risk of developing RA. In these patients, it was shown that prior to diagnosis, lower apolipoprotein A1 and HDL cholesterol levels were predictive for the development of arthritis. A recent study demonstrated that women with a diagnosis of RA during the follow-up had higher total cholesterol levels at baseline compared with controls. This association remained statistically significant in multivariate models adjusted for smoking and a history of early menopause. In contrast, cholesterol levels in men did not have a significant impact on the risk of RA. Furthermore, it was shown that triglycerides did not predict RA in either men or women [8].

7. **Which are the early synovial pathology findings in rheumatoid arthritis patients?**

- A band-like mucoid swelling of the synovial adventitia, with increased acid glycosaminoglycans
- More frequent occurrence of vasculitis
- Less marked infiltration of lymphocytes and plasma cells
- Absence of gross fibrin infiltration and granulocyte infiltration
- Absence of diffuse fibrosis and hyalinosis

8. **What are fibrillar collagen type II (CII) antibodies, and in which rheumatoid arthritis phenotype can they be found?**

Fibrillar collagen type II (CII) is a major protein of the hyaline cartilage. Antibodies to CII (anti-CII) form immune complexes and induce the production of pro-inflammatory cytokines from mononuclear and polymorphonuclear granulocytes. Increased anti-CII levels are detected in a subgroup of rheumatoid arthritis (RA) patients mainly at the time of diagnosis. In these patients, the presence of anti-CII antibodies has been shown to associate with an acute inflammation (increased C-reactive protein, erythrocyte sedimentation rate) and clinically relevant markers (swollen joint count and disease activity score (DAS)28), which nevertheless is transient and lasts up to 6 months after diagnosis, in contrast to anti-citrullinated peptide antibody (ACPA)-positive RA patients. Anti-CII antibodies are positively associated with HLA-DRB1*01 and HLA-DRB1*03 and negatively with smoking, opposite associations as compared to ACPA. Although anti-CII antibodies are not yet diagnostically useful, the early anti-CII detection predicts a more favorable RA phenotype regarding inflammatory outcome [9].

9. **What is pannus?**

The synovium is the primary site of the inflammatory process in rheumatoid arthritis (RA). In normal joints, it is a thin (only 1–3 cells thick) lining that serves as a source of nutrients for cartilage since cartilage itself is avascular. In RA, the inflammatory cytokine milieu causes the synovial lining cells (fibroblast-like and macrophage-like synoviocytes) to proliferate. The inflamed synovium becomes greatly hypertrophied (8–10 cells thick) and develops villous projections that invade and erode the cartilage and bone, leading to destruction of the joint. This inflamed, hypertrophied synovium is called pannus.

10. What are the characteristics of rheumatoid arthritis synovial fluid?

The synovial fluid in rheumatoid arthritis (RA) is an exudate, with white blood cell counts ranging from 5000 to 50,000/mm^3 and with a neutrophil predominance. The protein level is elevated, while the fluid glucose level may be lower than that of the serum. Crystals are absent and cultures are negative. Synovial fluid rheumatoid factor can be positive, and complement (C3, C4) levels can be lower than the serum complement levels. The presence of cells called "ragocytes," which are granulocytes that have phagocytized immune complexes, can be found in the inflammatory synovial fluid from RA patients and may indicate an unfavorable disease prognosis.

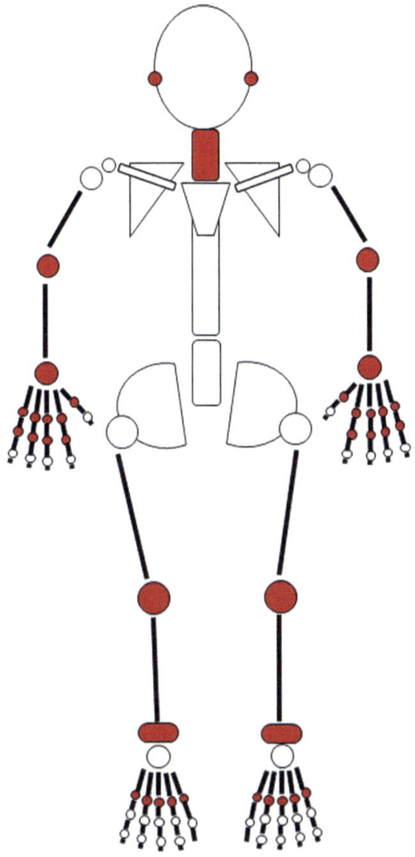

Fig. 3.1 Rheumatoid arthritis: schematic representation of the affected joints (*Figure created by Evangelia Zampeli, MD*)

11. Which joints are more commonly affected in rheumatoid arthritis? (Fig. 3.1)

Most patients with rheumatoid arthritis have symmetrical arthritis involving primarily the metacarpophalangeal (MCP) joints, the proximal interphalangeal (PIP) joints, the wrists (with a predilection for ulnar styloid and triquetrum), and the metatarsophalangeal (MTP) joints. Larger joints tend to become involved after the involvement of the small joints. The cervical spine can be involved with the C1–C2 (atlantoaxial) joint being the most commonly affected level.

12. How can disease activity score (DAS) 28 be calculated in rheumatoid arthritis?

The number 28 refers to the joints assessed: shoulders, elbows, wrists, metacarpophalangeal joints, proximal interphalangeal joints, and knees.

- Count the number of swollen joints (out of the 28)
- Count the number of tender joints (out of 28)
- Measure erythrocyte sedimentation rate and/or C-reactive protein levels
- Global assessment of health by the patient in a scale from 1 (very good) to 10 (very bad)
- Feed this information into a mathematical formula
- DAS28 $\leq$2.6 = disease in remission, DAS28 >2.6 to $\leq$3.2 = low disease activity, DAS28 >3.2 to $\leq$5.1 = moderate disease activity, and DAS28 >5.1 = severe disease activity

13. Which are the typical radiographic features of rheumatoid arthritis-affected joints? (Fig. 3.2)

The radiographic hallmarks of rheumatoid arthritis are:

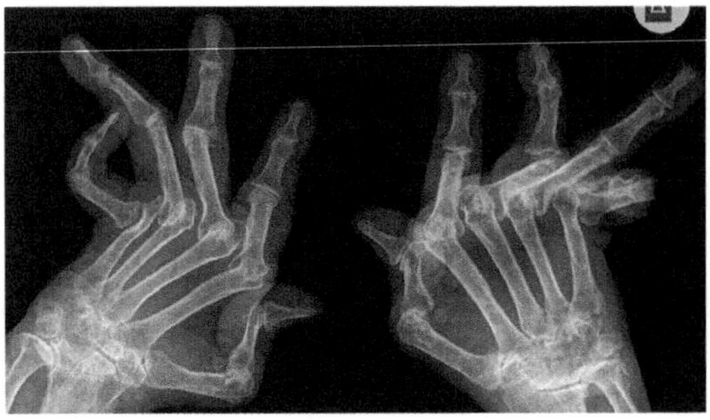

Fig. 3.2 Advanced seropositive rheumatoid arthritis: hand X-ray showing marked subluxation of the fingers with ulnar deviation of the metacarpophalangeal joints, bone cysts, and diffuse osteopenia. Hitchhiker's thumb deformity is best seen on the left hand. The carpal bones are fused with cystic lesions and sclerosis (*Figure courtesy of Professor Alexandros A. Drosos, MD*)

- Soft tissue swelling: Fusiform and periarticular. It represents a combination of joint effusion, edema, and tenosynovitis, and it can be the very early sole radiographic finding
- Osteoporosis: Initially juxta-articular and later generalized (affected additionally by corticosteroid therapy and limited joint movement)
- Joint space narrowing: Typically symmetrical
- Marginal erosions: Due to erosion by pannus

Late changes include:

- Subchondral cyst formation: Destruction of the cartilage presses synovial fluid into the bone
- Subluxation causing:
  - Ulnar deviation of the metacarpophalangeal joints
  - Boutonnière and swan neck deformities
- Deformities: Hitchhiker's thumb deformity, hammertoe deformity, and hallux valgus
- Carpal instability: Scapholunate dissociation and ulnar translocation
- Radiographic findings in cervical spine involvement include:
  - Atlantoaxial subluxation
  - Erosion and fusion of apophyseal and facet joints
  - Erosion of spinous processes
  - Osteoporosis and osteoporotic fractures

14. What are telescopic fingers in inflammatory arthritis?

In long-lasting inflammatory arthritis (rheumatoid or psoriatic arthritis), destructive erosive arthritis of hand joints (arthritis mutilans) may cause bone resorption of interphalangeal joints resulting in collapse of the joints over themselves giving an X-ray image of a sliding telescope tubes into each other, termed "telescope fingers." Fingers appear shortened and are unstable. Nowadays, with early diagnosis and treatment, these severe destructive forms of arthritis are becoming extremely rare.

15. Is joint ultrasound better than clinical examination to evaluate treat-to-target efficacy in patients with early rheumatoid arthritis?

To date no study has clearly demonstrated a beneficial effect of targeting ultrasound remission over clinical remission in rheumatoid arthritis (RA) patients. A recent study investigated whether management of early RA by a tight control strategy, incorporating ultrasound information in treatment decision making, would lead to reduced Magnetic Resonance Image (MRI) inflammation or less MRI structural damage compared to a conventional tight control strategy. Two hundred and thirty early RA patients that had not received treatment with disease-modifying drugs (DMARD) were randomized either to an ultrasound tight control strategy or conventional strategy (both targeting DAS <1.6). Patients in both arms were treated similarly. Evaluation of bone marrow edema, synovitis, and tenosynovitis was examined with MRI. During a 2-year MRI follow-up, no difference between an ultrasound-guided treat-to-target strategy and a conventional clinically guided treat-to-target strategy in the MRI outcomes for inflammatory activity and structural damage was demonstrated. These findings support the notion that adding ultrasound information to strategic treatment decisions and targeting therapy toward ultrasound remission does not lead to improved outcomes and may cause overtreatment [10].

16. Asymptomatic patients with autoantibodies to immunoglobulins (rheumatoid factor) and citrullinated peptides (ACPA). What is the probability that they develop rheumatoid arthritis?

A study of healthy relatives of rheumatoid arthritis patients has shown that the positive predictive value was 64% when both ACPA and rheumatoid factor were positive and 58% when only ACPA autoantibodies were present [11].

17. Which are (according to incidence) the extra-articular manifestations of rheumatoid arthritis?

Extra-articular manifestations can develop prior or during the clinical course of the disease. Anemia (of chronic disease), Sjögren's syndrome, pleurisy, pericarditis, and subcutaneous and lung nodules are some of the extra-articular manifestations of rheumatoid arthritis (RA). B-cell lymphoma development occurs in RA patients three times more frequently than in age-, sex-, and race-matched healthy individuals. In untreated or poorly responding to therapy RA patients, AA amyloidosis can develop. AA amyloidosis, vasculitis, and Felty's syndrome these days are seen very infrequently.

18. What are the clinical and laboratory findings of pleurisy in rheumatoid arthritis patients?

Pleurisy in rheumatoid arthritis (RA) occurs more commonly in seropositive men than female patients, usually sometime during the course of the disease. The pleural RA effusion can be transitory, recurring, or may persist for years. Pleurisy in these patients is usually asymptomatic and unilateral predominantly on the left pleural space. Less commonly it is bilateral and produces chest pain. Examination of the pleural fluid reveals an exudate in which during early disease phases the majority of cells in the fluid are neutrophils and later on lymphocytes predominate with low pH and low glucose levels.

19. Which are the most common mortality causes of patients with rheumatoid arthritis?

- Cardiovascular disease
- Interstitial lung disease
- Infections
- Lymphoproliferative disorders
- Treatment/drug related, e.g., nonsteroidal anti-inflammatory drugs causing upper gastrointestinal tract bleeding

20. Which clinical manifestation(s) in rheumatoid arthritis patients can lead to sudden death?

- Subluxation of the odontoid process into medulla oblongata
- Unrecognized coronary artery disease leading to sudden cardiac death

21. Is the incidence of cardiovascular disease increased in patients with rheumatoid arthritis, and if so, what are the underlying causes?

Rheumatoid arthritis (RA) by itself is considered an independent risk factor for cardiovascular disease (CVD), associated with at least 1.5-fold increased risk for a fatal coronary event compared to age- and sex-matched general population. RA patients present evidence of advanced preclinical carotid atherosclerosis compared to healthy controls, to a magnitude similar to that observed in diabetes mellitus patients. RA patients present an increased burden of traditional CVD risk factors including hypertension, dyslipidemia, smoking, insulin resistance, obesity/altered body composition, and physical inactivity, but all these accounts only partly for the excess CVD mortality. The systemic inflammatory burden and chronic activation of the immune system present in RA play a major role in the atherosclerotic process. The extent to which traditional CVD risk factors and RA-related parameters (inflammatory burden, activity/remission, and treatment modalities) interact and/or contribute to increased CVD incidence remains inconclusive. Nevertheless, besides effectively inducing RA remission, it is of equal importance to optimally control classical CVD risk factors in RA patients.

22. Should statins be used in rheumatoid arthritis patients without risk factors for cardiovascular disease?

It is known that rheumatoid arthritis (RA) patients have an increased prevalence of coronary artery disease (CAD). It is not known, however, if statins can be used in RA patients without the classical risk factors for CAD for its primary prevention. In a recent randomized double-blind, placebo-controlled trial of over 3000 adults, >50-years old with RA and no history of CAD or diabetes, there was a non-significant trend toward reduction in composite cardiovascular risk compared to placebo; the study was discontinued prior termination due to a lower-than-anticipated number of cardiovascular events [12]. Thus, statins are not indicated for CAD prevention in RA patients.

23. Which are the cutaneous manifestations of rheumatoid arthritis patients, and do these patients constitute a particular disease subgroup?

- Raynaud's phenomenon is present in around 5–10% of rheumatoid arthritis (RA) patients and can predict an aggressive disease course
- Rheumatoid nodules are subcutaneous nodules found in 10–20% of RA patients, who are typically seropositive and have severe disease (Fig. 3.3)
- Small-vessel vasculitis can develop when the RA articular disease is in remission and can present with a clinical picture ranging from purpuric lesions to ulcerative-necrotic cutaneous lesions
- Pyoderma gangrenosum and Sweet's syndrome are both infrequent neutrophilic dermatoses that can be seldom seen in RA patients

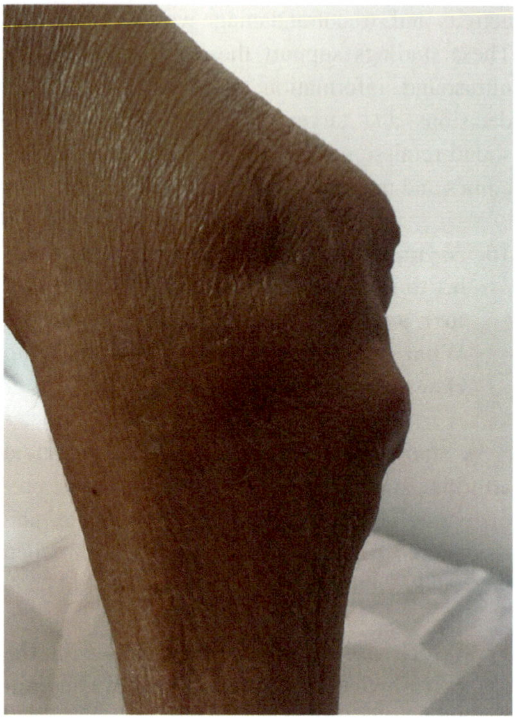

Fig. 3.3 Rheumatoid nodules: subcutaneous nodules on the extensor surface of the elbow in a 58-year-old female patient with long-standing seropositive rheumatoid arthritis

24. Which organs (according to incidence) rheumatoid vasculitis affects?

Primarily the skin. Major manifestations include palpable purpura, ischemic ulcers, and digital gangrene. Digital infarctions may accompany other manifestations of vasculitis or may occur alone as isolated digital arteritis, in which case the prognosis is relatively favorable. Mononeuritis multiplex is another classic presentation of rheumatoid vasculitis. Weight loss, pleurisy, pericarditis, ocular inflammation, splenomegaly, hepatomegaly, and Felty's syndrome have also been reported in association with rheumatoid vasculitis.

25. In which rheumatoid arthritis patient subpopulation rheumatoid nodules can be seen in the lungs?

Lung nodules are seen in rheumatoid arthritis (RA) patients that have worked as coal miners (Caplan's syndrome/rheumatoid pneumoconiosis) as well as in RA patients exposed to silica dust or asbestos. Drugs such as methotrexate, leflunomide, or anti-tumor necrosis factor (anti-TNF) agents can cause the appearance of rheumatoid nodules. Regression has been reported following treatment with tocilizumab and/or rituximab.

26. Which are the clinical, laboratory, and other characteristics of rheumatoid arthritis patients demonstrating anti-Ro/SSA antibody positivity?

Anti-Ro/SSA positive rheumatoid arthritis (RA) patients have the same articular and extra-articular manifestations as anti-Ro/SSA negative patients. However, they are predominantly females with lower rheumatoid factor titers in their sera and a higher incidence of round cell infiltrates in the minor salivary gland biopsy specimens compared to RA patients without anti-Ro/SSA. Finally, anti-Ro/SSA positive RA patients more frequently experience side effects with D-penicillamine treatment [13].

27. What is the kidney pathology which can develop in rheumatoid arthritis patients?

Rheumatoid arthritis (RA) has been associated with a variety of kidney disorders principally due to chronic inflammation and drug exposure/toxicity. From kidney biopsies performed on RA patients, the most commonly observed renal pathologies are mesangial proliferative glomerulonephritis, membranous nephropathy, immunoglobulin A nephropathy, minimal change disease, pauci-immune glomerulonephritis, analgesic nephropathy, interstitial nephritis, and AA amyloidosis.

28. How common is Felty's syndrome? In which rheumatoid arthritis patient subgroup does this syndrome develop?

Felty's syndrome is rheumatoid arthritis (RA) in combination with splenomegaly and leukopenia. It is seen in less than 1% of RA patients who are seropositive (rheumatoid factor positive) and have subcutaneous nodules and other extra-articular manifestations. It has been shown that in most of these RA patients there is an association with the alloantigen HLA-DR4.

29. Is the risk of breast cancer development higher or lower in women patients with rheumatoid arthritis?

Several studies had shown that the risk of breast cancer is decreased in women patients with rheumatoid arthritis (RA). In a recent study, it was shown again that the risk of breast cancer before and after RA development was indeed reduced, finding which further pointed that this association could not be readily explained by traditional breast cancer risk factors, but rather by other factors not related to RA. In addition, this study showed that tamoxifen and aromatase inhibitors did not appear to increase the risk of future RA development [14].

30. Is the risk for periodontitis increased in rheumatoid arthritis patients?

Yes. According to the nation-wide studies from the United States, individuals who fulfill the rheumatoid arthritis classification criteria present four times higher risk to develop periodontitis compared to individuals who do not fulfill the criteria [15].

31. Is there a link between osteoporosis and rheumatoid arthritis?

Rheumatoid arthritis (RA) has been found to be associated with osteoporosis, not only because RA patients are treated with corticosteroids but also because the RA-related inflammatory burden can by itself add to the risk of developing osteoporosis. When RA synovitis becomes persistent, then the bones around the joints become thinned, and this is known as localized secondary osteoporosis.

32. How does pregnancy affect the course of rheumatoid arthritis?

Clinical symptomatology of rheumatoid arthritis (RA) improves during pregnancy in 50–70% of patients. Disease relapse, however, can be often seen some months postpartum. RA with an active disease during the third trimester are more likely to have preterm births and small-for-gestational-age babies. Infertility is not increased in RA patients, and there is no significant increase in maternal or fetal complications except for risks related to RA therapy [16].

33. Do children of mothers with rheumatoid arthritis have greater risk for development of autoimmune diseases?

Rheumatoid arthritis (RA) affects three times more women than men, primarily in the childbearing age. The consequences of maternal RA are not only limited to perinatal outcomes. Is known from previous work that babies born from RA mothers have low birth weight, preterm birth, and spontaneous abortions. Since genetic predisposition is a significant pathogenetic factor for the pathogenesis of autoimmune disorders the long sequelae of the offsprings from RA mothers was studied in a carefully designed Danish Nationwide cohort study which showed that: children of Caucasian mothers with RA have threefold risk for Juvenile Idiopathic Arthritis (JIA), more than twofold greater risk for RA and thyroid disease and 40% greater risk for Diabetes Mellitus type I, and 30% greater risk for asthma [17].

34. Palindromic rheumatism. What is the clinical picture and which disease will these individuals develop eventually?

Palindromic rheumatism is a type of recurrent episodes of inflammatory arthritis. The arthritis symptoms disappear between attacks and the affected joints return to normal. Men are equally affected with women between the ages of 20 and 50 years. Over time 35–50% of the affected individuals will evolve to rheumatoid arthritis (RA), particularly those who possess in their serum rheumatoid factor and/or anti-citrullinated peptide antibodies (ACPA) positivity. It is worth noting though that recognition of ACPA epitopes and isotypes in patients with palindromic rheumatism is different than those in RA [18].

35. What is the remitting, seronegative, symmetrical synovitis with pitting edema (RS3PE) syndrome?

It is a syndrome that affects mostly men above the age of 60 years. It has an acute onset and a benign course, since it remits by less than 36 months and does not relapse. It presents with edema of the dorsum of the hands and feet, symmetrical synovitis of small joints, and flexor tendinitis. Rheumatoid factor is negative, and the patients respond quickly to low-dose corticosteroids. X-rays of the affected joints do not present any pathological signs.

36. What did we learn from the genetic studies of ankylosing spondylitis?

The genetic background confers an over 90% risk for the development of ankylosing spondylitis (AS). Genetic studies strongly suggest that AS develops from the interaction of the mucosal immune system with the intestinal microbiome, an interplay which leads to excess IL-23 production and initiation of the inflammatory process. Genetics also play a significant role in AS parameters such as disease activity, joint fusion rate, and the development of extra-articular manifestations [19].

37. What is the hypothesis regarding the role of human leukocyte antigen (HLA)-B27 in the pathogenesis of ankylosing spondylitis?

A genetically susceptible (HLA-B27 alloantigen-positive) individual, when exposed to microbial triggers, is postulated to clinically express ankylosing spondylitis. There are four different related hypotheses:

- *Arthritogenic peptide hypothesis*: suggests that the HLA-B27-specific autoimmune

response may be directly initiated for structurally unique peptide–MHC complexes, depending on the amino acid composition of the antigen peptides
- *Molecular mimicry hypothesis*: suggests that a cross-reactive peptide derived from an infecting bacterial pathogen stimulates T cells, which subsequently respond to an HLA-B27-associated "self-peptide" or to peptides derived from HLA-B27 directly
- *Free heavy-chain hypothesis*: HLAB-27 heavy chain can form stable homodimers without associated β2 microglobulin on the cell surface. These homodimers can trigger a direct activation of natural killer cells causing IL-17 and TNF-α release
- *Unfolded protein hypothesis*: HLA-B27 appears to exhibit a tendency to misfold and a predilection for forming dimers or multimers in the endoplasmic reticulum. This causes a stress response, resulting in the release of inflammatory cytokines (IL-23) and stimulation of Th17 cells. Furthermore, endoplasmic reticulum aminopeptidase 1 (ERAP-1) is involved in the loading of MHC molecules in the endoplasmic reticulum, and abnormal loading may contribute to misfolding of HLAB-27. Both ERAP-1 and IL-23 receptor polymorphisms have been implicated in the genetic risk for developing ankylosing spondylitis

38. Which peripheral joints are affected by ankylosing spondylitis?

Ankylosing spondylitis (AS) affects primarily the sacroiliac joints and the joints of the spine. However, approximately 30% of AS patients will develop peripheral arthritis. The hips, the shoulders, and the knees are most commonly involved (Fig. 3.4). Rarely, arthritis of the sternoclavicular, temporomandibular, and cricoarytenoid joints or the pubic symphysis occurs. Involvement of the thoracic, costovertebral, sternocostal, and manubriosternal joints can also rarely occur.

39. Which are the causes of Achilles tendinitis? (Fig. 3.5)

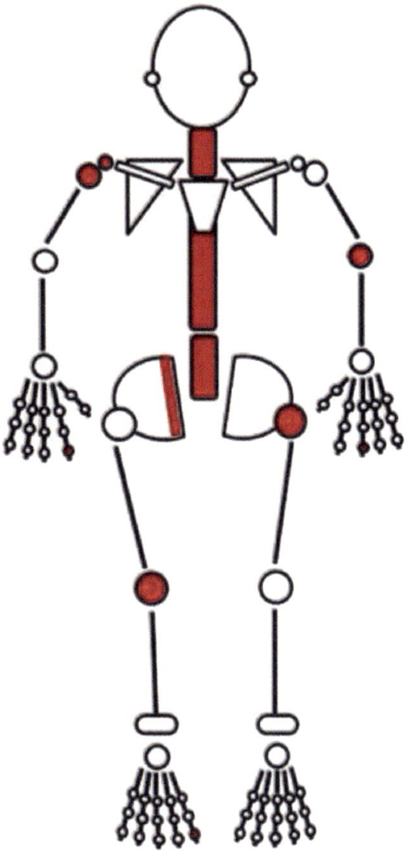

Fig. 3.4 Ankylosing spondylitis: schematic representation of the affected joints (*Figure created by Evangelia Zampeli, MD*)

The commonest cause of Achilles tendinitis is repetitive and intense tension on the tendon as occurs in men with flat foot (pes planus), who exercise strenuously. Inflammation of the tendon enthesis is another etiology of Achilles tendinitis. Patients with HLA-B27-related diseases like ankylosing spondylitis, reactive arthritis, and psoriatic arthritis can manifest Achilles tendinitis. Patients with hereditary connective tissue disorders can also develop Achilles tendinitis.

40. Which are the spine and pelvis radiological findings in patients with ankylosing spondylitis?

Sacroiliac joints: involvement is usually bilateral and symmetric. Initially the synovial-lined

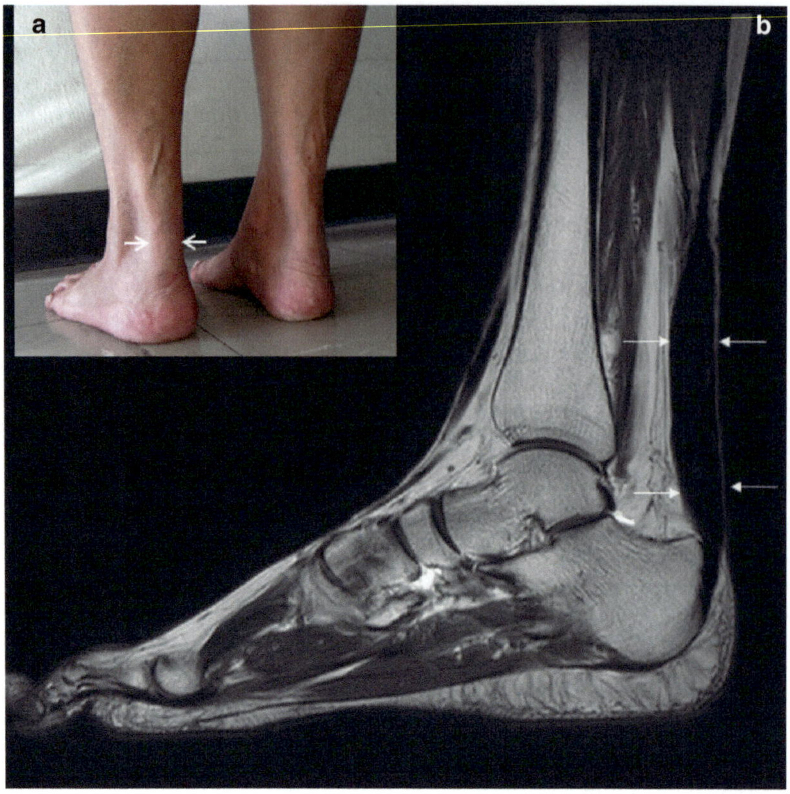

Fig. 3.5 Achilles tendinitis: (**a**) in a 55-year-old female with psoriatic arthritis who presented with a painful left foot. On clinical examination, a painful and swollen Achilles tendon was palpated (white arrows). (**b**) Magnetic resonance imaging (proton density, modified Dixon) revealed diffuse fusiform thickening in the whole length of the Achilles tendon (anteroposterior diameter 15 mm, normal <6 mm) with no tear or enthesitis (white arrows) (*Figure courtesy of Professor Alexandros A. Drosos, MD*)

upper two-thirds of the sacroiliac joint become involved. The earliest radiographic change is erosion of the iliac side of the sacroiliac joint. Progression results in an initial "pseudo-widening" of the sacroiliac joint space with bony sclerosis eventually followed by complete bony fusion of the joint (Fig. 3.6a). In early sacroiliitis when plain X-rays may appear normal, magnetic resonance imaging (MRI) will show inflammation and edema.

Spine: an early MRI finding is the so-called shinny corners (Romanus lesion) which represent the insertion of the annulus fibrosus to the corners of the vertebral bodies. Andersson lesion is the inflammatory involvement of the intervertebral discs by spondyloarthritis that presents as non-infectious spondylodiscitis in a few ankylosing spondylitis patients and can mimic infection. Gradual ossification of the outer layers of the annulus fibrosus forms intervertebral bony bridges called syndesmophytes. Squaring of the vertebral bodies, bilateral syndesmophytes, fusion of the apophyseal joints, and calcification of the spinal ligaments result in the complete fusion of the vertebral column giving the appearance of "bamboo spine" (Fig. 3.6b). In advanced stages of the disease—especially if poorly treated—these changes result in loss of natural spinal curvature, thoracic kyphosis, loss of lumbar lordosis, buttock atrophy, and forward bending of the neck (Fig. 3.6c).

41. Which are the magnetic resonance imaging findings seen in patients with sacroiliitis?

The presence on magnetic resonance imaging (MRI) of bone marrow edema in subchondral bone is considered to be the finding that determines the presence of active sacroiliitis (Fig. 3.7). If structural lesions are seen in the sacroiliac joints on MRI, these may further contribute toward the diagnosis of inflammatory lesions of ankylosing spondylitis.

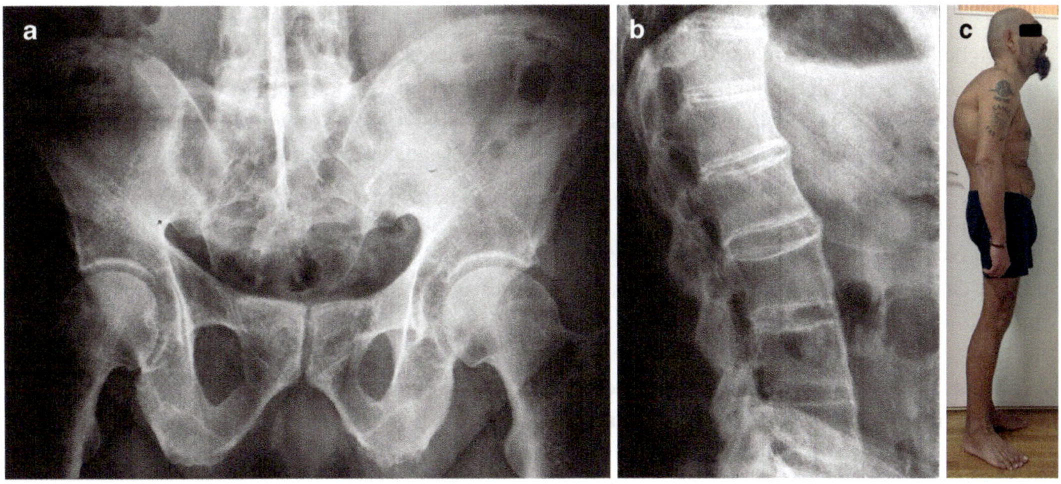

Fig. 3.6 Fused sacroiliac joints in a 48-year-old male patient with advanced untreated ankylosing spondylitis. (**a**) Plain pelvis X-ray showing complete bony fusion of both sacroiliac joints. (**b**) Lateral X-ray view of lumbar spine of the same patient showing large syndesmophytes and calcification of the anterior longitudinal ligament giving the appearance of "bamboo spine." (**c**) The patient's clinical picture shows loss of lumbar lordosis, buttock atrophy, and exaggerated thoracic kyphosis with a forward neck bending

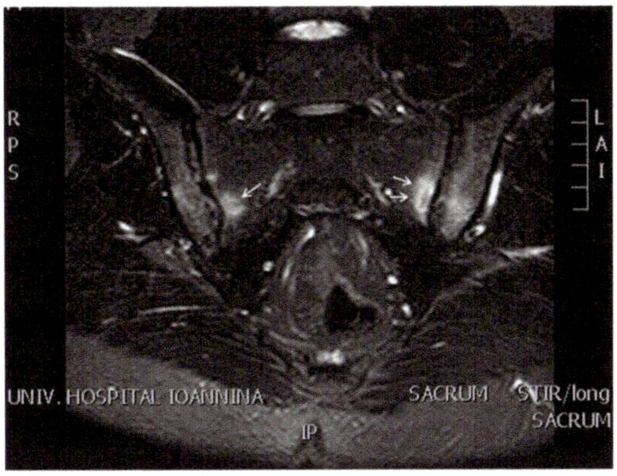

Fig. 3.7 Sacroiliitis: magnetic resonance imaging (STIR sequences in coronal view) of the sacroiliac (SI) joints in a 28-year-old male with low back pain. Diffuse bone edema with high signal of the SI joints bilaterally (arrows) is evident, more prominent on the left side (*Figure courtesy of Professor Alexandros A. Drosos, MD*)

42. Which are the differences between magnetic resonance imaging and radiography in detecting structural lesions of the sacroiliac joints in patients with axial spondyloarthritis?

Magnetic resonance imaging (MRI) appears to be superior to radiography in detecting erosions and joint space narrowing. In contrast, MRI is inferior to radiography in detecting joint sclerosis [20].

43. Are bone marrow edema and fatty lesions on spinal magnetic resonance imaging specific diagnostic signs of axial spondyloarthritis?

In a recent community-based cohort study the spinal and sacroiliac MRIs of 793 volunteers less than 45-years old were evaluated. In 27% of them, bone marrow edema was evident while 81% had fatty lesions. Logistic regression analysis showed that bone marrow edema and fatty lesions, especially of vertebral corners on spinal MRI, were related to increasing age. This study shows that inflammatory and fatty lesions that could be suggestive of axial spondyloarthritis are not infrequent in the ageing general population [21].

44. What is non-radiographic axial spondyloarthritis, what are its clinical characteristics and outcome?

The term non-radiographic axial spondyloarthritis (nrAxSpA) is used to describe patients who have a clinical picture of ankylosing spondylitis (AS) but do not exhibit radiographic sacroiliitis. Patients with nrAxSpA, compared to AS patients, are usually younger in age, more frequently females, with shorter disease duration. They present more often involvement of peripheral joints, have higher inflammatory markers (C-reactive protein) and more frequently inflammatory bowel disease. Albeit, nrAxSpA patients are less often HLAB27 positive. The rate of radiographic progression of nrAxSpA patients varies greatly among studies, from 10 to 40% during 2–10 years of follow up. Nonetheless, it seems that baseline radiographic damage, male gender and smoking are risk factors for future radiographic progression [22].

45. What is the lung pathology which can be seen in ankylosing spondylitis patients?

Ankylosing spondylitis (AS) patients can rarely present with pulmonary apical fibrocystic disease. In the early phase of the disease, lung involvement may be unilateral. In the majority of cases though, as disease progresses, involvement becomes bilateral and fibrobullous nodules coalesce to form cysts and cavities, while fibrosis and bronchiectasis are also common. Fungal or mycobacterial superinfection of the cysts and cavities is not uncommon. *Aspergillus fumigatus* is the most common pathogen isolated. Moreover, a restrictive ventilatory impairment can also be seen in patients with AS due to restricted thoracic cage expansion (ankylosis of the thoracic spine, fusion of the costovertebral joints, and anterior chest wall involvement).

46. Which cardiovascular manifestations can be seen in ankylosing spondylitis patients?

Cardiovascular manifestations are more frequently seen in ankylosing spondylitis (AS) patients with long-standing disease and with peripheral joint involvement. They are observed in around 5% of patients, as conduction defects (atrioventricular block, or branch block) and aortic insufficiency. Aortitis of the ascending aorta can be seen infrequently.

47. Which are the pregnancy outcomes in women with ankylosing spondylitis?

Although there are few reports regarding birth outcomes and ankylosing spondylitis (AS), disease manifestations and pharmacological treatment could possibly contribute to adverse pregnancy outcomes in women with AS. Vaginal delivery in women with AS can be problematic particularly in those with hip arthritis and spinal anesthesia can't be delivered in those with lumbar spine syndesmophytes. A nationwide Swedish study showed that pregnant women with AS, compared to general population controls, after adjusting for smoking, age, level of education, parity and excluding women with comorbidities, had lower point estimates of risk, while they had almost twice more frequently Caesarean sections. The offsprings of women with AS were two times more frequently preterm and small-for-gestational-age compared to offsprings of the general population controls [23].

48. How can one differentiate, based on symptomatology, low back pain due to degenerative arthritis versus spondyloarthritis?

The low back pain of spondyloarthritis (inflammatory) is usually characterized by morning stiffness, subsides with movement, and worsens with rest in contrast to low back pain of degenerative arthritis which worsens with movement.

49. What is osteitis condensans ilii and how does it differ from sacroiliitis?

Both entities can present with low back pain, but radiologically they have quite different appearances. Osteitis condensans ilii is a disorder seen in multiparous women. Firm sclerosis, in a triangular shape, usually bilaterally, is seen at the iliac part of the sacroiliac joint, while the sacrum and joint space are intact (Fig. 3.8). In patients with sacroiliitis erosions and sacroiliac joint space narrowing, bilaterally or unilaterally are the cardinal X-ray manifestations.

50. How does physical strain, (e.g., sports) affect the appearance of bone marrow edema of the sacroiliac joints seen by magnetic resonance imaging?

Low grade bone marrow edema is reported in the sacroiliac joints of up to 25% of healthy individuals and mechanical back pain patients, chal-

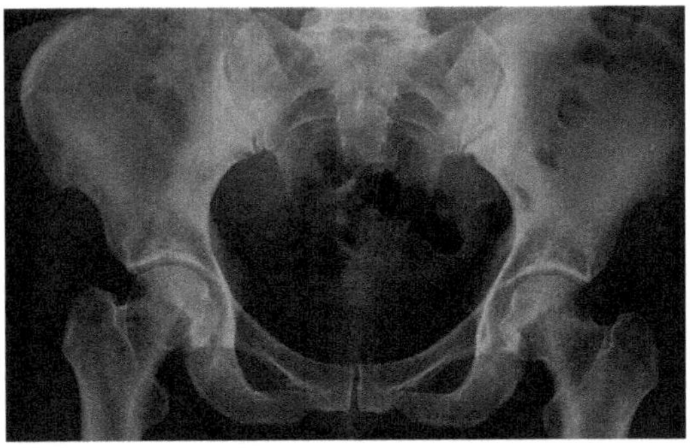

Fig. 3.8 Osteitis condensans ilii: a multiparous 41-year-old female presented with low back pain. X-rays of the pelvis showed sclerosis of the iliac side of the sacroiliac (SI) joints bilaterally (more pronounced on the left side) without joint space narrowing of the SI joints. This finding is considered diagnostic for osteitis condensans ilii (*Figure courtesy of Professor Alexandros A. Drosos, MD*)

lenging the imaging discrimination from early spondyloarthritis. In a recent study comparing two cohorts of healthy hobby runners and professional ice hockey players, the frequency of bone marrow edema on magnetic resonance imaging (MRI) was determined before and after a competitive run and before and after a competitive season respectively. Bone marrow edema was identified in 3–4 quadrants on average for both groups of athletes and the posterior lower ilium was the most affected region in all of these athletes, followed by the anterior upper sacrum.

Therefore, it should be noted that physical strain can cause the presence of low-grade bone marrow edema, especially clustered in the posterior lower ilium or anterior upper sacrum, and this is not sufficient to confirm axial spondyloarthritis in these individuals [24].

51. What is diffuse idiopathic skeletal hyperostosis?

Diffuse idiopathic skeletal hyperostosis (DISH) also known as Forestier's disease is characterized by ossification of ligaments of the spine, especially the anterior longitudinal ligament of the spine. It is a non-inflammatory disease that commonly occurs in obese, diabetic males over 50 years of age. Plain X-ray of the spine shows large osteophytes, flowing hyperostosis, and calcification of the anterolateral aspect of at least four continuous vertebral bodies (Fig. 3.9). The absence of ankylosis of facet joints and erosions of sacroiliac joints differentiate DISH from ankylosing spondylitis.

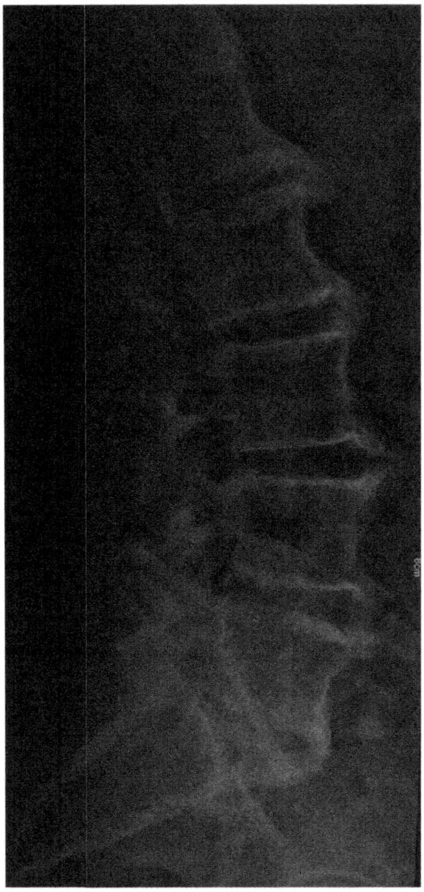

Fig. 3.9 Diffuse idiopathic skeletal hyperostosis: lateral X-ray view of the lumbar spine from a 70-year-old patient revealing flowing ossification along the anterior aspects of more than four contiguous vertebrae, while disc spaces are preserved

52. Which are the common pathogenetic pathways in psoriasis and rheumatoid arthritis (RA)?

Studies which sequence the RNA of peripheral blood mononuclear cells from psoriasis and RA patients and healthy controls, showed that a cytokine imbalance is operating in both psoriasis and RA patients. More specifically the common characteristic molecular mechanisms include the extracellular signal-regulated kinase 2 (ERK1/2),[1] mitogen-activated protein kinase (MAPK),[2] tumor necrosis factor, colony-stimulating factor 3, interleukin-6, interferon, and canonical signaling pathways [25].

53. Which joints can be affected in patients with psoriatic arthritis?

Psoriatic arthritis can affect any joint (large and small) of the body. Large joints of the lower extremities are more often affected. One joint, e.g., the knee (monoarthritis), small number of joints (<3 joints, oligoarthritis) (Fig. 3.10), or multiple joints (polyarthritis) can be affected simultaneously. Fingers or toes can be affected and resemble the appearance of sausages, a condition called dactylitis. Sacroiliitis, more often asymmetric, can also be a psoriatic arthritis manifestation.

54. What is the relation between the onset and flares of psoriasis with the development of psoriatic arthritis?

In the majority (70%) of patients, psoriasis precedes arthritis by an average of 7 years. Arthritis precedes or occurs simultaneously with psoriasis in one-third of the patients. In patients with simultaneous onset of skin and joint disease, flares of both diseases are usually coexisting. However, for the majority of patients, the skin and arthritis run non-synchronous courses.

[1] ERK1/2 are widely expressed protein kinase intracellular signaling molecules, which are stimulated by growth factors, cytokines, viral infections, transforming agents, and carcinogens. They are involved in different steps of differentiating cells.

[2] Mitogen-activated protein kinases (MAPK or MAP kinase) are protein kinases specific to amino acids serine and threonine. They are involved in guiding cellular responses to stimuli like pro-inflammatory cytokines, osmotic stress, and heat shock. They also control cell proliferation, gene expression, differentiation, mitosis, cell survival, and apoptosis.

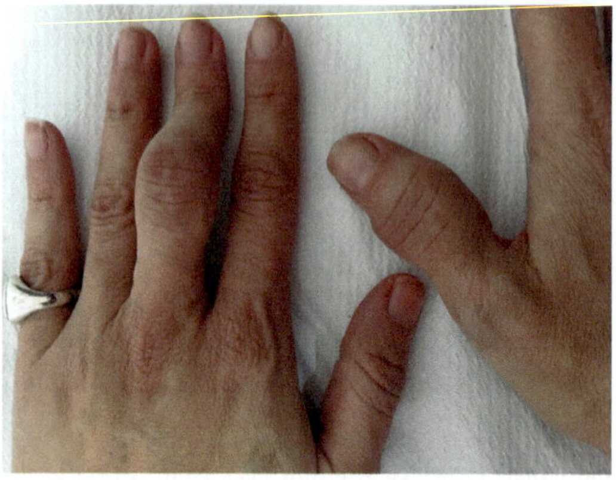

Fig. 3.10 Oligoarticular psoriatic arthritis: a 42-year-old female patient with arthritis affecting the left third proximal interphalangeal joint and the first right distal interphalangeal joint

55. How do structural structural entheseal lesions in patients with psoriasis influence the risk of progression to psoriatic arthritis?

In a recent prospective cohort study, 114 psoriasis patients without clinical evidence of psoriatic arthritis (PsA) were assessed at baseline for structural entheseal lesions and volumetric bone mineral density (vBMD) at entheseal sites by high-resolution peripheral quantitative computed tomography. After a follow-up period of 28 months, 24 patients developed PsA. It was shown that psoriasis patients with structural entheseal lesions were at higher risk of developing PsA compared to patients without such lesions. With respect to vBMD, it was shown that an increased entheseal vBMD was associated with a 30% reduction of risk to PsA progression [26].

56. Which are the characteristic nail changes in patients with psoriatic disease?

- Oil drop or salmon patch: translucent yellow-red discoloration in the nail bed which resembles a drop of oil under the nail plate
- Pitting: loss of parakeratotic cells from the surface of the nail plate

- Beau's lines: transverse lines in the nails due to intermittent inflammation causing growth arrest lines
- Leukonychia: areas of white nail plate due to foci of parakeratosis within the body of the nail plate
- Subungual hyperkeratosis: excessive proliferation of the nail bed and hyponychium. This may lead to onycholysis (Fig. 3.11a)
- Onycholysis: the nail plate separates from its underlying attachment to the nail bed. The nail plate whitens and may detach. Secondary infection may occur
- Nail plate crumbling: the nail plate weakens due to disease of underlying structures (Fig. 3.11b)

57. What is Koebner phenomenon?

Koebner phenomenon occurs in patients with an underlying cutaneous disease, like psoriasis, vitiligo, or lichen planus. It consists of new skin lesions on previously unaffected skin secondary to skin injury, even if trivial. The new lesions are clinically and histologically identical to the patient's pre-existing cutaneous disease (also termed isomorphic phenomenon). The incidence of Koebner phenomenon is higher in psoriasis with a prevalence ranging from 11 to 75%.

58. Which parameters predict radiologic disease progression in psoriatic arthritis?

Severe disease at presentation and elevated C-reactive protein levels.

59. Which medical conditions coexist commonly with psoriatic arthritis?

Obesity, type II diabetes mellitus, hyperuricemia, hypertension, fatty liver, increased incidence of metabolic syndrome, and risk of premature atherosclerosis and cardiovascular disease.

60. Which clinical entities can lead to arthritis mutilans?

Psoriatic arthritis and rarely systemic lupus erythematosus, mixed connective tissue disease, juvenile idiopathic arthritis, as well as multicentric reticulohistiocytosis.

61. In which rheumatic disorders dactylitis can be a manifestation?

Dactylitis occurs in seronegative arthritis, psoriatic arthritis, ankylosing spondylitis, and post-infectious (reactive) arthritis.

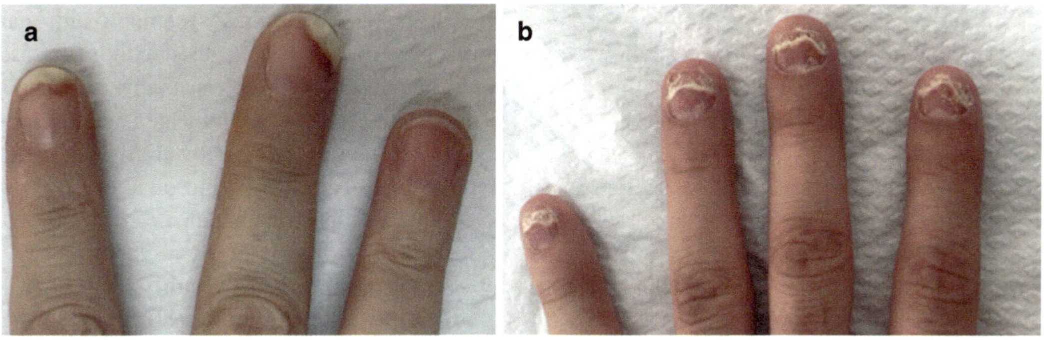

Fig. 3.11 Nail psoriasis: (**a**) a 48-year-old female patient with psoriatic arthritis presents separation of the nail plate from the underlying nail bed and hyponychium affecting the nails of the second and third right fingers, a form of nail psoriasis termed onycholysis. (**b**) A 31-year-old male patient with psoriatic arthritis presents with nail plate crumbling in all fingernails

62. What are the differences in the synovial fluid findings between patients with rheumatoid arthritis and seronegative arthritis?

In the synovial fluid from an inflamed joint of a rheumatoid arthritis patient, in contrast to synovial fluid from a joint of a patient with seronegative arthritis, rheumatoid factors, and decreased complement (C3 and C4) levels may be found.

63. Which are the rheumatologic manifestations in patients with inflammatory bowel disease?

In inflammatory bowel disease, rheumatologic manifestations are frequent and include peripheral arthritis, axial involvement, and peripheral enthesitis. Secondary osteoporosis and hypertrophic osteoarthropathy may also occur. Axial involvement ranges from low back pain to true ankylosing spondylitis. Two types of peripheral arthritis can be seen in inflammatory bowel disease patients: type I, pauciarticular usually nondestructive arthritis affecting large joints and usually associated with active bowel disease, and type II, polyarticular affecting small joints and tending to run a course independent of the bowel disease.

64. What is the course of arthritis in patients with inflammatory bowel disease?

Typically, the course of arthritis follows that of the inflammatory bowel disease; flares and remission of both pathologies coincide.

65. Which bowel diseases are associated with inflammatory arthritis?

- Inflammatory bowel disease (Crohn's disease and ulcerative colitis)
- Microscopic colitis
- Whipple disease
- Gluten-sensitive enteropathy (celiac disease)

66. What extraintestinal manifestations can occur in patients with inflammatory bowel disease and inflammatory arthritis?

- Pyoderma gangrenosum
- Erythema nodosum
- Sweet syndrome
- Anterior uveitis, episcleritis, and scleritis
- Aphthous stomatitis
- Primary sclerosing cholangitis
- Sensorineural hearing loss

67. Which are the major and minor diagnostic criteria for adult-onset Still's disease?

- Major criteria: fever (>39 °C) lasting for more than 7 days, arthralgias/arthritis of more than 2-week duration, characteristic salmon-like rash, and leukocytosis (>10 × 10^9/L with >80% neutrophils)
- Minor criteria: sore throat, lymphadenopathy, hepatosplenomegaly, abnormal liver function tests, negative rheumatoid factor, and antinuclear antibodies

Diagnosis requires at least five diagnostic criteria, two of which being major.

68. Which are poor prognostic factors for adult-onset Still's disease course?

Patients with chronic polyarticular disease generally have worse prognosis and more disability than patients with only systemic manifestations. Nevertheless, adult-onset Still's disease could be life-threatening, especially in patients with systemic disease complicated with hemophagocytic (macrophage activation) syndrome, acute respiratory distress syndrome, or disseminated intravascular coagulation.

69. Which are the different subtypes of arthritis in juvenile idiopathic arthritis (JIA)?

- Systemic JIA: is characterized by recurrent high fever, evanescent erythematous rash, mainly during the periods of fever and arthritis. Generalized lymph node enlargement and/or hepatomegaly and/or splenomegaly, serositis, arthralgia lasting 2 weeks or longer (in the absence of arthritis) and leukocytosis ($\geq$15,000/mm^3) with neutrophilia can also be present

- Rheumatoid factor (RF)-positive JIA: resembles adult rheumatoid arthritis, presents with symmetric arthritis, is RF and anti-citrullinated peptide positive, and has worse prognosis
- Enthesitis/spondylitis-related JIA: is characterized by peripheral arthritis and/or enthesitis, or inflammatory back pain and sacroiliitis on imaging. In these patients HLA-B27 antigen can be present, acute, anterior uveitis can occur and history of a spondyloarthropathy in a first-degree relative is not uncommon
- Early-onset ANA-positive JIA: occurs mostly in young children ($\leq$6 years), has a female predominance, is characterized by arthritis (mainly oligoarthritis), chronic iridocyclitis, and ANA positivity [27]

70. Which are the types of sarcoid arthropathy?

Around 15–25% of patients with sarcoidosis develop arthritis (mostly of small hand and feet joints), which can either be of the acute, transient type or of the persistent, chronic type. The acute or transient type is more common, often being the presenting manifestation of the disease. It generally has a favorable outcome. It affects male patients, younger than 40 years of age, who usually manifest erythema nodosum and subsequently develop, within 2 months, symmetrical ankle arthritis. The next most commonly affected joints are the knees, wrists, and metacarpophalangeal joints. Fever is present in 1/3 to 2/3 of patients according to different reports. The only laboratory finding is elevated erythrocyte sedimentation rate. All patients with sarcoid arthritis have hilar adenopathy. The chronic type of arthritis appears either early or late during the course of sarcoidosis, which is generally active in other organ systems.

71. What are the radiological findings of chronic sarcoid arthropathy?

Radiological findings include soft tissue swelling, periarticular osteopenia, joint space narrowing, cyst formation, punched-out erosions, sclerosis and periosteal reactions, pathologic fractures, and phalangeal fragmentation. The phalanges in chronic sarcoid bone involvement demonstrate a reticulated trabecular pattern.

72. Which microbial species are responsible for the development of post-infectious arthritis?

- Urogenital: *Chlamydia trachomatis* and *Ureaplasma urealyticum*
- Enterogenic: *Salmonella* species, *Shigella* species, *Yersinia* species, and *Campylobacter* species
- Others: *Clostridium difficile*, *Neisseria gonorrhoeae*, *Streptococcus* (post-streptococcal reactive arthritis), *Giardia lamblia*, mycoplasma, and *Borrelia burgdorferi*

73. Which are the rheumatologic manifestations of Whipple disease?

Whipple disease is a chronic, multisystem infection caused by *Tropheryma whipplei*. The disease usually affects middle-aged men. The most common symptoms arise from the gastrointestinal tract and are expressed with diarrhea and weight loss. In three-quarters of patients, arthritis is the initial manifestation and can precede by a mean of 6 years the other disease symptoms. The classic disease scenario is long-term, unexplained, seronegative oligoarthritis or polyarthritis with a palindromic or relapsing course, although chronic destructive polyarthritis and spondyloarthritis have been repeatedly reported. The diagnosis of the disease in the majority of patients is set with periodic acid-Schiff staining of the proximal small bowel biopsy specimens which reveals the bacterial structures as inclusions within the tissue macrophages. Today polymerase chain reaction for *T. whipplei* DNA from tissue or blood is the diagnostic tool used in patients in the early stages of the disease or with atypical Whipple disease.

74. Migratory arthritis. In which medical disorders is it observed?

Migratory arthritis is the arthritis which affects, over a period of days, one joint after the other. Disorders which present with migratory arthritis are systemic gonococcal infection, rheumatic fever, sarcoidosis, systemic lupus erythematosus, Lyme disease, bacterial endocarditis, and neoplasia (paraneoplastic syndrome).

75. Which are the three phases of Lyme disease?

Lyme disease is caused by the pathogenic spirochete Borrelia burgdorferi via a tick vector. It has three stages:

- The early localized disease phase; it starts days to weeks after the tick bite. At the site of the bite, erythema migrans (Fig. 10.2) initially appears as a small red papule that gradually enlarges to form an annular lesion
- The early disseminated disease phase; it occurs after hematogenous or lymphatic dissemination of the disease. It is characterized by secondary annular lesions accompanied by headache, neck stiffness, fever, chills, arthralgias, muscle aches, and profound malaise. In this stage neurologic abnormalities may present as meningitis, subtle encephalitis, cranial neuritis, neuropathy, ataxia, or myelitis. Cardiac complications rarely occur and present as atrioventricular blocks of varying degrees, myopericarditis, or cardiomegaly
- The late disease phase; it occurs months after *Borrelia burgdorferi* infection. In this phase, recurrent episodes of arthritis affecting large joints (mostly the knees) can present and last weeks to months in a single joint. Chronic neurologic sequelae may occur as another manifestation of late-stage disease, which may present as memory, mood, or sleep disorders

76. What is the clinical picture of gonococcal arthritis?

Gonococcal arthritis results from the bacteremic spread of *Neisseria gonorrhoeae*, a sexually transmitted pathogen. It is more commonly seen in young healthy individuals although it may occur in any age group. Host risk factors, such as complement deficiencies particularly the membrane attack complex, menstruation, pregnancy, history of pelvic surgery, and intrauterine devices are associated with disseminated gonococcal infection. Furthermore, specific strains of *N. gonorrhoeae* have virulence factors that promote dissemination, while it is also hypothesized that the pathogenesis of disseminated gonococcal infection may be partly immune-mediated. Gonococcal arthritis may occur in two different clinical forms: localized septic arthritis and arthritis-dermatitis syndrome. Localized septic arthritis presents as monoarthritis or asymmetric oligo- or polyarthritis with pain and swelling of one or more joints. Most patients do not present with systemic symptoms such as fever or chills. Joints that are commonly affected include knees, ankles, wrists, and elbows.

77. What is the arthritis-dermatitis gonococcal syndrome?

The arthritis-dermatitis syndrome comprises the triad of tenosynovitis, dermatitis, and polyarthritis. Tenosynovitis affects multiple tendons, more commonly the fingers, wrists, toes, and ankles. Polyarthritis is migratory, asymmetric and may affect both large and small joints. Pustular or vesicular skin lesions appear on the trunk and extremities, sparing the face, in almost 75% of cases. They are typically transient and may disappear after several days even without treatment. Constitutional symptoms (fever, rigors, and malaise) are common.

78. Which are manifestations of post-infectious arthritis (reactive arthritis)?

- Fever and shaking chills (rigors)
- Increased frequency and discomfort during urination may occur, as well as inflammation of the prostate gland or cervix
- Joint pain and stiffness, typically of the knees, ankles, and feet. Wrists, fingers, and other joints are affected less often. Spondylitis and dactylitis can also develop
- Warmth and redness around the joint
- Commonly inflammation of the tendons (tendinitis) or at places where tendons attach to the bone (enthesitis)
- Mild conjunctivitis sometimes difficult to detect and more infrequently anterior uveitis can develop
- Painless oral and/or genital mucosa ulcers
- Keratoderma blennorrhagica (prominent hyperkeratotic scaling lesions of the palms and soles, Fig. 3.12a, b)
- Balanitis circinata

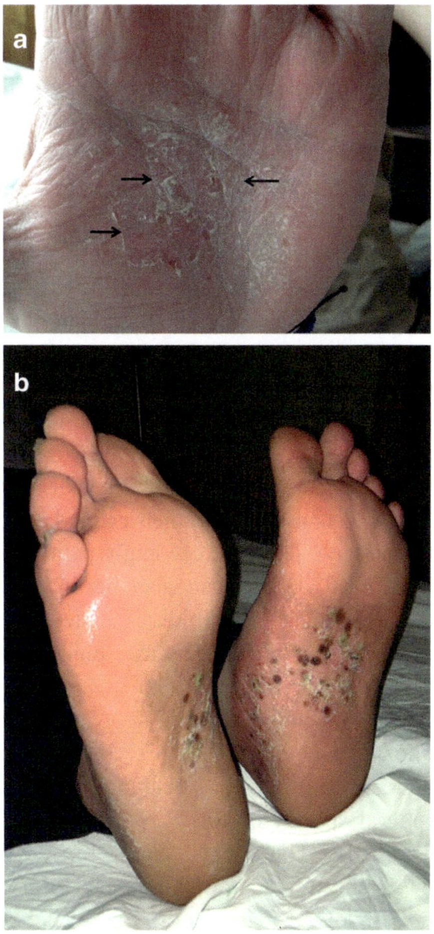

Fig. 3.12 Keratoderma blennorrhagica: a 27-year-old male patient with chronic post-infectious arthritis. Vesicopustular waxy lesions coalescing to form larger crusty plaques with desquamating edges are evident (**a**) on palms (arrows) and (**b**) soles

79. Which viral infection, in the initial phase, can give the picture (arthralgias, fever, urticarial rash, and low complement levels) of serum sickness?

Hepatitis B infection.

80. Which are the rheumatologic manifestations of parvovirus 19 infection?

In adults, the virus can cause inflammatory arthritis that is difficult to be differentiated from rheumatoid arthritis. Arthritis affects symmetrically the wrists, hands, knees, and ankles. Joint symptoms last usually for 1–3 weeks, although in 20% or more of the affected individuals, arthritis may persist for months to years. Adults, in contrast to infected children, often do not experience fever nor do they develop cutaneous rashes. In some patients, the arthritis can be debilitating and requires prednisone to control symptoms. The presence of circulating IgM antiviral antibodies connotes an acute viral infection. The IgM antibody should eventually clear and convert entirely over to IgG antibody. If arthritis does not get better, other types of inflammatory arthritis should be considered.

81. What is the cause, clinical/laboratory findings of patients with Chikungunya arthritis?

Chikungunya arthritis is caused by a mosquito-borne arbovirus, the chikungunya virus (CHIK). Outbreaks of CHIKV had been reported since the mid-2000s in Africa, Asia, and the Indian and Pacific Oceans. However, increasing tourism, population migration, infection of naive individuals and viral mutations have led to the global CHIKV epidemic which from 2004 to 2011 affected around 6.5 million individuals worldwide.

Chikungunya infection has an acute phase (<3 months) and a chronic phase (>3 months). The acute phase is characterized by sudden onset of high-grade fever (often >39 °C), severe polyarthralgia/polyarthritis, myalgias, conjunctivitis, and skin rash. The skin rash may be diffuse or focal, it is pruritic, appears as vesicles or purpura and is often accompanied by skin hyperesthesia. Polyarthritis is usually symmetrical and involves small and large joints. Exceedingly painful tenosynovitis and bursitis can also occur. Patients with concomitant comorbidities (osteoarthritis, heart failure, respiratory disease, renal disease, and diabetes) are likely to have more severe manifestations of acute infection.

The chronic phase of the disease may follow a pattern similar to rheumatoid arthritis, peripheral spondyloarthritis, and undifferentiated arthritis. The ankles, knees, hips, wrists, elbows, and metacarpophalangeal joints are mainly involved. The reported prevalence of CHIKV arthritis patients progressing to a chronic stage (>3 months) ranges from 4.1 to 78.6%. The severity of acute illness, high viral titers during acute infection, and age >45 years are predictors of progression to chronic CHIKV arthritis.

During the initial stages of the disease anemia, leukopenia, lymphopenia, mild thrombocytopenia, raised liver enzymes, and serum creatinine levels are common. Chikungunya virus can be detected by the reverse transcription (RT)-PCR method only in the early (<7 days) phase of the infection. Thereafter PCR detection becomes unreliable and it can only be diagnosed by detecting immunoglobulins (IgM and IgG).

82. What is the management of Chikungunya arthritis?

At present no specific antiviral therapy is available for CHIKV infection. Most CHIKV infections are self-limiting. Analgesia with paracetamol may be required for a few weeks until pain resolves for non-complicated acute cases, while aspirin should be avoided. Ibuprofen, diclofenac, naproxen, or aceclofenac are the nonsteroidal anti-inflammatory drugs (NSAIDs) that can be taken along with paracetamol for intractable symptoms. In the subacute phase, for persistent synovitis and tenosynovitis, low dose oral prednisolone can be used, at a dose of 10 mg daily for 5 days and further tapering over the next 10 days. The maximum dose of steroids recommended is 0.5 mg/kg and steroids are not advised for more than 4 weeks. For peripheral neuropathy symptoms, pregabalin or amitriptyline should be used. Chloroquine phosphate or hydroxychloroquine in the acute phase can be used at doses 300 mg or 200 mg, respectively, once daily for 4 weeks for resistant musculoskeletal symptoms. Disease-modifying antirheumatic drugs (DMARDs) such as methotrexate, sulfasalazine, and hydroxychloroquine have shown benefits in the chronic phase of CHIKV arthritis with ongoing synovitis or tenosynovitis. Biologic DMARDs such as tumor necrosis factor-α inhibitors can be used in resistant cases [28, 29].

83. Which rheumatic manifestations can be seen in patients with chronic hepatitis C?

Hepatitis C virus (HCV) is lymphotropic and can trigger a B-cell expansion, which causes a wide spectrum of autoimmune/lymphoproliferative disorders. These extrahepatic manifestations become clinically manifest in 40–70% of the HCV-infected patients and can be classified as rheumatic. These include arthralgias, arthritis, fatigue, fibromyalgia, cryoglobulinemic vasculitis, and chronic sialadenitis (Sjögren's-like syndrome).

84. What is the clinical picture of arthritis occurring in patients with rheumatic fever versus the clinical picture seen in patients with rheumatoid arthritis?

Arthritis in patients with rheumatic fever is acute and migratory. Typically it affects large joints like knees, ankles, elbows, and wrists. The affected joints can be red, hot, or swollen. Arthritis responds usually well to aspirin and does not leave any cartilage or bone defects. In adult rheumatic fever patients, tenosynovitis is common and sometimes severe and resembles disseminated gonococcal disease. In contrast, rheumatoid arthritis is a chronic polyarthritis which affects symmetrically small and large joints and can cause permanent joint destruction and deformity.

85. Which parts of the heart are affected by rheumatic fever and which are the sequelae?

In patients with rheumatic fever, all parts of the heart (endocardium, pericardium, and myocardium) can be affected. The hallmark of rheumatic carditis is valvular lesions. The most commonly affected valve is the mitral either alone or together with the aortic valve. The early valvular damage is usually valve regurgitation. After repeated recurrences of rheumatic fever, the valvular leaflets get thickened, scarred, and calcified, pathologies which lead to valvular stenosis.

86. Which are the clinical/pathological characteristics of multicentric reticulohistiocytosis?

Multicentric reticulohistiocytosis is a rare disease affecting more females than males (3:1). Constitutional symptoms such as fever, malaise, weight loss, and itching are commonly present. Mucocutaneous manifestations typically manifest with reddish-brown papules and nodules in the hands, fingers (Fig. 3.13a), around the nails, as well as in the oropharyngeal and nasal mucosal surface. Biopsy of the lesions characteristically shows eosinophilic histiocytes and multinuclear giant cell infiltrates with opalescent appearance, fine vacuoles, and PAS-positive granules (Fig. 3.13b). In some patients, arthritis remits spontaneously, while in 1/3 of the patients, it can progress to destructive (mutilans) arthritis. In the latter group of patients, arthritis can be symmetrical and debilitating, usually affecting the interphalangeal finger joints but also the hips and knees. The diagnosis of multicentric reticulohistiocytosis can be easily suspected when a patient presents with the typical skin lesions associated with erosive arthritis.

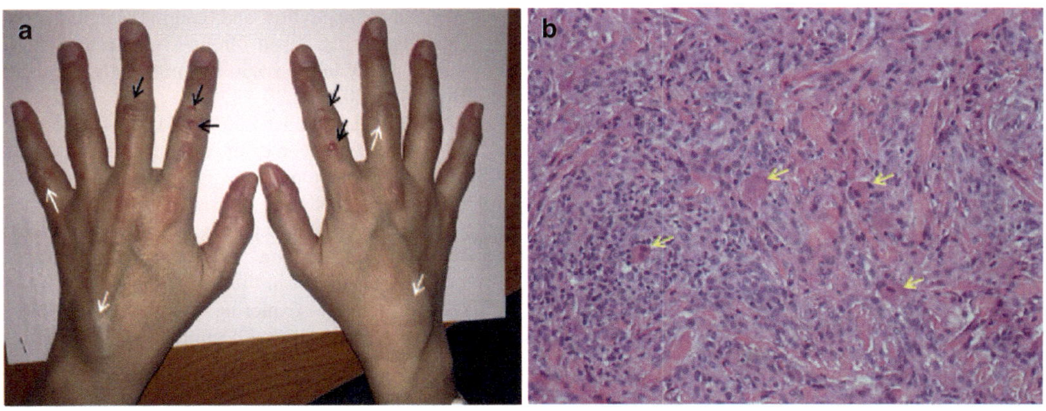

Fig. 3.13 Multicentric reticulohistiocytosis: (**a**) a 33-year-old female presented with fever, joint pain, morning stiffness, and multiple, red-brown, non-tender, cutaneous nodules ranging from 1 to 5 mm, localized on both hands (*black arrows*) along with symmetrical arthritis of the proximal interphalangeal and wrist joints (*white arrows*). (**b**) Biopsy of the nodules demonstrated abundant infiltration of the dermis by histiocytes and scattered multinucleated giant cells (large histiocytes) with finely granulated eosinophilic cytoplasm (H&E ×200, yellow arrows)

References

1. Giannini D, Antonucci M, Petrelli F, et al. One year in review 2020: pathogenesis of rheumatoid arthritis. Clin Exp Rheumatol. 2020;38:387–97.
2. Karami J, Aslani S, Jamshidi A, et al. Genetic implications in the pathogenesis of rheumatoid arthritis: an updated review. Gene. 2019;702:8–16.
3. Di Giuseppe D, Discacciati A, Orsini N, Wolk A. Cigarette smoking and risk of rheumatoid arthritis: a dose-response meta-analysis. Arthritis Res Ther. 2014;16:R61.
4. Balk EM, Earley A, Avendano EA, Raman G. Long-term health outcomes in women with silicone gel breast implants: a systematic review. Ann Intern Med. 2016;164:164–75.
5. Orellana C, Saevarsdottir S, Klareskog L, Karlson EW, Alfredsson L, Bengtsson C. Oral contraceptives, breastfeeding and the risk of developing rheumatoid arthritis: results from the Swedish EIRA study. Ann Rheum Dis. 2017;76:1845–52.
6. Konig MF, Abusleme L, Reinholdt J, Palmer RJ, Teles RP, Sampson K, Rosen A, Nigrovic PA, Sokolove J, Giles JT, Moutsopoulos NM, Andrade F. Aggregatibacter actinomycetemcomitans-induced hypercitrullination links periodontal infection to autoimmunity in rheumatoid arthritis. Sci Transl Med. 2016;8:369ra176.
7. van de Stadt LA, van Sijl AM, van Schaardenburg D, et al. Dyslipidaemia in patients with seropositive arthralgia predicts the development of arthritis. Ann Rheum Dis. 2012;71:1915–6.
8. Turesson C, Bergström U, Pikwer M, et al. High serum cholesterol predicts rheumatoid arthritis in women, but not in men: a prospective study. Arthritis Res Ther. 2015;17:285–93.
9. Manivel VA, Mullazehi M, Padyukov L, Westerlind H, Klareskog L, Alfredsson L, et al. Anticollagen type II antibodies are associated with an acute onset rheumatoid arthritis phenotype and prognosticate lower degree of inflammation during 5 years follow-up. Ann Rheum Dis. 2017;76:1529–36.
10. Sundin U, Aga AB, Skare Ø, et al. Conventional versus ultrasound treat to target: no difference in magnetic resonance imaging inflammation or joint damage over 2 years in early rheumatoid arthritis. Rheumatology. 2020;59:2550-5.
11. Ramos-Remus C, Castillo-Ortiz JD, Aguilar-Lozano L, Padilla-Ibarra J, Sandoval-Castro C, Vargas-Serafin CO, et al. Autoantibodies in prediction of the development of rheumatoid arthritis among healthy relatives of patients with the disease. Arthritis Rheumatol. 2015;67:2837–44.
12. Kitas GD, Nightingale P, Armitage J, et al. A multicenter, randomized, placebo-controlled trial of atorvastatin for the primary prevention of cardiovascular events in patients with rheumatoid arthritis. Arthritis Rheumatol. 2019;71:1437.
13. Skopouli FN, Andonopoulos AP, Moutsopoulos HM. Clinical implications of the presence of anti-Ro (SSA) antibodies in patients with rheumatoid arthritis. J Autoimmun. 1988;1:381–8.
14. Wadström H, Pettersson A, Smedby KE, et al. Risk of breast cancer before and after rheumatoid arthritis, and the impact of hormonal factors. Ann Rheum Dis. 2020;79:581-6.
15. Chou YY, Lai KL, Chen DY, Lin CH, Chen HH. Rheumatoid arthritis risk associated with periodontitis exposure: a nationwide, population-based cohort study. PLoS One. 2015;10:e0139693.
16. Hazes JM, Coulie PG, Geenen V, Vermeire S, Carbonnel F, Louis E, et al. Rheumatoid arthritis and pregnancy: evolution of disease activity and pathophysiological considerations for drug use. Rheumatology (Oxford). 2011;50:1955–68.
17. Rom AL, Wu CS, Olsen J, et al. Parental rheumatoid arthritis and long-term child morbidity: a nationwide cohort study. Ann Rheum Dis. 2016;75:1831–7.
18. Mankia K, Emery P. Palindromic rheumatism as part of the rheumatoid arthritis continuum. Nat Rev Rheumatol. 2019;15:687–95.
19. Brown MA, Kenna T, Wordsworth BP. Genetics of ankylosing spondylitis—insights into pathogenesis. Nat Rev Rheumatol. 2016;12:81–91.
20. Diekhoff T, Hermann KA, Greese J, Schwenke C, Poddubnyy D, Hamm B, et al. Comparison of MRI with radiography for detecting structural lesions of the sacroiliac joint using CT as standard of reference: results from the SIMACT study. Ann Rheum Dis. 2017;76:1502–8.
21. Baraliakos X, Richter A, Feldmann D, et al. Frequency of MRI changes suggestive of axial spondyloarthritis in the axial skeleton in a large population-based cohort of individuals aged <45 years. Ann Rheum Dis. 2020;79:186–92.
22. Chimenti MS, Conigliaro P, Navarini L, et al. Demographic and clinical differences between ankylosing spondylitis and non-radiographic axial spondyloarthritis: results from a multicentre retrospective study in the Lazio region of Italy. Clin Exp Rheumatol. 2020;38:88–93.
23. Jakobsson GL, Stephansson O, Askling J, Jacobsson LT. Pregnancy outcomes in patients with ankylosing spondylitis: a nationwide register study. Ann Rheum Dis. 2016;75:1838-42.
24. Weber U, Jurik AG, Zejden A, et al. Frequency and Anatomic Distribution of Magnetic Resonance Imaging Features in the Sacroiliac Joints of Young Athletes: Exploring "Background Noise" Toward a Data-Driven Definition of Sacroiliitis in Early Spondyloarthritis. Arthritis Rheumatol. 2018;70:736-745.
25. Tan Y, Qi Q, Lu C, et al. Cytokine imbalance as a common mechanism in both psoriasis and rheumatoid arthritis. Mediators Inflamm. 2017;2017:2405291.
26. Simon D, Tascilar K, Kleyer A, et al. Structural entheseal lesions in patients with psoriasis are associated with an increased risk of progression to psoriatic arthritis [published online ahead of print, 2020 Feb 26]. Arthritis Rheumatol. 2020;10.1002/art.41239.

27. Martini A, Ravelli A, Avcin T, et al. Toward new classification criteria for juvenile idiopathic arthritis: first steps, Pediatric Rheumatology International Trials Organization International Consensus. J Rheumatol. 2019;46:190–7
28. Zaid A, Gérardin P, Taylor A, et al. Chikungunya arthritis: implications of acute and chronic inflammation mechanisms on disease management. Arthritis Rheumatol. 2018;70:484–95.
29. Pathak H, Mohan MC, Ravidran V. Chikungunya arthritis. Clin Med (Lond). 2019;19:381–5.

Suggested Reading

Hochberg M, Silman AJ, Smolen J, Weinblatt M, Weisman M. Rheumatology, 2-volume set. 7th ed. Mosby Ltd; 2018.

Watts RA, Conaghan PG, Denton C, Foster H, Isaacs J, Müller-Ladner U. Oxford textbook of rheumatology. 4th ed. Oxford: Oxford University Press; 2018.

4 Systemic Lupus Erythematosus, Mixed Connective Tissue Disease and Antiphospholipid Syndrome

Haralampos M. Moutsopoulos
and Evangelia Zampeli

Abstract

This chapter presents essential knowledge on systemic lupus erythematosus (SLE), mixed connective tissue disease (MCTD) and antiphospholipid syndrome (APS). These diseases share common features in the sense that they are systemic, can be overlapping, and present with non-destructive arthritis.

SLE is the prototype immune complex-mediated disease in humans. There is a strong but not absolute, genetic predisposition for its development. Patients' serum contains autoantibodies against nuclear antigens (ANA) as well as other autoantibodies (e.g., anti-dsDNA, anti-Ro/SSA, anti-La/SSB, anti-U1RNP or anti-Sm, antiphospholipids, anti-ribosomal proteins). Some of them are diagnostic biomarkers, while others predict particular clinical manifestations. Such examples are anti-Ro/SSA antibodies which are associated with a photosensitive, annular/polycyclic, and psoriasiform/papulosquamous rash, anti-dsDNA antibodies with SLE nephritis, anti-ribosomal P with psychosis, antiphospholipids with thromboses and recurrent abortions, and anti-histones with drug-induced SLE. IgG anti-Ro/SSA or anti-La/SSB antibodies cross the placenta and affect the fetus which develops anti-Ro-related rashes, thrombocytopenia, and rather infrequently cardiomyopathy which leads to complete heart block (neonatal lupus).

MCTD is a disease characterized by Raynaud's phenomenon, puffy hands, and arthritis/arthralgias. Acrosclerosis, esophageal dysmotility, myositis, lung fibrosis, and pulmonary hypertension can manifest in patients with MCTD, along with high titers of anti-U1RNP antibodies. The outcome is unpredictable, yet the majority of MCTD patients remain stable, while a minority evolves to another systemic autoimmune disorder (rheumatoid arthritis, SLE, systemic sclerosis, and anti-synthetase syndrome).

APS is an acquired, autoimmune thrombophilia, characterized by the presence of antiphospholipid antibodies and expressed mainly by thrombotic events, pregnancy morbidity, autoimmune hemolytic anemia, or thrombocytopenia. Thrombotic events reoccur usually in the same vascular bed (arterial or venous) and can range from isolated thromboses to massive pulmonary emboli or concurrent thromboses in many organs (catastrophic APS). The heart is involved in terms of coronary artery disease or valvular, non-infectious vegetations (Libman-Sacks endocarditis), while the kidney by thrombotic microangiopathy of the glomeruli or chronic renal vascular lesions.

H. M. Moutsopoulos (✉)
Athens Academy, Athens, Greece
e-mail: hmoutsop@med.uoa.gr

E. Zampeli
Bioclinic General Hospital of Athens and Institute for Autoimmune Systemic and Neurological Disorders, Athens, Greece
e-mail: ezampeli@bioclinic.gr

H. M. Moutsopoulos, E. Zampeli (eds.), *Immunology and Rheumatology in Questions*,
https://doi.org/10.1007/978-3-030-56670-8_4

1. Does inheritance play a role in the development of systemic lupus erythematosus?

Population-based studies have shown two to three times increased relative risk to develop systemic lupus erythematosus (SLE) in individuals with particular HLA class II genes (HLA-DR2 and HLA-DR3). The strongest evidence that SLE is genetically determined comes from familial aggregation studies. An identical twin of a patient with SLE carries a 25–50% chance of developing SLE, while a non-identical twin has a risk of 2–5%, the latter still being greater than that in the general population. First-degree relatives of a patient with SLE carry a six times higher risk of developing SLE. Furthermore, inherited deficiencies of early complement components (C1q, C2, and C4) increase five to ten times the risk of SLE development. A recent meta-analysis at the genome-wide level identified five new loci associated with SLE: GRB2, SMYD3, ST8SIA4, LAT2, and ARHGAP27. Furthermore, pathway analysis revealed several biological processes significantly associated with SLE risk: B cell receptor signaling, CTLA4 co-stimulation during T cell activation, interleukin-4 signaling, and cell surface interactions at the vascular wall [1].

2. Which are the major pathogenic aspects of systemic lupus erythematosus?

Genetic predisposition (as described in the above question) is a *sine qua non* factor for the disease genesis. This, in addition to certain environmental factors (viruses, medications, ultraviolet radiation, and stress), as well as the patients' hormonal milieu, are important triggers for the disease development. The interplay of genetic and environmental factors lead to defective immune regulatory mechanisms, such as the impaired clearance of apoptotic cells, increased auto-antigenic load from the apoptotic cells, altered innate immune responses, excessive T cell help, defective T regulatory cell function, shifting of T helper 1 (Th1) to Th2 function, B cell hyperreactivity, and formation of immune complexes. Activated immunocytes, release of cytokines, autoantibodies, immune complexes and activation of complement components, all lead to tissue injury and disease development.

3. Which cytokines are detected in the sera of active systemic lupus erythematosus patients?

Serum interferon (IFN)- α, interleukin (IL)-6, IL-8, IL-17, and IL-18 levels are elevated in active systemic lupus erythematosus (SLE) patients and correlate with SLE Disease Activity Index (SLEDAI).

4. Which clinical or laboratory manifestations predict that a patient not fulfilling diagnostic criteria will evolve to systemic lupus erythematosus, and when?

The presence of malar rash, oral ulcers, elevated anti-dsDNA, and decreased serum C4 complement levels predict that an individual not fulfilling at that time systemic lupus erythematosus (SLE) diagnostic criteria will evolve to SLE within the next 2–5 years, but not necessarily with major organ involvement.

5. Which are the most common autoantibodies encountered in patients with systemic lupus erythematosus, and what are their main clinical associations?

- Antinuclear antibodies (ANA): are not specific for systemic lupus erythematosus (SLE), and less than 5% of individuals presenting ANA positivity will actually develop SLE. Yet, 98% of SLE patients will demonstrate elevated ANA titers
- Anti-dsDNA: highly diagnostic for SLE and correlate with disease activity, in particular lupus nephritis
- Anti-Sm (Smith): highly diagnostic for SLE and do not correlate with disease activity
- Anti-Ro/SSA: SLE patients have mostly combined anti-Ro52/anti-Ro60 autoantibodies in their sera, which associates strongly with anti-La and/or anti-dsDNA autoantibody positivity. Solo anti-Ro60

reactivity often coexists with autoantibodies to Sm or U1RNP. Anti-Ro/SSA are also encountered in patients with subacute cutaneous lupus erythematosus (SCLE, mainly anti-Ro60), Sjögren's syndrome, neonatal lupus (especially anti-Ro60), neuromyelitis optica spectrum disorders, and photosensitivity
- Anti-La/SSB: encountered primarily in patients with Sjögren's syndrome and patients with SCLE
- Anti-ribosomal P: highly specific for SLE with psychiatric disease (lupus psychosis, epilepsy)
- Antiphospholipids: associated with inhibition of in vitro coagulation tests (lupus anticoagulant), thrombosis, recurrent fetal loss, and thrombocytopenia
- Anti-histones: encountered in SLE and drug-induced lupus erythematosus patients

6. Which medications the physicians should be aware that may be responsible for the development of cutaneous (CLE) or systemic lupus erythematosus (SLE)?

More than 100 drugs have been suspected, up to now, to be responsible for the development of drug-induced lupus erythematosus. In a recently published Danish study the use of drugs that preceded the development of CLE or SLE was evaluated. The study included, from 2000–2017, 1298 patients with CLE and 1850 with SLE, from the National Patient Register and 31 480 matched controls (1:10) for age and sex, from the general population. It was found that the use of Fexofenadine hydrochloride (anti-histamine, H1 selective inhibitor), levothyroxine sodium, metoclopramide hydrochloride (for symptomatic treatment of nausea and vomiting), and metronidazole hydrochloride preceded the development of CLE or SLE. It is evident from the results of this study that the reported associations of drug-induced lupus in published case reports most probably reflects publication bias [2].

7. In a febrile systemic lupus erythematosus patient, which simple lab test(s) will point to fever being due to bacterial infection and not to disease exacerbation?

- White blood cell count: leukocytosis
- Elevated serum C-reactive protein levels (more than 15–20 times above normal value)
- Elevated serum procalcitonin levels

8. A patient with arthralgias, skin rash, leukopenia (WBC < 4000/mm^3), and negative antinuclear antibodies (ANA). What is the possibility that this patient has another autoantibody, which one, and why?

Anti-Ro/SSA autoantibodies. Patients in whom the only autoantibodies present are anti-Ro antibodies may have a falsely negative ANA test using the traditional human epithelial cell line-2 (HEp-2) substrate, because Ro60 immunoreactivity may be lost during the preparation of the cells and because Ro52 is a cytoplasmic, rather than a nuclear autoantigen. This patient might also have positive antithyroid peroxidase or anti-thyroglobulin antibodies.

9. Which laboratory parameters should be periodically evaluated in order to follow systemic lupus erythematosus disease activity?

Laboratory parameters used to follow disease activity in systemic lupus erythematosus patients include complete blood count, erythrocyte sedimentation rate, serum creatinine, liver enzymes, urine analysis, serum C3 and C4 levels, and anti-dsDNA autoantibody levels.

10. Which are the demographic and clinical findings which predict that an acute exacerbation (flare) will occur in a systemic lupus erythematosus patient?

Young age of systemic lupus erythematosus onset (<25 years), proliferative lupus nephritis at diagnosis, oral ulcers, acute malar rash, leukopenia, thrombocytopenia, increased anti-dsDNA levels, and anti-Sm antibody positivity are all factors that can predict a lupus flare, while the patient is on immunosuppressive therapy.

11. Which are the commonest morbidity and mortality causes in patients with systemic lupus erythematosus?

The commonest causes of *morbidity* in patients with systemic lupus erythematosus (SLE) are infections, hypertension, cardiovascular disease, osteoporosis, cytopenias due to immunosuppressive agents, and malignancies. The most frequent causes of *mortality* in patients with SLE are active SLE, cardiovascular disease, thromboses, and serious infections.

12. Which are the most common infections seen in immunosuppressed systemic lupus erythematosus patients?

Microbial septicemia, *Pneumocystis jiroveci* pneumonia, varicella zoster virus infection, and tuberculosis.

13. When does varicella zoster infection develop in systemic lupus erythematosus patients, and which are the risk factors for generalized infection?

Varicella zoster virus infection can occur in systemic lupus erythematosus (SLE) patients treated with immunosuppressive agents, when the disease is in remission. Usually the course of varicella zoster virus infection is benign; however, seldomly, and especially in cases of sciatic nerve involvement, generalized varicella zoster virus infection can develop. Varicella zoster virus infection by itself does not seem to exacerbate. Discontinuation of immunosuppressive agents is recommended, and antiviral therapy should be instituted.

14. Which are common causes of anemia in systemic lupus erythematosus patients?

Anemia is found in about 50% of systemic lupus erythematosus (SLE) patients, with anemia of chronic disease being the most common one. Autoantibodies against erythropoietin may play a role in the pathogenesis of this type of anemia. Autoimmune hemolytic anemia in SLE patients usually belongs to a distinct category. It is associated with antiphospholipid antibodies, thrombosis, thrombocytopenia, and renal disease, often in the context of secondary antiphospholipid syndrome. In addition, autoantibodies, T lymphocytes, and upregulated cytokine network can affect bone marrow erythropoiesis, leading to anemia.

15. Which conditions usually coexist with autoimmune hemolytic anemia in systemic lupus erythematosus patients?

Renal involvement, thrombocytopenia, and less often antiphospholipid syndrome.

16. What is the incidence of systemic lupus erythematosus in patients with idiopathic thrombocytopenic purpura?

Idiopathic thrombocytopenic purpura (ITP) can either be a primary disorder or it can occur as early-stage manifestation of autoimmune diseases, in particular systemic lupus erythematosus (SLE). In a recent population-based retrospective cohort study of newly diagnosed ITP patients, matched 1:2 for age and sex with non-ITP patients, followed for an average of 80 months revealed that patients with ITP had 26 times greater risk of SLE development compared to the control population. An excess risk was demonstrated in those ITP patients for development of Sjögren's syndrome as well. Thus patients presenting with ITP should be monitored for development of systemic autoimmune disease [3].

17. What is the clinical picture of Jaccoud's arthropathy? In which autoimmune patients can it be seen?

Jaccoud's arthropathy was first described in patients with rheumatic fever, but it can be seen in patients with systemic lupus erythematosus and Sjögren's syndrome as well as in patients with other connective tissue diseases and pyrophosphate crystals deposition disease. It presents with correctable deformities of the metacarpophalangeal and interphalangeal joints which is the result of soft tissue abnormalities such as laxity of ligaments, fibrosis of the capsule, and muscular imbalance, rather than joint bony destructions (Fig. 4.1).

18. What is lupus band test? In which skin area is it performed? What is its diagnostic and prognostic uses?

The lupus band test is a diagnostic procedure performed on a skin biopsy specimen that detects, with direct immunofluorescence staining, deposits of immunoglobulins, and various complement components along the dermo-epidermal junction in lupus erythematosus patients. Detection of these deposits in the skin of patients with systemic lupus erythematosus (SLE) demonstrates a linear band at the basement membrane zone, hence the name lupus band test. Biopsy tissue is taken from clinically healthy skin of SLE patients preferably unexposed to sun. It is positive in 70–80% of sun-exposed non-lesional skin specimens obtained from patients with SLE and in 55% of SLE patients if sun-protected non-lesional skin is analyzed. In contrast to SLE patients where the lupus band test is frequently positive in both involved and uninvolved skin, in patients with cutaneous lupus, only the lesional skin shows a positive lupus band test (Fig. 4.2). Moreover, a positive lupus band test may serve as a prognostic indicator in patients with an established diagnosis of SLE, as it correlates with severe extracutaneous disease, mainly lupus nephritis, and with anti-dsDNA antibodies.

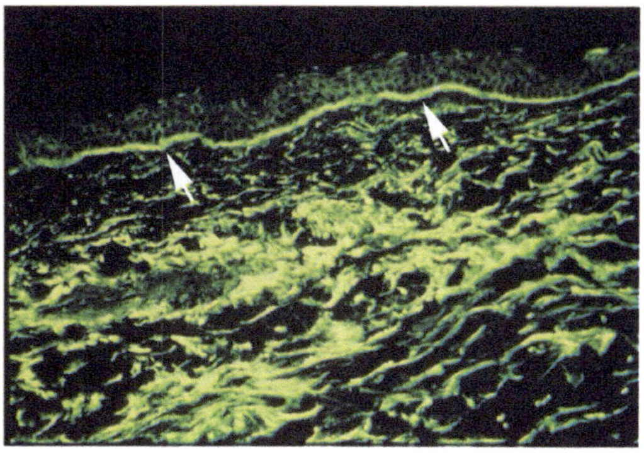

Fig. 4.2 Lupus band test: Direct immunofluorescence staining of clinically healthy and unexposed to sun skin from systemic lupus erythematosus patient revealed deposits of immunoglobulins and complement components along the dermo-epidermal junction (arrows)

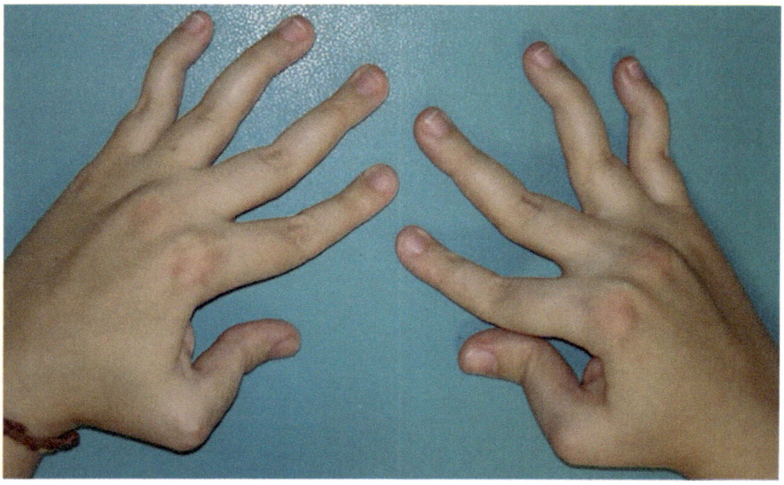

Fig. 4.1 Jaccoud's arthropathy: A 28-year-old female with long-standing systemic lupus erythematosus presents with correctable deformities of the metacarpophalangeal and proximal interphalangeal joints which is the result of soft tissues abnormalities such as laxity of ligaments, fibrosis of the capsule, and muscular imbalance, rather than joint bony destructions

19. Which are non-specific (non-diagnostic) cutaneous manifestations of systemic lupus erythematosus?

The skin manifestations of systemic lupus erythematosus (SLE) can be divided into non-specific (non-diagnostic) and specific (diagnostic). Non-diagnostic SLE skin manifestations include:

- Raynaud's phenomenon (Fig. 4.3)
- Non-scarring alopecia (Fig. 4.4)
- Livedo reticularis (Fig. 4.5)
- Skin vasculitis

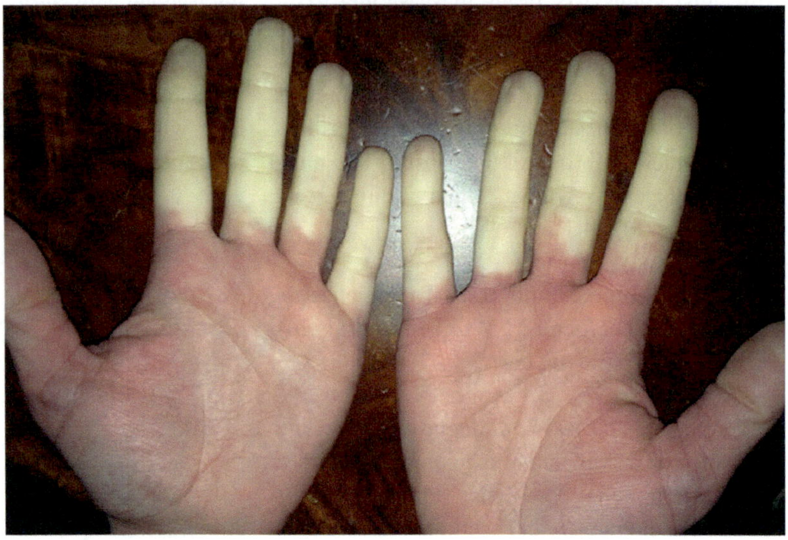

Fig. 4.3 Raynaud's phenomenon in a 40-year-old male patient with systemic lupus erythematosus who upon stress develops white coloring of the fingers

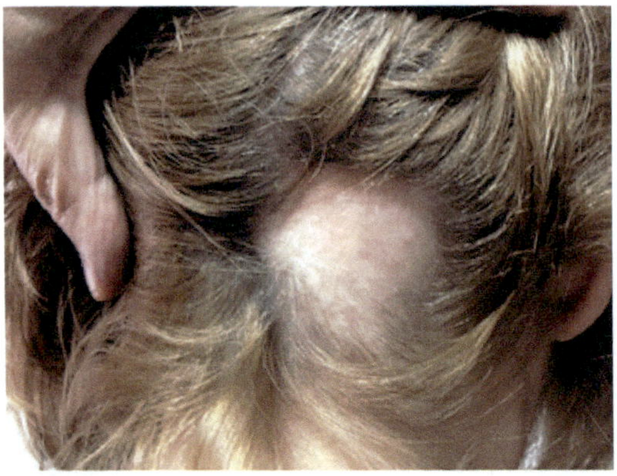

Fig. 4.4 Non-scarring scalp alopecia in a 52-year-old female patient with systemic lupus erythematosus

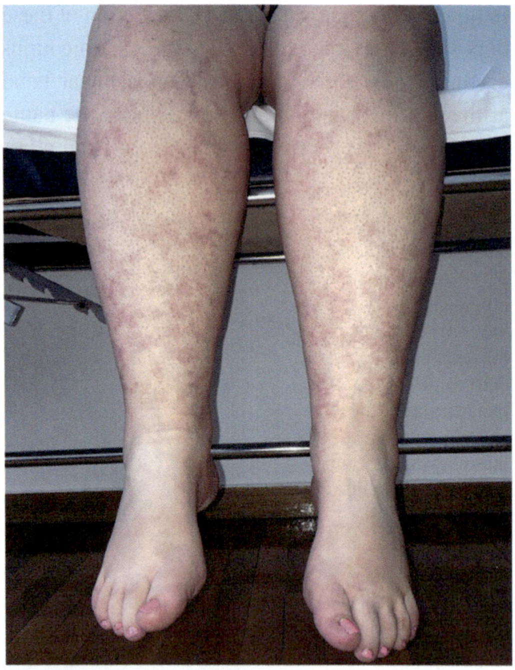

Fig. 4.5 Livedo reticularis in a 20-year-old female with systemic lupus erythematosus and antiphospholipid syndrome

20. Which are the cutaneous manifestations of acute systemic lupus erythematosus?

- Butterfly rash (maculopapular eruption in the central face area around the nose) (Fig. 4.6)
- Photosensitivity eruptions in sun-exposed areas
- Papular erythematous rashes in the arms and legs

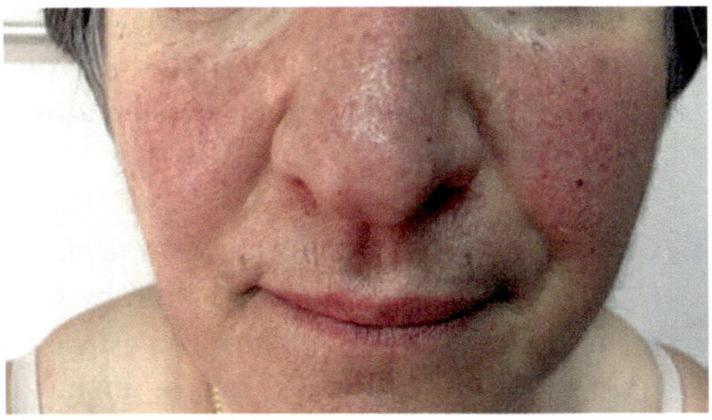

Fig. 4.6 Butterfly rash in a 50-year-old woman with systemic lupus erythematosus

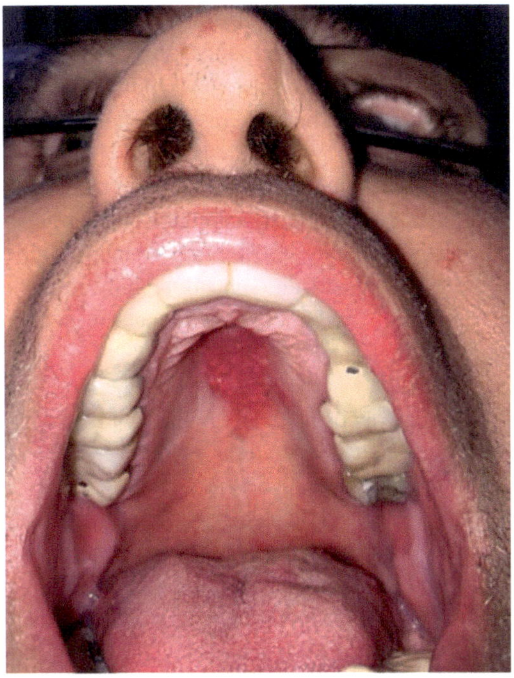

Fig. 4.7 Painless hard palate ulcer in a 40-year-old lady with exacerbating systemic lupus erythematosus

- Bullous eruptions with erosions and mouth/hard palate ulcers (Fig. 4.7)

21. Which are the cutaneous manifestations of subacute cutaneous lupus erythematosus (SCLE)?

Annular/polycyclic and psoriasiform/papulosquamous rashes (Fig. 4.8). The lesions typically occur in a photosensitive distribution. Common locations of SCLE rash include the neck, the shoulders, the upper chest, the upper back, and the extensor surface of the hands. In the majority of patients, sun exposure exacerbates the disease.

22. Which are the chronic cutaneous manifestations of systemic lupus erythematosus?

Chronic cutaneous manifestations in systemic lupus erythematosus patients include discoid rashes which are painless disc-shaped erythematous plaques with areas of follicular hyperkeratosis. When the lesions progress, they result in cutaneous atrophy, either in loss or increase of skin pigmentation (Fig. 4.9), and depressed scars can develop. If the discoid lesions are on the scalp, they result in scarring alopecia (Fig. 4.10).

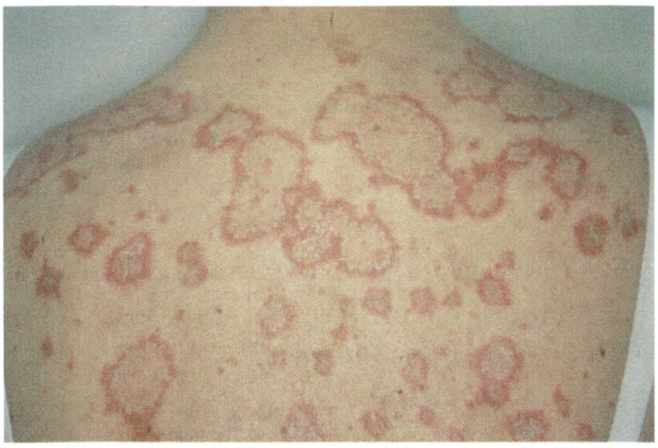

Fig. 4.8 Subacute cutaneous lupus erythematosus in a 21-year-old female patient with an annular/polycyclic and psoriasiform/papulosquamous rash on the back after sun exposure

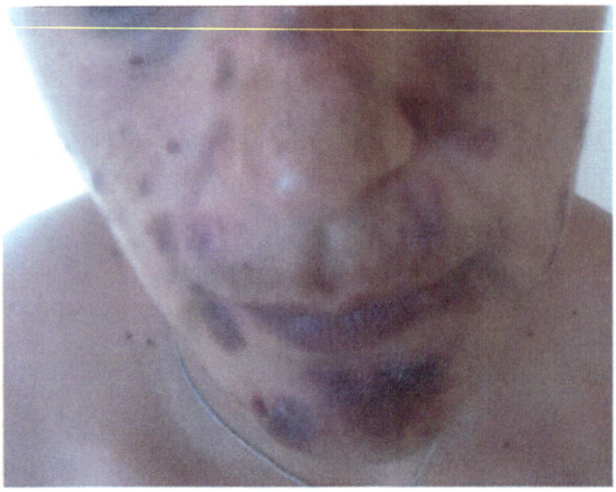

Fig. 4.9 Discoid lupus erythematosus: A 36-year-old female patient with multiple chronic hyperpigmented discoid lesions on the face

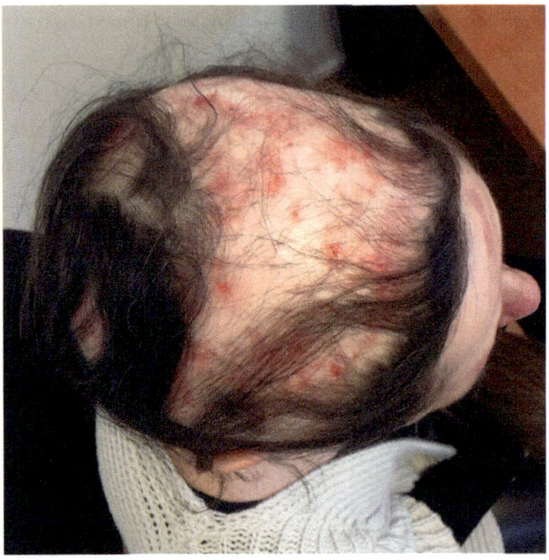

Fig. 4.10 Scarring scalp alopecia: A 34-year-old female with systemic lupus erythematosus and multiple discoid scarring scalp lesions

23. Which are the clinical and laboratory findings of pleurisy in systemic lupus erythematosus patients?

Pleurisy is infrequently one of the first clinical manifestations in patients with systemic lupus erythematosus (SLE), but it can develop during the course of the disease in almost half of the patients. In addition, drug-induced lupus can present with pleurisy. Pleurisy in SLE patients can be bilateral or unilateral, with or without pericarditis. It usually presents with fever, chest pain cough, and dyspnea. Rarely, it can be asymptomatic. The amount of pleural effusion ranges mostly from small to moderate, but it can be massive. The effusions are exudates with leukocyte count ranging between 500 and 15,000/μL. High titers of antinuclear autoantibodies and low complement levels are characteristic findings of SLE lupus pleural effusions. Pleural biopsy should be performed when malignancy or tuberculosis is suspected.

24. What is the histopathologic classification used for systemic lupus erythematosus renal biopsies?

- *Class I: minimal mesangial lupus nephritis (LN)* — normal appearing glomeruli by light microscopy (LM) with immune deposits confined to the mesangium visible by immunofluorescence (IF)
- *Class II: mesangial proliferative LN* — mesangial proliferation (of any degree) visible by LM and mesangial deposits by IF. Minute subendothelial or subepithelial immune deposits may rarely be visible by IF or electron microscopy (EM), but not by LM, whether or not there is endocapillary proliferation
- *Class III: focal LN* — focal, segmental, or global endo- or extracapillary glomerulonephritis involving <50% of all glomeruli, typically with focal subendothelial immune deposits, with or without mesangial alterations
- *Class IV: diffuse LN* — subendothelial immune deposits visible by LM with or without mesangial alterations involving ≥50% of all glomeruli

Class IV is subdivided into diffuse segmental (IV-S, segmental defined as a glomerular lesion that involves less than half of the glomerular tuft) when ≥50% of the involved glomeruli has segmental lesions, and diffuse global (IV-G) when ≥50% of the involved glomeruli have global lesions.

Lesions in classes III and IV are further characterized as purely active (A), as purely chronic (C), and as a combination of active and chronic lesions (A/C).

- *Class V: membranous LN* — global or segmental subepithelial immune deposits involving ≥50% of the glomerular tuft in ≥50% of glomeruli. Class V lupus nephritis may occur in combination with class III or IV
- *Class VI: advanced sclerosing LN* — ≥90% of glomeruli are globally sclerotic with no evidence of ongoing activity

25. Where do immune complexes deposit in proliferative lupus nephritis and where in the membranous lupus nephritis?

In the proliferative lupus nephritis (class III, class IV), the immune complexes deposit subendothelially, while in the membranous lupus nephritis subepithelially (Fig. 4.11).

26. Which lupus patients have lower incidence of lupus nephritis?

Drug-induced lupus and subacute cutaneous lupus erythematosus patients.

27. Which are the adverse predictors of remission and relapse of lupus nephritis?

Adverse predictors of remission are severe proteinuria and delayed initiation of therapy from the time nephritis was clinically diagnosed. Predictors of earlier relapse for patients entering remission include a longer time to remission and a history of central nervous system involvement.

28. Which are poor prognostic factors for lupus nephritis?

Hypertension, renal failure, massive proteinuria, and high activity score of lupus nephritis on renal biopsy specimen are all associated with poor renal prognosis.

29. Do we have changes in clinical–histological presentation and renal outcome of lupus nephritis over the last five decades?

Lupus nephritis (LN) can be one of the most serious disease manifestations either at the time

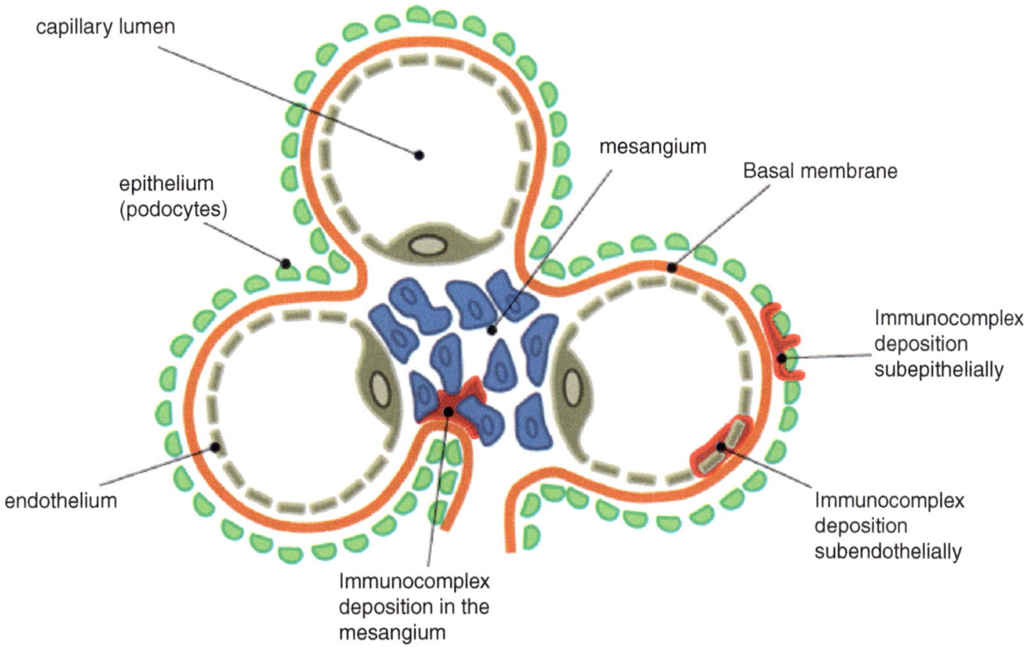

Fig. 4.11 Lupus nephritis: A schematic representation of the renal pathology. Deposition of immune complexes (ICs) in the mesangium occurs in patients with mesangial glomerulonephritis (GMN), and deposition of ICs under the endothelium is observed in patients with proliferative GMN, while deposition under the epithelium is found in patients with membranous GMN (*Figure created by Evangelia Zampeli, MD*)

of diagnosis or during the disease course. It can manifest with a wide clinical spectrum from asymptomatic urinary abnormalities to chronic irreversible renal insufficiency. Renal involvement in systemic lupus erythematosus (SLE) patients is considered a strong predictor of death and end-stage renal disease. In the last few decades, however, the rate of renal flares has considerably decreased as well as the improvement of LN prognosis due to earlier and more effective therapeutic interventions as well as the effective treatment of comorbidities like hypertension, infections and cardiovascular diseases. A recent multicenter study included 499 patients who were diagnosed with LN from 1970 to 2016. Changes in demographic, clinical, and histological features at the time of LN presentation were studied in three time periods: 1970–1985, 1986–2001, and 2002–2016. From the first period of observation to the last the following were noted: the mean age of LN diagnosis was increased; as well as the time of SLE diagnosis to LN development; In contrast, the incidence of end-stage renal disease decreased while the isolated renal abnormalities increased. Furthermore, histologic activity did not change while chronicity indexes decreased. Survival without end-stage renal disease improved from 87% in the first time period to 99% in the third time period. It appears from these findings that renal involvement in SLE has become milder with a better prognosis [4].

30. Does renal transplantation improve survival of systemic lupus erythematosus patients with end-stage renal disease?

It is known that systemic lupus erythematosus (SLE) patients with end-stage renal disease (ESRD) have high mortality rates. The question is if renal transplant improves survival rates in this patient population. This question was answered from the results of a nationwide cohort USA study in which 9659 SLE patients with ESRD who were waiting for a renal transplant were included. 5738 (59%) patients (female 82%) underwent renal transplantation. The transplantation resulted in decrease of all causes mortality from cardiovascular diseases, coronary artery disease, infection, and septicemia. These results suggest that an SLE patient with ESRD should be transplanted as soon as possible in order to improve survival benefit [5].

31. Which are the clinical and laboratory findings distinguishing toxemia of pregnancy from lupus nephritis flare?

The distinction between severe toxemia of pregnancy (pre-eclampsia/eclampsia) and active lupus nephritis can be difficult, since both conditions may present with hypertension, thrombocytopenia, hemolytic anemia, and compromised renal function with proteinuria. The absence of other clinical manifestations indicative of systemic lupus erythematosus activity (arthritis, rash, pleurisy, leukopenia, etc.), as well as the lack of white blood cells, red cells, and casts in the urine and stable anti-dsDNA autoantibodies, decreased urine calcium, and increased serum uric acid levels, makes the diagnosis of eclampsia more likely. Serum complement levels are not helpful in distinguishing the two conditions, since they can be decreased during a lupus flare as well as in patients with pregnancy toxemia.

32. Which are the transient and which are the permanent lesions in newborns with neonatal lupus?

Neonatal lupus is associated with the transplacental passage of maternal anti-Ro/SSA and anti-La/SSB antibodies. The most frequent manifestations seen in affected neonates are skin rash (lesions of discoid lupus or subacute cutaneous lupus), hepatic dysfunction, and thrombocytopenia. The cutaneous, hepatic, and hematologic manifestations are transient, generally resolving in 2–6 months after delivery. The most serious manifestation of neonatal lupus is cardiomyopathy that leads to a complete heart block (CHB). Heart block typically begins in utero during the second or third trimester initially as first- or second-degree atrioventricular block and then can progress to third-degree block. CHB, if established, appears to be irreversible, and the neonate may require a permanent pacemaker. The long-term prognosis of children with neonatal lupus is guarded since some of them will develop later in their life other autoimmune disorders.

33. Have outcomes of pregnant systemic lupus erythematosus women improved in the last years for the mother and the fetus?

Studies have shown that the best time for a systemic lupus erythematosus (SLE) patient to become pregnant is when SLE is in remission for at least 6 months. Since our knowledge on clinical and therapeutic interventions in SLE has improved the question which arises is if in the last decades the outcome of pregnant women has improved. This question is answered in a retrospective cohort study which was performed in the United States from 1998 to 2015. Database from hospitalizations of adult pregnant women with and without SLE of the National Inpatient Sample (NIS) were used. In this period of time, 93820 pregnant women with SLE and 78045 without SLE were hospitalized in the United States. Outcome measures were in-hospital maternal mortality, fetal mortality, preeclampsia or eclampsia, cesarean sections, non-delivery-related admissions, and length of stay. It was noted that maternal deaths (per 100,000 admissions) were 442 versus 13 among patients with SLE versus non-SLE during the years 1998–2000 and <50 SLE versus 10 non SLE for the years 2013–2015. The decrease in maternal deaths was much greater in women with SLE. This large study clearly points out that maternal mortality, particularly in women with SLE, over the years and overall outcomes improved markedly [6]. Attempts however should be placed to further improve the outcomes of pregnant SLE women.

34. Which anatomic heart sites can be affected by systemic lupus erythematosus?

Pericardium, coronary arteries, heart valves, myocardium, and endocardium.

35. Is atrial fibrillation common in patients with systemic erythematosus?

Myocarditis presents with tachycardia, conduction disturbances, systolic, and/or diastolic dysfunction, with or without heart failure, and arrhythmias. Until recently the development of atrial fibrillation (AF) in systemic lupus erythematosus (SLE) was not commonly reported. A recent study showed that the risk of AF is around three times higher in SLE patients compared to age sex and race controls. SLE patients under the age of 40 years showed a higher incidence of AF. SLE patients with AF had a higher mortality rate compared with patients with AF, without SLE and SLE patients without AF. Conditions that appear to be responsible for the development of AF in SLE patients are disease activity, drug toxicity (intravenous pulse steroid therapy, immunosuppressive medications), hypertension, atherosclerosis, and obesity. Another recent study, using phenome-wide association studies, showed that AF is more common in male than in female SLE patients. Hydroxychloroquine appears to be protective against the development of AF. Thus, in SLE patients at risk to develop AF, hydroxychloroquine can be used not only as disease-modifying agent but also in order to reduce the risk of AF [7, 8].

36. Which valves are commonly affected by Libman-Sacks endocarditis and what are the sequelae?

Libman-Sacks endocarditis is a non-infectious endocarditis, also called verrucous or marantic, that can occur in systemic lupus erythematosus and antiphospholipid syndrome patients with active disease of long duration. The valvular vegetations (Fig. 4.12) are composed of fibrin, neutrophils, lymphocytes, and histiocytes and more frequently produce valvular regurgitation, while stenosis occurs infrequently. The ventricular and atrial surface of the mitral valve is typically and more often affected. These vegetations infrequently embolize. Verrucous endocarditis is also seen in patients with hypercoagulable states and malignancy.

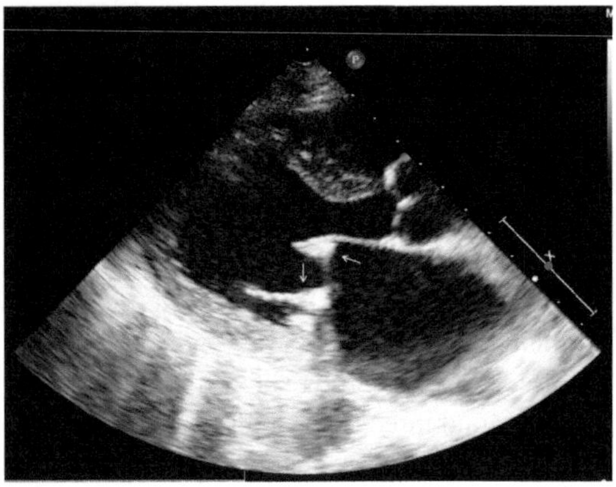

Fig. 4.12 Libman-Sacks vegetations: A 40-year-old woman with systemic lupus erythematosus and antiphospholipid syndrome demonstrating serious mitral valve insufficiency. Transthoracic two-dimensional echocardiogram revealed thickening and calcification of the posterior mitral valve leaflet (white arrow) and Libman-Sacks vegetation (yellow arrow) (*Figure courtesy of Ioannis Moyssakis, MD*)

37. Pulmonary arterial hypertension is a serious complication of systemic lupus erythematosus. Which risk factor(s) can predict this complication in systemic lupus erythematosus patients?

Early recognition of pulmonary arterial hypertension (PAH) is not easy due to lack of specific symptoms. Recent meta-analyses showed that the presence of anti-U1RNP, anti-Sm, and antiphospholipid antibodies in the sera of systemic lupus erythematosus patients (SLE)-especially Asian in origin- is a risk factor for PAH development, warranting careful monitoring and screening for PAH of SLE patients with these autoantibody reactivities [9, 10].

38. Which neurologic manifestations can be seen in systemic lupus erythematosus patients?

Cognitive impairment is the most frequent manifestation, followed by seizures. Additional manifestations include peripheral neuropathies, acute confusional state, headache, and depression. Central nervous system involvement can also manifest as lupus retinopathy. Lupus retinopathy is a microangiopathy of retinal vessels, particularly associated with vasculitis or anti-cardiolipin antibodies; it is associated with active systemic disease (mostly lupus nephritis), and retinal lesions during fundus examination (Fig. 4.13) are of critical importance, both visually and prognostically.

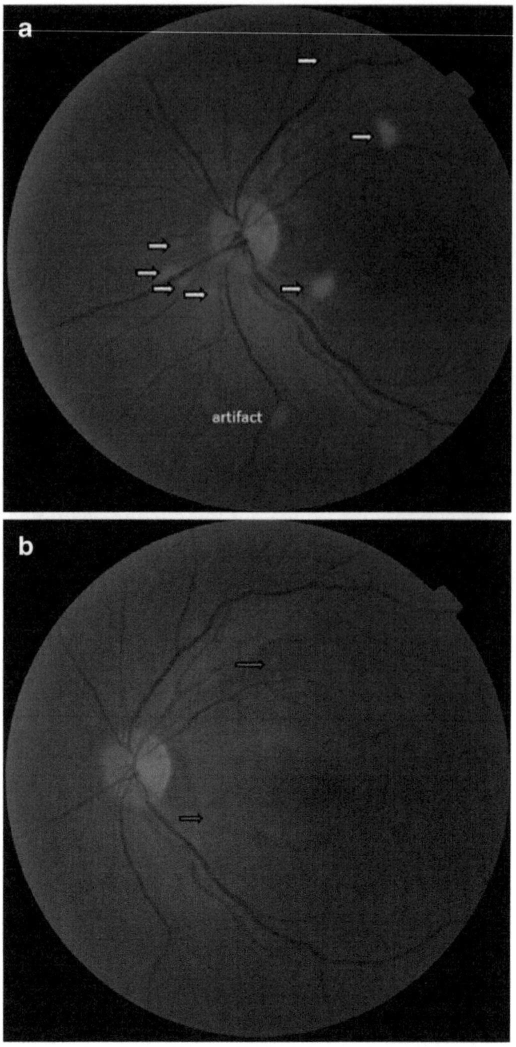

Fig. 4.13 Lupus retinopathy: A 58-year-old non-hypertensive, non-diabetic female patient with systemic lupus erythematosus and lupus nephritis who presented with fever, microscopic hematuria, and a generalized vasculitic rash. (**a**) Funduscopic examination revealed cotton wool spots (grayish-white slightly elevated lesions which look like clouds) in the superficial retina (arrows) in both eyes. (**b**) Cotton wool spots regressed after treatment with methylprednisolone and cyclophosphamide intravenous pulses (*Figure courtesy of Professor Athanasios G. Tzioufas, MD*)

Less common manifestations are psychosis, movement disorders, myelopathy, optic neuritis, cerebrovascular accidents, cranial neuropathies, and aseptic meningitis.

39. How common are strokes in systemic lupus erythematosus patients?

Strokes in systemic lupus erythematosus (SLE) patients are twice more common compared to the incidence of strokes in the general population. Usually, strokes occur within the first year after SLE diagnosis. Thus, as soon as the diagnosis of systemic lupus erythematosus is established, the physicians should search for stroke risk factors such as hypercoagulable state, hypertension, cerebral vasculopathy, atherosclerosis, thrombosis, and emboli of Libman-Sacks endocarditis and apply the necessary measures to eliminate them [11].

40. In which systemic lupus erythematosus patients posterior reversible encephalopathy syndrome (PRES) can occur, and what is its clinical course?

This syndrome has been rarely described in systemic lupus erythematosus (SLE) patients. Several risk factors have been postulated for the development of PRES in SLE, such as younger age, high disease activity, lymphopenia, hypertension, dyslipidemia, renal function impairment, and immunosuppressive therapy (including high doses of corticosteroids alone or in combination with cyclophosphamide). The onset of the neurologic symptomatology can be acute or subacute. The patients present with altered mental status and headaches and can develop seizures or vision loss. Magnetic resonance imaging findings are characteristic and reveal white matter changes mostly in the parieto-occipital areas bilaterally. These findings differentiate posterior reversible encephalopathy syndrome from other central nervous system complications of SLE. The clinical and imaging abnormalities of the syndrome resolve within 1–4 weeks without any sequelae [12].

41. Which are the cerebrospinal fluid findings in a systemic lupus erythematosus patient with central nervous system disease?

Examination of cerebrospinal fluid (CSF) from a systemic lupus erythematosus (SLE) patient primarily aims to rule out central nervous system (CNS) infection. However, the presence in the CSF of high immunoglobulin (Ig) G index (connotes intrathecal IgG production), oligoclonal Ig bands, low complement C4 component, and normal sugar levels all attest toward the diagnosis of CNS involvement from SLE.

42. Which are the predictors of poor outcome in systemic lupus erythematosus patients with neuropsychiatric manifestations?

Systemic lupus erythematosus patients with neuropsychiatric manifestations have an increased rate of organ damage and a high degree of working incapacity. The number of previous neuropsychiatric events and the coexistence of antiphospholipid syndrome are predictors of poor outcome in these patients.

43. Which are the clinical and laboratory findings in patients with mixed connective tissue disease?

Patients with mixed connective tissue disease (MCTD) express manifestations of different systemic autoimmune connective tissue diseases but do not fulfill classification criteria for any of them. The most common clinical manifestations include Raynaud's phenomenon, puffy (swollen) hands (Fig. 4.14), and arthritis/arthralgias. Acrosclerosis, esophageal dysmotility, myositis, interstitial lung disease, and pulmonary hypertension can manifest in patients with MCTD, while severe renal and CNS diseases are uncommon. High levels of anti-U1RNP antibodies are the laboratory hallmark of MCTD, and these patients characteristically lack other specific autoantibodies (e.g., anti-Sm, anti-dsDNA).

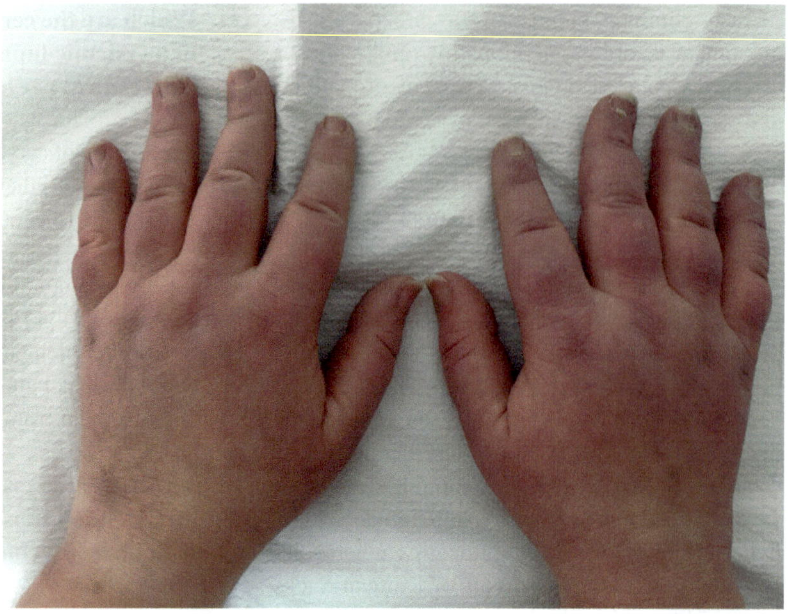

Fig. 4.14 Mixed connective tissue disease: Puffy (swollen) hands in a 33-year-old female patient diagnosed with high titers of anti-U1RNP antibodies

44. Mixed connective tissue disease: Is it evolving?

Previous studies which attempted to answer the question if mixed connective tissue disease (MCTD) is an undifferentiated, transient, or stable disease failed to provide a solid answer primarily due to the fact that different diagnostic criteria were used and the definition of the criteria of MCTD evolution were not clear. In a recent study of a Norwegian nationwide cohort of MCTD patients ($n = 147$), the disorder phenotype stability was studied by longitudinal analyses of clinical manifestations and autoantibody presence. Disease activity and remission were evaluated using disease indexes for systemic sclerosis (SSc) and for systemic lupus erythematosus (SLE). Furthermore, MCTD manifestations that can predict disease evolution were identified. In the long follow-up period (7 years), 71% of the originally diagnosed as MCTD remain stable, only 9% evolved to another systemic autoimmune disorder (rheumatoid arthritis, SLE, SSc, and anti-synthetase syndrome), 11% died during follow up and 9% refused to participate. The results of this study clearly showed that MCTD is a relatively stable disease; particularly patients with swollen hands run a mild disease, its course is milder compared to SLE or SSc and infrequently (around 1/10 patients) evolves to another systemic autoimmune disorder [13].

45. Undifferentiated connective tissue disease: What are the clinical characteristics and the differences from mixed connective tissue disease?

Undifferentiated connective tissue disease (UCTD) is a term used to describe those patients with clinical features and antibodies compatible with an autoimmune rheumatic disease, who nevertheless do not fulfil diagnostic criteria for any well-defined individual autoimmune rheumatic disease. According to several UCTD cohort studies arthritis, Raynaud's phenomenon, malar rash and photosensitivity are common clinical manifestations. Pulmonary disease is not described as frequently as in the mixed connective tissue disease (MCTD) cohorts, but UCTD cohorts have a shorter follow-up time. In contrast, in studies evaluating patients with interstitial lung disease (ILD), more of them are described as UCTD patients than MCTD patients. Thus, pulmonary disease in UCTD may have a higher incidence than that described in UCTD cohorts, yet more studies are needed. Anti-U1RNP antibodies are reported in the UCTD cohorts, with no consistent clinical significance. Evolution to well-established autoimmune rheumatic diseases ranges from rare to frequent according to several studies, depending on antibody positivity at presentation or new autoantibody appearance during follow-up [14].

46. In which medical situations should the suspicion of antiphospholipid syndrome be raised?

Antiphospholipid syndrome should be ruled out as a possible underlying diagnosis in patients with:

- Arterial thrombosis in an individual younger than 50 years of age
- Recurrent miscarriages not explained by other causes (anatomic, hormonal, and genetic)
- Recurrent venous thromboses, when genetic factors are ruled out
- Simultaneous arterial and venous thromboses
- Thromboses at unusual vascular sites

47. What is termed primary and secondary antiphospholipid syndrome?

Primary antiphospholipid syndrome (Hughes syndrome) is defined by the presence of antiphospholipid autoantibodies, thrombotic events, and/or pregnancy morbidity in the absence of another associated autoimmune disease. Up to 10% of individuals with primary antiphospholipid syndrome will evolve to systemic lupus erythematosus (SLE) within 10 years of diagnosis. SLE or patients with other autoimmune diseases and antiphospholipid autoantibodies who develop a thrombotic event are defined as having secondary antiphospholipid syndrome.

48. Does the concomitant diagnosis of systemic lupus erythematosus in patients with positive antiphospholipid antibodies influence their clinical and/or laboratory manifestations?

Approximately one-third of systemic lupus erythematosus (SLE) patients exhibit positivity for one or more antiphospholipid antibodies (lupus anticoagulant, anti-cardiolipins IgG/IgM, and/or anti-β_2GPI IgG/IgM). Of those, around 30% have clinically apparent manifestations of antiphospholipid syndrome. A recent retrospective cross-sectional international multicenter study aimed to examine the impact of SLE on the clinical phenotype and prognosis of persistently antiphospholipid-positive patients by comparing clinical and laboratory characteristics of antiphospholipid-positive patients with or without SLE. The frequency of isolated and/or recurrent thrombotic episodes and pregnancy morbidity was similar between antiphospholipid-positive patients with or without SLE. However, concomitant SLE diagnosis in persistently antiphospholipid-positive patients was associated with an increased frequency of thrombocytopenia, hemolytic anemia, low complement levels, and IgA anti-β_2GPI positivity compared to antiphospholipid-positive patients without SLE. Interestingly, prevalence of cognitive dysfunction was higher in persistently antiphospholipid-positive patients without SLE [15].

49. Which are the clinical and renal histological lesions in antiphospholipid syndrome patients with nephritis?

Renal involvement occurs in as many as 25% of patients with primary antiphospholipid syndrome (APS). Clinically APS-associated nephropathy presents with hypertension, microscopic hematuria, and proteinuria (usually mild) and if untreated leads to renal insufficiency. The spectrum of renal pathology in APS includes renal artery thrombosis, renal infarction, renal vein thrombosis, and a small vessel vaso-occlusive nephropathy defined as "antiphospholipid antibody-associated nephropathy." This nephropathy is characterized by acute lesions, thrombotic microangiopathy, and chronic lesions such as fibrous intimal hyperplasia, organizing thrombi with or without recanalization, fibrous occlusions of arteries or arterioles, and focal cortical atrophy [16].

50. Which clinical or laboratory findings can predict that an antiphospholipid syndrome patient will run a serious clinical course?

Initial presentation of antiphospholipid syndrome (APS) with arterial thrombosis, autoimmune hemolytic anemia, and antibodies to β_2GPI will run a more serious course compared to APS patients with recurrent abortions.

51. What is the clinical presentation of catastrophic antiphospholipid syndrome?

Infection usually precedes the catastrophic antiphospholipid syndrome (cAPS). cAPS is a very infrequent medical condition. It affects only 1% of the antiphospholipid syndrome patient population. The clinical highlights of cAPS are simultaneous multiple organ (e.g., brain, kidneys, and lungs) involvement, high titers of circulating antiphospholipid antibodies, and histopathologic confirmation of multiple—in different body sites—vessel occlusions.

52. How common is asymptomatic aseptic bone necrosis in antiphospholipid syndrome, and which patient population is more prone to develop it?

Antiphospholipid syndrome (APS) patients who had never received steroids and were asymptomatic for aseptic bone necrosis have been evaluated with magnetic resonance imaging (MRI), and aseptic (avascular) bone necrosis (Fig. 4.15) was found in one out of five patients tested. Younger APS patients and those with clinically apparent livedo reticularis tend to develop aseptic bone necrosis more often than older patients and patients without livedo reticularis [17].

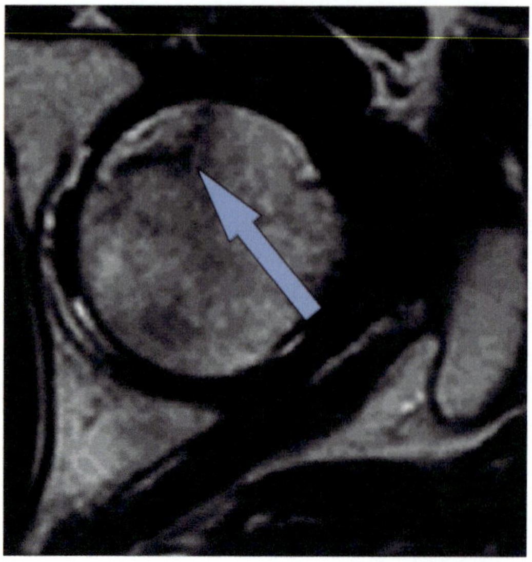

Fig. 4.15 Avascular femoral head necrosis in a 39-year-old female patient with primary antiphospholipid syndrome. Magnetic resonance of the femoral head reveals an early low-intensity band in the subchondral zone of the femoral head (the band sign, blue arrow)

53. An antiphospholipid syndrome patient develops an arterial thrombosis. Which is the commonest vascular area of recurrence when this patient will have another thrombotic episode?

Usually arterial thrombosis is followed by arterial thrombosis and vein thrombosis by vein thrombosis.

54. Which is the pregnancy morbidity in antiphospholipid syndrome?

Antiphospholipid syndrome-related pregnancy morbidity includes:

- Fetal loss—either as miscarriage, intrauterine fetal death, or stillbirth
- Obstetric complications, such as intrauterine growth restriction, uteroplacental insufficiency, pre-eclampsia, and preterm birth delivery

55. Which antiphospholipid syndrome patients demonstrate an increased risk for cognitive dysfunction?

Cognitive dysfunction (mainly complex attention and verbal fluency) is often found in patients with antiphospholipid syndrome (APS), regardless of any history of central nervous system involvement. Livedo reticularis and the presence of white matter lesions on brain magnetic resonance imaging is associated with an increased risk for cognitive dysfunction in patients with APS [18].

References

1. Julià A, López-Longo FJ, Pérez Venegas JJ, et al. Genome-wide association study meta-analysis identifies five new loci for systemic lupus erythematosus. Arthritis Res Ther. 2018;20:100.
2. Haugaard JH, Kofoed K, Gislason G, Dreyer L, Egeberg A. Association between drug use and subsequent diagnosis of lupus erythematosus. JAMA Dermatol. Published online September 02, 2020.
3. Zhu FX, Huang JY, Ye Z, et al. Risk of systemic lupus erythematosus in patients with idiopathic thrombocytopenic purpura: a population-based cohort study. Ann Rheum Dis. 2020;79:793-9.
4. Moroni G, Vercelloni PG, Quaglini S, et al. Changing patterns in clinical–histological presentation and renal outcome over the last five decades in a cohort of 499 patients with lupus nephritis. Ann Rheum Dis. 2018;77:1318–25.
5. Jorge A, Wallace ZS, Lu N, et al. Renal transplantation and survival among patients with lupus nephritis: a cohort study. Ann Intern Med. 2019;170:240–7.
6. Mehta B, Luo Y, Xu J, et al. Trends in maternal and fetal outcomes among pregnant women with systemic lupus erythematosus in the United States: a cross-sectional analysis. Ann Intern Med. 2019;171:164–71.
7. Lim S, Bae EH, Han K-D, et al. Systemic lupus erythematosus is a risk factor for atrial fibrillation: a nationwide, population-based study. Clin Exp Rheumatol. 2019;37:1019–25.
8. Barnado A, Carroll RJ, Casey C, et al. Phenome-wide association studies uncover a novel association of increased atrial fibrillation in males with systemic lupus erythematosus. Arthritis Care Res. 2018;70:1630–6.
9. Wang J, Qian J, Wang Y, et al. Serological biomarkers as risk factors of SLE-associated pulmonary arterial hypertension: a systematic review and meta-analysis. Lupus. 2017;1:961203317702255.
10. Zuily S, Domingues V, Suty-Selton C, et al. Antiphospholipid antibodies can identify lupus patients at risk of pulmonary hypertension: a systematic review and meta-analysis. Autoimmun Rev. 2017;16:576–86.
11. Arkema EV, Svenungsson E, Von Euler M, Sjöwall C, Simard JF. Stroke in systemic lupus erythematosus: a Swedish population-based cohort study. Ann Rheum Dis. 2017;76:1544–9.
12. Merayo-Chalico J, Apodaca E, Barrera-Vargas A, Alcocer-Varela J, Colunga-Pedraza I, González-Patiño A, et al. Clinical outcomes and risk factors for posterior reversible encephalopathy syndrome in systemic lupus erythematosus: a multicentric case-control study. J Neurol Neurosurg Psychiatry. 2016;87:287–94.
13. Reiseter S, Gunnarsson R, Corander J, et al. Disease evolution in mixed connective tissue disease: results from a long-term nationwide prospective cohort study. Arthritis Res Ther. 2017;19:284.
14. Alves MA, Isenberg DA. "Mixed connective tissue disease": a condition in search of an identity. Clin Exp Med. 2020;20:159–66.
15. Unlu O, Erkan D, Barbhaiya M, et al. The impact of systemic lupus erythematosus on the clinical phenotype of antiphospholipid antibody-positive patients: results from the antiphospholipid syndrome alliance for clinical trials and international clinical database and repository. Arthritis Care Res (Hoboken). 2019;71:134–41.
16. Tektonidou MG. Identification and treatment of APS renal involvement. Lupus. 2014;23:1276–8.
17. Tektonidou MG, Malagari K, Vlachoyiannopoulos PG, Kelekis DA, Moutsopoulos HM. Asymptomatic avascular necrosis in patients with primary antiphospholipid syndrome in the absence of corticosteroid use: a prospective study by magnetic resonance imaging. Arthritis Rheum. 2003;48:732–6.
18. Tektonidou MG, Varsou N, Kotoulas G, Antoniou A, Moutsopoulos HM. Cognitive deficits in patients with antiphospholipid syndrome: association with clinical, laboratory, and brain magnetic resonance imaging findings. Arch Intern Med. 2006;166:2278–84.

Inflammatory Muscle Disease

5

Haralampos M. Moutsopoulos
and Evangelia Zampeli

Abstract

The main types of idiopathic inflammatory myopathies (IIM) are dermatomyositis (DM), polymyositis (PM), overlap myositis which includes the anti-synthetase syndrome, immune-mediated necrotizing myopathy (IMNM), and sporadic inclusion body myositis (sIBM). Major clinical and laboratory manifestations of IIMs are proximal muscle weakness, skin manifestations (Gottron's sign, heliotropic rash, mechanic's hands, and calcinosis cutis), lung involvement, elevated muscle enzymes, as well as myositis-specific and/or myositis-associated autoantibodies. These autoantibodies can be biomarkers for certain disease features: (a) anti-PM/Scl for interstitial lung disease (ILD), inflammatory arthritis, Raynaud's phenomenon (RP), mechanic's hands and overlap manifestations with systemic sclerosis (sclerodactyly, telangiectasias, esophageal reflux disease, subcutaneous edema, puffy hands, and calcinosis); (b) anti-U1snRNP for myositis in the context of mixed connective tissue disease (MCTD); (c) anti-Ku for overlap myositis with other autoimmune systemic diseases; (d) anti-Ro52 frequently co-occur with anti-Jo1 antibodies and connote an increased risk for severe ILD; (e) antibodies to aminoacyl-tRNA synthetases (anti-Jo1, anti-PL7, anti-PL12, anti-OJ, anti-EJ, anti-KS, anti-Zo, anti-SC, anti-JS, and anti-YRS) for the subtype of anti-synthetase syndrome characterized by mechanic's hands, arthritis, ILD, and RP; (f) anti-SRP (signal recognition particle), for severe muscle and heart involvement; (g) anti-HMGCR (3-hydroxy-3-methylglutaryl-coenzyme A reductase) for statin use-related necrotizing myopathy; (h) anti-MDA5 (melanoma differentiation-associated gene 5) for amyopathic myositis with ILD; and (i) anti-cN1A (cytosolic 5′ nucleotidase 1A) for sIBM. Paraneoplastic myositis is characterized by autoantibodies to TIF-1 (transcriptional intermediary factor 1) antigen. In terms of histopathology, DM is characterized by prominent perivascular and perifascicular inflammation, PM by endomysial inflammation, and sIBM by a combination of inflammation and degeneration of muscle fibers with internal rimmed vacuoles. IMNM is considered a macrophage-mediated inflammatory process. Scattered necrotic muscle fibers surrounded by sparse inflammatory cells (pre-

H. M. Moutsopoulos (✉)
Athens Academy, Athens, Greece
e-mail: hmoutsop@med.uoa.gr

E. Zampeli
Bioclinic General Hospital of Athens and Institute for Autoimmune Systemic and Neurological Disorders, Athens, Greece
e-mail: ezampeli@bioclinic.gr

H. M. Moutsopoulos, E. Zampeli (eds.), *Immunology and Rheumatology in Questions*,
https://doi.org/10.1007/978-3-030-56670-8_5

dominantly lymphocytes) are characteristic. Endocrine conditions (Cushing's disease, thyroid dysfunction, and diabetes mellitus) as well as genetic abnormalities (mitochondrial myopathies) induce muscle diseases, which have to be distinguished from IIMs. Furthermore, recently a distinct nosological entity has been described, which encompasses patients who present radiological and/or histological features of interstitial pneumonia along with clinical manifestations that could suggest an autoimmune process but do not meet established criteria for a particular connective tissue disease. These patients are categorized as having interstitial pneumonia with autoimmune features (IPAF). Follow-up of these patients is necessary for possible evolution to a definite autoimmune disease.

1. Which are the main types of idiopathic inflammatory myopathies?

The main types of idiopathic inflammatory myopathies (IIM) are dermatomyositis (DM), polymyositis (PM), overlap myositis—including anti-synthetase syndrome—, immune-mediated necrotizing myopathy (IMNM), sporadic inclusion body myositis (sIBM), and clinically amyopathic dermatomyositis (CADM) [1–3].

2. Which are the major clinical and laboratory manifestations of dermatomyositis?

- Proximal muscle weakness: Occurs insidiously and is more prominent in the shoulder and pelvic girdle muscles. In more severe disease, pharyngeal and esophageal muscles may also be involved
- Characteristic skin manifestations:
  - Gottron's sign (Fig. 5.1): Red-to-violaceous papules over the dorsal surface of the metacarpophalangeal and interphalangeal joints. It can also occur on the extensor surfaces of the knees and elbows
  - Heliotrope rash (Fig. 5.2): Purple-red rash occurring around the eyelids, forehead, and nasolabial folds
  - V-sign rash: Violaceous rash occurring on the anterior chest wall and the neck
  - Shawl sign: Redness occurring over the shoulders
  - Mechanic's hands: Hyperkeratotic papules along with fissured and cracked palmar and finger-pad skin (Fig. 5.3)

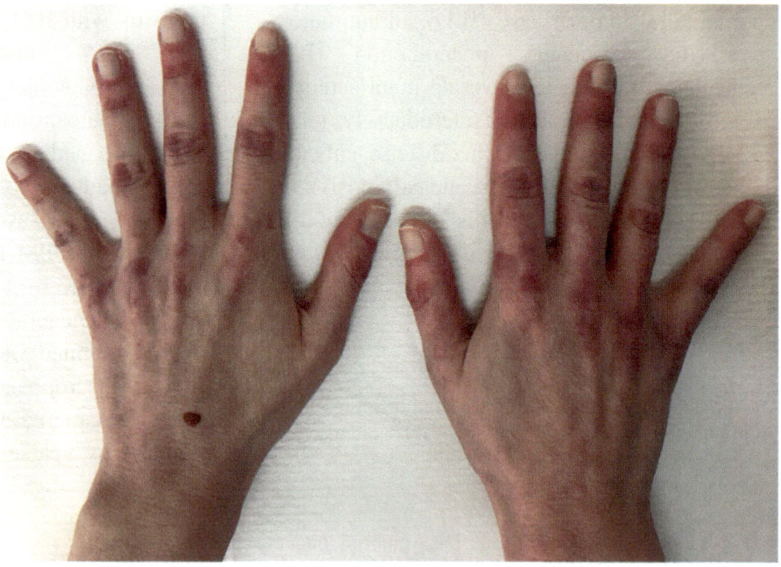

Fig. 5.1 Gottron's sign: Red-violaceous papules over the metacarpophalangeal and interphalangeal joints of a 45-year-old woman with dermatomyositis

– Calcinosis cutis: Deposition of insoluble calcium salts in the cutaneous and subcutaneous tissue (Fig. 5.4a, b). It is more commonly seen in the juvenile form of DM

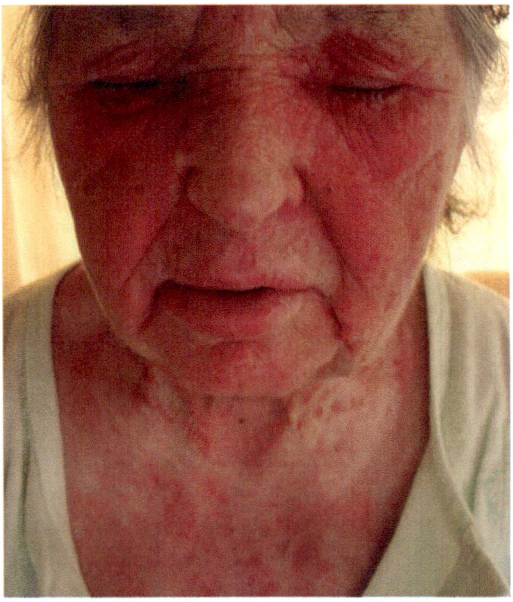

Fig. 5.2. Heliotrope rash: Purple-red rash occurring around the eyelids and nasolabial folds as well as erythroviolaceous rash on the "V" of the chest in a 74-year-old female with dermatomyositis

– Extra-muscular manifestations: Constitutional symptoms, arthralgias/ arthritis, interstitial lung disease, electrocardiographic abnormalities, myocarditis, and Raynaud's phenomenon
- Laboratory abnormalities:
  – Elevated serum muscle enzymes: Creatine phosphokinase, aspartate and alanine aminotransferase, and lactate dehydrogenase
  – Acute-phase reactants may be elevated or within normal levels
  – Presence of myositis-associated and myositis-specific autoantibodies

3. **Which are the myositis-specific autoantibodies and with what particular clinical manifestations do they correlate?**

Autoantibodies have been identified in over 50% of patients with inflammatory myopathies (myositis-associated and/or myositis-specific autoantibodies). They are important biomarkers, aiding in diagnosis, predicting additional clinical complications and response to treatment, and helping classify patients into more homogeneous groups.

Fig. 5.3 Mechanics hands: Hyperkeratotic, fissuring eruptions on the palmar side of fingers reminiscent of hands of manual workers, seen in a 56-year-old male patient who was diagnosed with anti-synthetase syndrome

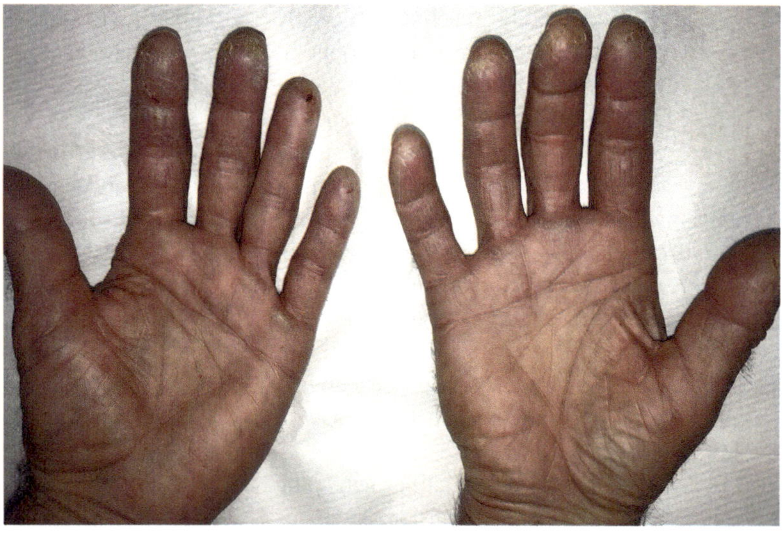

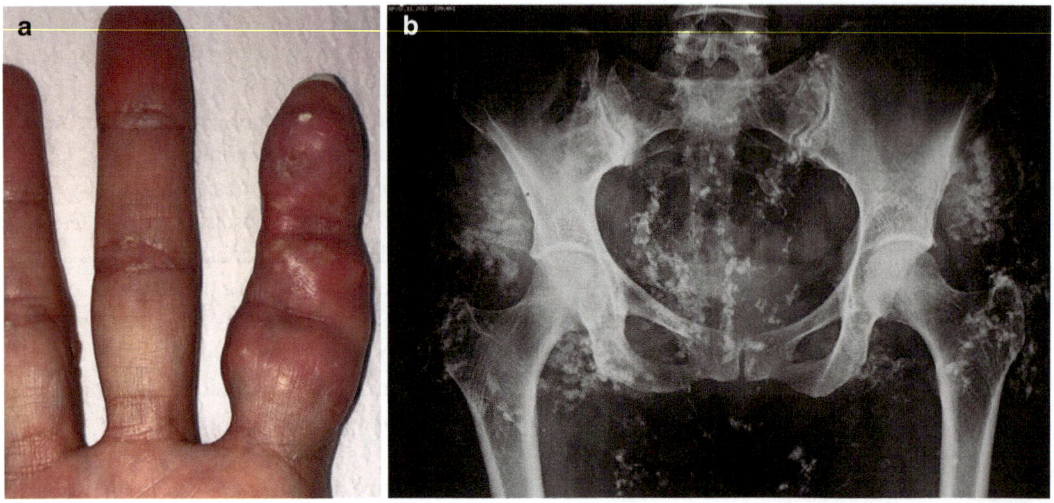

Fig. 5.4 Calcinosis cutis: Hard calcified subcutaneous nodules have developed in various areas (knees, elbows, gluteal areas, and fingers) in a 56-year-old female patient with long-standing, ineffectively treated dermatomyositis. (**a**) Extensive subcutaneous calcifications are evident on the index finger, (**b**) on pelvis X-ray, of the same patient, extensive calcinosis of the gluteal and hip areas is apparent

Myositis-specific are autoantibodies to:

- *ASA* (aminoacyl-tRNA synthetases: anti-Jo1, anti-PL7, anti-PL12, anti-OJ, anti-EJ, anti-KS, anti-Zo, anti-SC, anti-JS, and anti-YRS): correlating clinical manifestations—interstitial lung disease, mechanic's hands, arthritis, and Raynaud's phenomenon [1–4]
- *SRP* (signal recognition particle): Patients with this autoantibody reactivity typically present highly elevated creatine phosphokinase (CPK), severe weakness and muscle pain, dysphagia, and cardiac involvement and have a poor response to treatment. Muscle histology can reveal signs of necrotizing autoimmune myopathy [1, 5, 6]
- *HMGCR* (3-hydroxy-3-methylglutaryl-coenzyme A reductase): These patients have highly elevated CPK and significant necrotizing myopathy, which correlates with statin use [5, 7]
- *Mi-2* (nucleosome-remodeling deacetylase complex): It is significantly associated with skin rash
- *SAE* (small ubiquitin-like modifier activating enzyme): Myositis in this subgroup of patients can be amyopathic at onset; nevertheless skin rash is typically present (Fig. 5.5)
- *MDA5* (melanoma differentiation-associated gene 5): Patients with this autoantibody typically present with amyopathic myositis and rapidly progressive interstitial lung disease
- *NXP2* (nuclear matrix protein 2): This autoantibody reactivity is significantly associated with skin rash, malignancy in adults, and calcinosis in juveniles
- *TIF1* (transcriptional intermediary factor 1): It is strongly associated with underlying malignancy
- *cN1A* (cytosolic 5′-nucleotidase 1A): It is associated with sporadic inclusion body myositis [1, 3, 5]

4. **Which are myositis-associated autoantibodies and with what particular clinical manifestations do they correlate?**

Myositis-associated are autoantibodies to:

- *PM/Scl*: A 75-kDa protein found in polymyositis (PM)–scleroderma (Scl) overlap. Correlating clinical manifestations: increased risk of interstitial lung disease (ILD), inflammatory arthritis, mechanics hands, and Raynaud's phenomenon
- *U1snRNP* (U1 small nuclear ribonucleoprotein particle): Found in patients with myositis and mixed connective tissue disease overlap

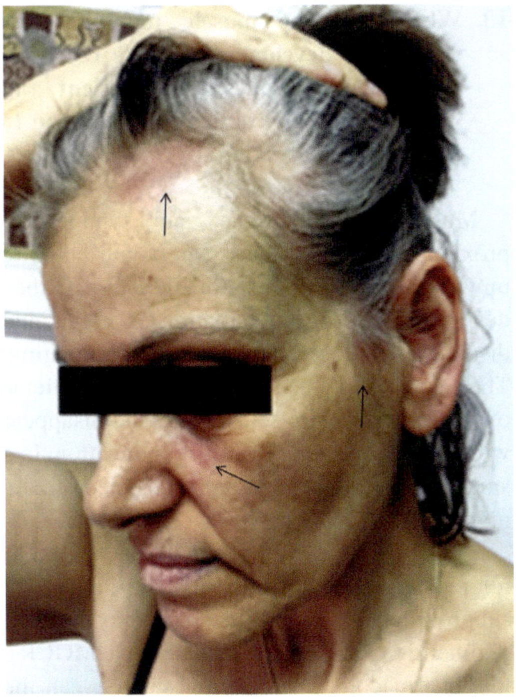

Fig. 5.5 A 52-year-old woman developed well-demarcated, non-scaling, non-pruritic erythroviolaceous plaques on her forehead, temporal and ante-auricular areas and below her eyes (arrows) and small violaceous papules over the bony prominences of the metcarpophalangeal and interphalangeal joints of her hands (Gottron' sign). Laboratory and serology testing revealed only positive antinuclear antibodies (ANA 1:640, fine speckled pattern) with normal serum muscle enzymes. Myositis specific autoantibodies showed the presence of anti-small ubiquitin-like modifier activating enzyme (anti-SAE) autoantibodies

- *Ku*: (composed of 70 and 80 kDa subunits, has a high affinity for DNA ends) found in 9–19% of myositis patients with overlap syndromes including systemic lupus erythematosus, scleroderma, as well as mixcd and undifferentiated connective tissue disease. These patients present with increased frequency of arthralgias, Raynaud's phenomenon, musculoskeletal manifestations, and ILD
- *Ro52*: Found in 56–72% of anti-Jo-1-positive patients. Patients with both anti-Jo-1 and anti-Ro-52 autoantibodies have an increased risk for severe ILD. They have a poorer outcome compared to patients with anti-Jo-1 alone [1, 2, 4]

5. Which are the nail findings in patients with dermatomyositis (DM)?

Thickened, hyperkeratotic, ragged cuticles, and telangiectasias of the proximal nail fold are the characteristic nail findings in patients with DM. These nail findings distinguish DM from other connective tissue disorders. Rare nail findings include complete loss of several toenails, red lunulae, and ventral pterygium. Ischemic nail lesions might predict underlying malignancy in patients with DM.

6. Which are the major clinical findings of patients with anti-synthetase syndrome?

Anti-synthetase syndrome (ASS) is a distinct subtype of idiopathic inflammatory myopathy (IIM) characterized by the presence of autoantibodies against one of many aminoacyl-tRNA synthetases with clinical features that include interstitial lung disease (ILD, 40–90%), arthritis (60%), myositis, Raynaud's phenomenon (60%), unexplained fever, and/or mechanic's hands [8, 9]. ASS patients present a higher prevalence of ILD compared to dermatomyositis (DM) and polymyositis (PM) patients, and ILD in these patients is often severe and rapidly progressive (mostly associated with anti-PL7 or anti-PL12 reactivity). Some ASS patients have also anti-Ro52 antibodies. These patients have more severe and fibrotic ILD, and their myositis is more resistant to therapy [10]. ASS patients rarely develop malignancy.

7. Which are the characteristics of interstitial lung disease (ILD) in inflammatory myopathy (IIM) patients?

In the sera of IIM patients with ILD, aminoacyl-tRNA synthetases (anti-synthetase syndrome, ASS) or anti-MDA-5 autoantibodies are usually present. In patients with ASS-ILD, the most frequent chest CT findings are ground glass opacities and reticulations, although consolidations are also common. As the disease progresses, consolidations typically resolve, whereas honeycombing and fibrosis become more common. The CT pattern most frequently ascribed to patients with ASS-ILD is non-specific interstitial pneumonia (NSIP) or NSIP with organizing pneumonia (OP). Patients with anti-MDA5 ILD have frequent ground glass opacities and consolidations and less reticulation. These patients more frequently have unclassifiable lung CT patterns.

8. Which are the symptoms and clinical signs of patients with sporadic inclusion body myositis?

Patients with sporadic inclusion body myositis (sIBM) are usually males over 50 years of age with insidious onset of proximal and later distal muscle weakness. Muscle atrophy is very prominent, especially in the thigh/pelvic muscles and the brachial/antebrachial muscles. sIBM patients present typically with difficulty in shaking hands and frequently suffer from recurrent falls. Besides myopathy, they can also have mild peripheral neuropathy with decreased deep tendon reflexes. sIBM is rarely associated with underlying malignancy and rarely exhibits lung, joint, or heart involvement.

9. What is the clinical picture of clinically amyopathic dermatomyositis (CADM, myositis sine myositis)?

The patients of this subcategory of dermatomyositis (DM) present with skin rashes (Fig. 5.5) characteristic of DM, yet without muscle weakness. Some patients develop rapidly progressive ILD. A small percentage of this patient population, particularly of Asian origin, may have in their sera anti-melanoma differentiation-associated gene 5 (MDA5) autoantibodies. DM-ILD patients with anti-MDA5 positivity are reported to have a worse prognosis compared to DM-ILD patients with anti-antisynthetase antibodies [11]. Furthermore, a high anti-MDA5 titer (>100 IU/mL) and high levels of serum ferritin levels in CADM patients seem to associate with the development of rapidly progressive ILD in the first 3 months after diagnosis [12]. Besides anti-MDA5 autoantibodies, patients with CADM may have myositis-associated autoantibodies (MAAs). Coexistent MAAs could be a marker of favorable prognosis in anti-MDA5-positive patients with CADM [12].

10. Which are the muscle manifestations which can develop in patients receiving statins? Which ones are transient and which persist and oblige the physician to discontinue statin therapy?

Muscle aches, fatigue, and symmetrical proximal muscle weakness can be attributed to unwanted effects of statin therapy if they develop 2 weeks after initiation of statins and disappear 2 weeks after statin discontinuation. The majority of muscle complaints in patients on statin therapy are self-limited and disappear without sequelae after their discontinuation. In a small portion of patients on statins, necrotizing myositis can develop which persists after discontinuation of statins and should be treated as idiopathic necrotizing myositis. In this patient subgroup autoantibodies to 3-hydroxy-3-methylglutaryl-coenzyme A reductase (HMGCR), the pharmacologic target of statins, can be detected.

11. In which patient age group myositis can be a paraneoplastic phenomenon?

It is seen in myositis patients over the age of 50 years with severe cutaneous and muscle manifestations as well as circulating antibodies to TIF-1 antigen. These individuals should be evaluated for underlying cancer. In patients with dermatomyositis ovarian, lung, pancreatic, non-Hodgkin lymphoma, stomach, colorectal, and breast cancer should be excluded. In patients with polymyositis non-Hodgkin lymphoma, lung, and bladder cancer are the commonest types of underlying malignancy.

12. Which are the major muscle histopathologic findings in patients with dermatomyositis, polymyositis, sporadic inclusion body myositis, and immune-mediated necrotizing myopathy?

Dermatomyositis: It is a complement-mediated vasculopathy of the muscle small vessels. The characteristic histological finding is perifascicular atrophy of muscle fibers with increased endomysial connective tissue and inflammatory infiltrates. Overexpression of type I interferon α/β by plasmacytoid dendritic cells, increased MHC-I antigens, and immunoglobulin gene transcripts can be also observed (Fig. 5.6a).

Polymyositis: It is a cell-mediated cytotoxic immune response, where CD8+ cytotoxic T cells and macrophages clonally expand and infiltrate the endomysium. The surrounded and invaded muscle cells express MHC class I molecules (Fig. 5.6b).

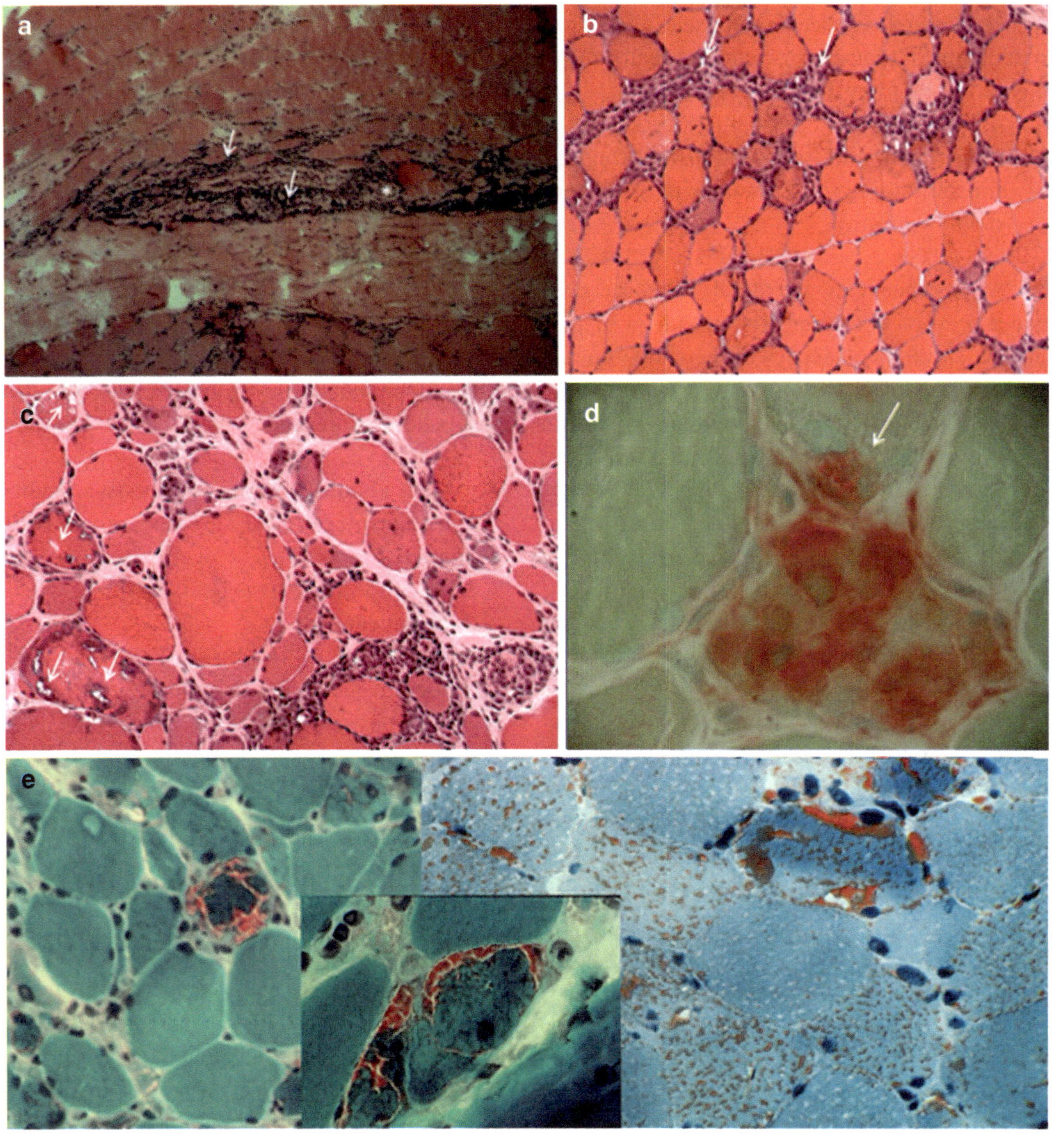

Fig. 5.6 Muscle histopathology: (**a**) Dermatomyositis: Inflammation is most prominent perivascularly (asterisk) and perifascicularly (arrows). (**b**) Polymyositis: Endomysial inflammation (arrows). (**c**) Sporadic inclusion body myositis: a combination of inflammatory and degenerative process. T cells invading healthy-appearing muscle fibers (asterisks) and vacuoles (in fibers not invaded by T cells, arrows). (**d**) Necrotizing autoimmune myositis: necrotic fibers are invaded by macrophages identified in red with alkaline phosphatase staining. (**e**) Mitochondrial myopathy: left—cross section of muscle biopsy stained with trichrome shows "ragged-red" fibers characterized by red stains in the periphery of the fibers due to accumulation of mitochondria. At high magnification, one such fiber also shows the cracks (ragged) parenchyma. Right—mitochondrial dysfunction indicative of defects in oxidative phosphorylation is accompanied by accumulation of fat visualized with oil red O stain (*Figures courtesy of Professor Marinos C. Dalakas, MD, FAAN*)

Sporadic inclusion body myositis: Atrophic and hypertrophic muscle fibers with internal rimmed vacuoles are the typical histopathologic findings (Fig. 5.6c).

Immune-mediated necrotizing myopathy: It is thought to be a macrophage-mediated immune response. Overexpression of MHC-I molecules in necrotic and regenerating muscle fibers, surrounded by T lymphocytes, are the major histopathologic findings (Fig. 5.6d) [13].

13. Which are the typical histopathologic muscle findings of patients with mitochondrial myopathy?

The presence of ragged red fibers. This ragged appearance of fibers sometimes can be seen in muscle specimen stained with hematoxylin and eosin. These fibers are typically recognized with modified Gomori-trichrome staining. This stain shows a red peripheral rim or granular red of the sarcoplasm. The red staining is the result of the increased amount of phospholipids in the membranes of proliferated mitochondria (Fig. 5.6e).

14. Which endocrine conditions can present with myopathy?

Thyroid dysfunction (hypothyroidism, myxedema, and thyrotoxic myopathy), vitamin D deficiency, adrenal dysfunction, parathyroid dysfunction (multiple endocrine neoplasia), pituitary dysfunction, and Langerhans islands dysfunction (ischemic infarction of the femoral muscles in diabetic myopathy).

15. Which drugs induce myopathies?

- Corticosteroids (mainly fluorinated preparations)
- Antithyroid drugs, e.g., Carbimazole
- Psychotropic drugs
- Combination of drugs such as fibrates and statins or colchicine and cyclosporine-A

16. On what grounds a physician should think that the patient has drug-induced myopathy?

- Lack of muscular complains prior to the initiation of therapy
- Lack of another cause accounting for the myopathy
- Complete or incomplete resolution of symptoms and signs after discontinuation of the medication

17. Which corticosteroid preparations mainly induce glucocorticoid-induced myopathy?

Steroid-induced myopathy is mostly associated with increased doses of fluorinated glucocorticoid preparations, which lead to type IIb muscle fiber atrophy.

18. When should immunosuppressive agents be considered for a dermatomyositis patient?

If the patient has:

- A poor response or is refractory to corticosteroid therapy or presents glucocorticoid-related side effects
- A rapidly progressively disease
- Severe internal organ involvement

19. What is the clinical picture of McArdle's syndrome?

McArdle's syndrome is a type V glycogen storage disease. It is caused by myophosphorylase deficiency. It starts in childhood, but the diagnosis is usually set in adulthood. It presents with muscle pain and painful cramps upon exercise which obligate the patient to rest. Upon strenuous exercise myoglobinuria can develop. The characteristic clinical sign observed in these patients is the second wind phenomenon. This phenomenon is characterized by the patient's better tolerance for aerobic exercise such as walking and cycling after resting for approximately 10 min.

20. Which are the muscle histopathologic findings in patients with McArdle's syndrome?

Muscle fibers of patients with McArdle's syndrome are characterized by subsarcolemmal storage of normal glycogen and by absent histochemical stain for phosphorylase reaction. In contrast, intramuscular vessels stain histochemically for phosphorylase.

21. What is interstitial pneumonia with autoimmune features?

Patients with radiological and/or histological features of interstitial pneumonia and without any underlying disease who additionally present clinical manifestations that could suggest an autoimmune process but do not meet established criteria for a particular connective tissue disease (CTD), are termed as having interstitial pneumonia with autoimmune features (IPAF). Classification criteria for IPAF take into consideration features from three domains: clinical, serological, and morphological. A diagnosis of IPAF is placed when the patient presents at least one feature from at least two of these domains [14] (Fig. 5.7).

22. Which are the clinical features characterizing patients with interstitial pneumonia with autoimmune features?

- Distal digital fissuring (i.e., "mechanic hands")
- Distal digital tip ulceration
- Inflammatory arthritis or polyarticular morning joint stiffness ≥60 min
- Palmar telangiectasia
- Raynaud's phenomenon
- Unexplained digital edema
- Unexplained fixed rash on the digital extensor surfaces (Gottron's sign) [14]

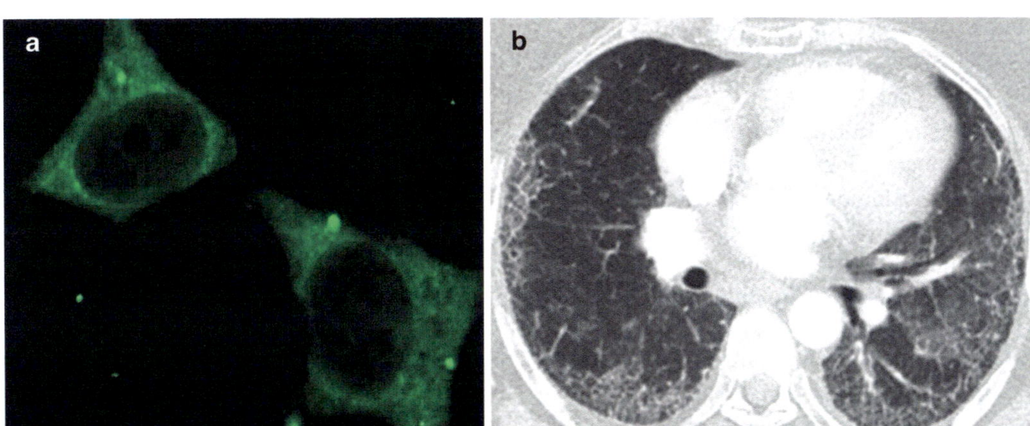

Fig. 5.7 A 53-year-old housewife, with arthralgias, Raynaud's phenomenon, edema of hands and progressively increasing dyspnea and dry cough. Physical examination revealed edematous hands with vasomotor changes and rales were audible upon auscultation on both lung bases. Oxygen saturation was decreased (92%) and blood gases showed hypoxemia (PO_2: 62 mmHg, PCO_2: 32 mmHg). Laboratory tests showed moderately increased C-reactive protein (32 mg/dL, normal value <5 mg/dL) and (**a**) positive ANA ≥ 1:320 (cytoplasmic pattern) and autoantibodies to signal recognition particle (anti-SRP). (**b**) High-resolution chest CT scan revealed honeycombing lesions in both lung bases while on the right lung base ground glass opacities. The clinical, laboratory, and chest CT findings are all compatible with interstitial pneumonia with autoimmune features

23. Which are the possible serological features of patients with interstitial pneumonia with autoimmune features?

- ANA ≥ 1:320 titer, diffuse, speckled, homogeneous patterns or ANA nucleolar pattern (any titer) or ANA centromere pattern (any titer)
- Seropositivity of any of the following autoantibodies: Rheumatoid factor (≥2× upper normal limit), anti-CCP, anti-dsDNA, anti-Ro, anti-La, anti-ribonucleoprotein, anti-Smith, anti-topoisomerase (Scl-70), anti-tRNA synthetases (e.g., Jo-1, PL-7, PL-12; others are: EJ, OJ, KS, Zo, and tRS), anti-PM-Scl, and anti-MDA-5 [14]

24. Which are the radiological and/or histological findings of patients with interstitial pneumonia with autoimmune features?

Morphological features include radiological patterns by high-resolution chest computed tomography and/or histological findings from lung biopsy suggestive of:

- Nonspecific interstitial pneumonitis (NISP)
- Organizing pneumonia (OP)
- NSIP/OP overlap
- Lymphocytic interstitial pneumonitis (LIP)
- Involvement of other pulmonary compartments (in addition to lung parenchyma), such as pleura effusion/thickening, pericardial effusion/thickening, unexplained intrinsic airways disease, or pulmonary vasculopathy [14]

25. What is the clinical picture and which are the causes of camptocormia?

Camptocormia is an acquired disease of body posture, presenting with forward bending of the thoracolumbar spine. The individual's forward bending of the body worsens when he/she walks or stands, while the posture is corrected when lying on supine position. Many neurological, muscular, and spine disorders may account for the development of camptocormia. Among them Parkinson's disease is the main etiology. Other causes include:

Myopathy (inclusion body myositis)
Alzheimer's disease
Motor neuron disease
Myasthenia gravis
Severe osteoporosis with multiple vertebral fractures
Spinal trauma/arthritis
Psychiatric syndromes
Paraneoplastic disorders [15]

References

1. Lundberg IE, Tjärnlund A, Bottai M, et al. 2017 European League Against Rheumatism/American College of Rheumatology classification criteria for adult and juvenile idiopathic inflammatory myopathies and their major subgroups. Ann Rheum Dis. 2017;76:1955–64.
2. Mariampillai K, Granger B, Amelin D, et al. Development of a new classification system for idiopathic inflammatory myopathies based on clinical manifestations and myositis-specific autoantibodies. JAMA Neurol. 2018;75:1528–37.
3. Selva-O'Callaghan A, Pinal-Fernandez I, Trallero-Araguás E, et al. Classification and management of adult inflammatory myopathies. Lancet Neurol. 2018;17:816–28.
4. Zampeli E, Venetsanopoulou A, Argyropoulou OD, et al. Myositis autoantibody profiles and their clinical associations in Greek patients with inflammatory myopathies. Clin Rheumatol. 2019;38:125–32.
5. Betteridge Z, McHugh N. Myositis-specific autoantibodies: an important tool to support diagnosis of myositis. J Intern Med. 2016;280:8–23.
6. Lundberg IE, Miller FW, Tjärnlund A, Bottai M. Diagnosis and classification of idiopathic inflammatory myopathies. J Intern Med. 2016;280:39–51.
7. Dalakas MC. Necrotising autoimmune myopathy (NAM): antibodies seem to be specific markers in aiding diagnosis. J Neurol Neurosurg Psychiatry. 2016;87:1037.
8. Solomon J, Swigris JJ, Brown KK. Myositis-related interstitial lung disease and antisynthetase syndrome. J Bras Pneumol. 2011;37:100–9.
9. Zampeli E, Moutsopoulos HM. Lesson of the month 2: Fever, arthralgias and hyperkeratotic, scaling and fissuring eruptions of the hands. Clin Med (Lond). 2019;19:255–6.
10. La Corte R, Lo Mo Naco A, Locaputo A, et al. In patients with antisynthetase syndrome the occurrence

of anti-Ro/SSA antibodies causes a more severe interstitial lung disease. Autoimmunity. 2006;39:249–53.
11. Kishaba T, McGill R, Nei Y, et al. Clinical characteristics of dermatomyosits/polymyositis associated interstitial lung disease according to the autoantibody. J Med Investig. 2018;65:251–7.
12. Yamaguchi K, Yamaguchi A, Kashiwagi C, et al. Differential clinical features of patients with clinically amyopathic dermato-myositis who have circulating anti-MDA5 autoantibodies with or without myositis-associated autoantibodies. Respir Med. 2018;140:1–5.
13. Dalakas MC. Inflammatory muscle diseases. N Engl J Med. 2015;372:1734–47.
14. Fischer A, Antoniou KM, Brown KK, et al. An official European Respiratory Society/American Thoracic Society research statement: interstitial pneumonia with autoimmune features. Eur Respir J. 2015;46:976–87.
15. Finsterer J, Strobl W. Causes of camptocormia. Disabil Rehabil. 2011;33:1702–3.

Sjögren's Syndrome, IgG4-Related Disorders

6

Haralampos M. Moutsopoulos
and Evangelia Zampeli

Abstract

Sjögren's syndrome (SS) is a chronic, systemic autoimmune disorder affecting predominantly middle-aged females. SS clinical manifestations can be related to glandular dysfunction (keratoconjunctivitis sicca, oral dryness, bronchitis sicca, parotid gland enlargement) and extra-glandular/systemic involvement. The latter is either due to peri-epithelial infiltrates in parenchymal organs (small airway disease, interstitial nephritis, and biliary cirrhosis) or due to immune complex deposition (palpable purpura, peripheral neuropathy, glomerulonephritis, and systemic vasculitis). In the majority of patients, SS runs an indolent benign course. In a small yet not negligible number of cases (5–10%), SS is complicated by lymphoid neoplasia. Sicca manifestations, increased fatigability, arthralgias/myalgias, non-erosive arthritis, Raynaud's phenomenon, and signs of renal tubular acidosis may be initial manifestations of SS. After excluding other causes of sicca symptomatology, patients should be assessed for lacrimal and salivary gland function (ocular staining with lissamine green or rose Bengal, Schirmer's test, and unstimulated saliva secretion, respectively), and a biopsy of labial minor salivary glands should be performed to evaluate the presence of lymphocytic infiltrate around salivary gland epithelium. SS patients presenting salivary gland enlargement, Raynaud's phenomenon, lymphadenopathy, anti-Ro/SSA or anti-La/SSB autoantibodies, rheumatoid factor positivity, monoclonality, and low serum C4 levels should be monitored closely, since these clinical, laboratory, and immunologic parameters have been shown to be independent predictors for non-Hodgkin's lymphoma development.

IgG4-related disease (IgG4-RD) has recently emerged as a new clinical entity. It comprises numerous conditions previously thought to be unrelated, such as sclerosing dacryoadenitis/orbital pseudotumor, sclerosing sialadenitis, autoimmune pancreatitis, retroperitoneal fibrosis/periaortitis, sclerosing cholangitis, Riedel thyroiditis, hypophysitis, and prostatitis. IgG4-RDs are clinically characterized by tumor-like lesions in affected organs. Histopathologically, they typically present lymphoplasmacytic infiltrates with increased IgG4+ plasma cells, storiform fibrosis, obliterative phlebitis, and tissue eosinophilia, while serum IgG4 concentration is usually increased. Typically IgG4-RD symptoms respond promptly to steroids.

H. M. Moutsopoulos (✉)
Athens Academy, Athens, Greece
e-mail: hmoutsop@med.uoa.gr

E. Zampeli
Bioclinic General Hospital of Athens and Institute for Autoimmune Systemic and Neurological Disorders, Athens, Greece
e-mail: ezampeli@bioclinic.gr

H. M. Moutsopoulos, E. Zampeli (eds.), *Immunology and Rheumatology in Questions*,
https://doi.org/10.1007/978-3-030-56670-8_6

1. **Which age group is primarily affected by Sjögren's syndrome?**

Females in the fourth and fifth decades of life are usually affected.

2. **Which are glandular and extra-glandular disease manifestations that present early before the full clinical picture of Sjögren's syndrome develops? How long does it take from the initial manifestations to full-blown disease?**

The initial manifestations of Sjögren's syndrome are usually nonspecific and include arthralgias, arthritis, fatigability, Raynaud's phenomenon, dry eyes and/or mouth, bronchitis sicca and infrequently parotid gland enlargement, purpura, and signs of renal tubular acidosis. Sjögren's syndrome is a slowly progressing disorder; 6–8 years may elapse from the initial manifestations to full-blown disease development. Glomerulonephritis, systemic vasculitis, and lymphoma are manifestations that develop years after Sjögren's syndrome diagnosis.

3. **What are the differences between arthritis seen in patients and rheumatoid arthritis and that seen in Sjögren's syndrome patients?**

Arthritis in both disease entities is symmetrical, accompanied by morning stiffness, and can affect primarily the wrists, metacarpophalangeal, and proximal interphalangeal joints. In contrast to rheumatoid arthritis, arthritis in Sjögren's syndrome is milder, usually transient, and does not lead to joint erosive changes. In some Sjögren's syndrome patients, Jaccoud's arthropathy may develop.

4. **Which histopathological findings in a labial minor salivary gland biopsy are characteristic for focal lymphocytic sialadenitis?**

Labial minor salivary gland biopsy (LMSGB) is one of the objective tests used in order to set the diagnosis of Sjögren's syndrome. Although it is an invasive procedure (Fig. 6.1), it is safe and

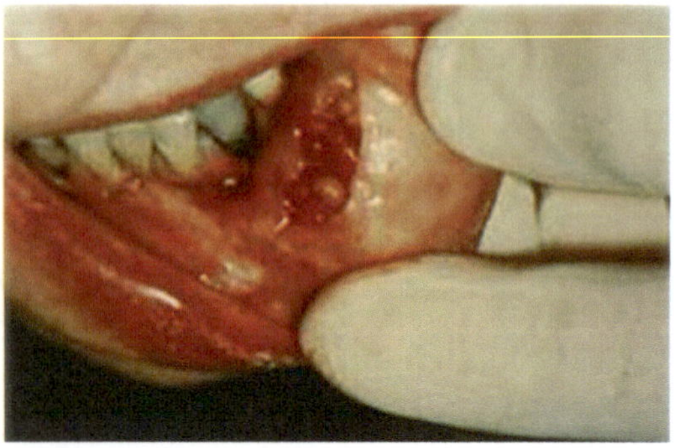

Fig. 6.1 Labial minor salivary gland biopsy: it is obtained by an approximately 1-cm wide incision of the lower lip mucosa

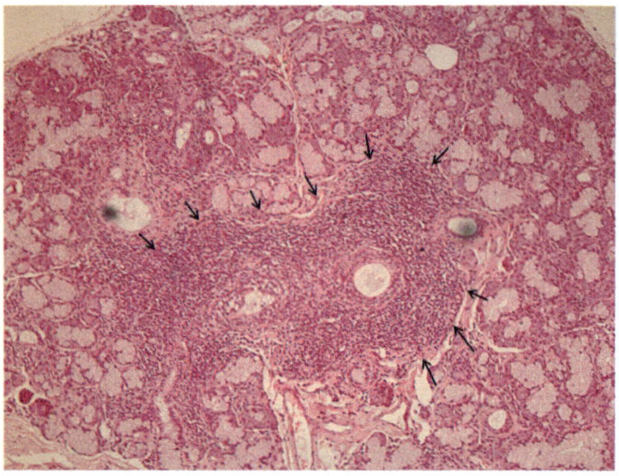

Fig. 6.2 Labial minor salivary gland histopathology: a cluster of round cells (at least 50 lymphocytes), called a focus, is seen (black arrows) in the salivary gland tissue specimen. The focal lymphocytic infiltrates are localized around ducts, and replace functional glandular epithelium

is associated with few local adverse effects. The key requirements for a correct histological evaluation of LMSGB include a minimum size of biopsy material of 4 mm^2 containing an adequate number—at least five—salivary gland lobules. A cluster of round cells with at least 50 lymphocytes is called a focus. Focal lymphocytic sialadenitis is diagnosed when in the biopsy specimen multiple, dense aggregates of ≥ 50 lymphocytes in peri-epithelial ductal areas in the majority of sampled glands are evident. This constitutes the characteristic histopathological feature of Sjögren's syndrome (Fig. 6.2). The severity of the histopathologic lesion of the labial minor salivary glands is graded according to the system described by Chisholm and Mason, which counts the number of lymphocytic foci per 4 mm^2 of the salivary tissue under investigation.

5. What is the cellular composition of the labial minor salivary gland focal round cell infiltrates from patients with Sjögren's syndrome?

In mild inflammatory lesions in labial minor salivary gland tissues from Sjögren's syndrome patients, T lymphocytes predominate, while in severe lesions B lymphocytes are more prominent than T lymphocytes. Furthermore, in severe lesions, increased numbers of macrophages and dendritic cells are present [1].

6. Which are the major pathogenetic steps leading to development of Sjögren's syndrome?

The interplay of endogenous (intracellular stress, inappropriate overexpression of endogenous nucleic acids) and exogenous triggers (viruses, hormones, stressful life events) in a background of a genetically determined hyperactive immune response seems to be crucial for the initiation and the perpetuation of Sjögren's syndrome. Ductal and acinar epithelial cells appear to play a significant role in the initiation and perpetuation of autoimmune injury. These cells: (1) express inappropriately co-stimulatory molecules, and the intracellular Ro and La autoantigens on the glandular epithelial cell membranes, acquiring the capacity to provide signals essential for lymphocytic activation, (2) produce pro-inflammatory cytokines and lymphocyte attracting chemokines necessary to attract immunocytes, sustaining the autoimmune lesion and allowing the formation of ectopic germinal centers, (3) express functional receptors of innate immunity -Toll-like receptors (TLRs) 3, 7, and 9-, molecules which may account for the initiation of the autoimmune reactivity, (4) express immunoregulatory molecules like intercellular adhesion molecules (ICAM) and CD40, (5) have also an active role in the production of BAFF (B cell-activating factor), which is induced after stimulation with type I and II interferons, and finally (6) die from apoptotic death which through apoptotic blebs release intracellular antigens that further fuels the autoimmune reactivity [2].

7. What clinical/laboratory and histological parameters are required to set the diagnosis of Sjögren's syndrome?

The parameters required include anti-Ro/SSA (primarily anti-Ro60) as well as anti-La/SSB antibody positivity and focal lymphocytic sialadenitis with a focus score of ≥1 foci/4 mm^2 (each scoring 3); an abnormal ocular staining score (with lissamine green or rose Bengal, measured by the van Bijsterveld scale and having a score of ≥4), a Schirmer's test result of ≤5 mm/5 min and an unstimulated salivary flow rate of ≤0.1 mL/min (each scoring 1). Individuals with signs and/or symptoms suggestive of Sjögren's syndrome who have a total score of ≥4 after adding the scores of the above items meet the criteria for primary Sjögren's syndrome [3].

8. What is keratoconjunctivitis sicca?

Keratoconjunctivitis sicca (KCS) is a condition commonly referred to as "dry eyes" syndrome, where damage of the cornea and/or conjunctival epithelium results in secondary inflammation. The patients complain of burning sensation, feeling of sand or grit in the eyes, eye fatigability, and pressure behind the eyes, symptoms which become worse as the day goes on. It is the result of meibomian gland dysfunction, allergies, Sjögren's syndrome, vitamin A deficiency, and drugs (antidepressants, antihistamines, and others). The diagnosis of KCS is placed with slit-lamp examination after the conjunctiva and cornea are stained either with lissamine green or rose Bengal.

9. How Schirmer's I test is performed?

Schirmer's I test measures the lacrimal flow. It is performed by placing a piece of Whatman filter paper under the inferior eyelid, usually without prior application of topical anesthetic, and measuring the amount of wetness over a specified time. Normal wetting is >15 mm in 5 min, whereas <5 mm is a strong indication of diminished tear production. It should be taken into account that lacrimal flow varies according to the time of the day measured, the hydration status of the individual, the phase of the menstrual cycle, and the environmental humidity.

10. Which are the therapeutic interventions for keratoconjunctivitis sicca of Sjögren's syndrome?

Artificial tears (preservative-free), stimulation of tear secretion (e.g., pilocarpine hydrochloride 5 mg t.i.d.), tear retention treatment (plugging of the lacrimal puncta and canaliculi), and local application of immunomodulatory agents with anti-inflammatory activity, like cyclosporine-A, may be used for keratoconjunctivitis sicca in Sjögren's syndrome according to disease severity.

11. Which are other causes of dry eyes except for Sjögren's syndrome?

- Aging
- Medical conditions, including diabetes mellitus, thyroid disease, and vitamin A deficiency
- Medications: Antihistamines, decongestants, hormone replacement therapy, antidepressants, and antihypertensives
- Laser eye surgery, though symptoms of dry eyes related to this procedure are usually temporary
- Lacrimal gland damage from inflammation or radiation
- Sarcoidosis
- Chronic hepatitis C, HIV, and HTLV infections
- Chronic graft-versus-host disease

12. Which are the main symptoms of a patient with xerostomia?

- Sticky, dry feeling in the mouth and in the throat
- Difficulty swallowing dry food
- Burning or tingling sensation in the mouth and especially on the tongue (Fig. 6.3)
- Change in taste sensation
- Frequently sipping water
- Frequent dental caries and predisposition to oral candidiasis
- Gastroesophageal reflux symptoms

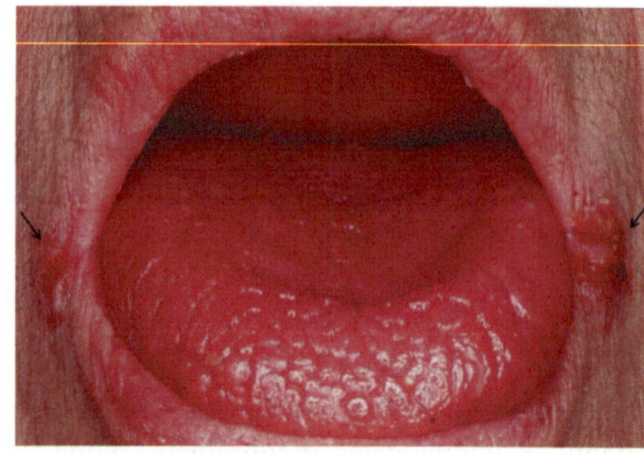

Fig. 6.3 Atrophic tongue papillae: a beefy-red, deeply fissured tongue with atrophic lingual papillae of a 45-year-old female with severe xerostomia. Angular cheilitis is also present (arrows)

13. What is the diagnostic value of major salivary between ultrasound and sialography in Sjögren's syndrome patients?

Major salivary (parotid) gland imaging with ultrasound can differentiate inflammatory from neoplastic disease and diffuse from focal suppurative syndromes, it can also identify sialoliths, and demonstrate salivary duct morphology. In the salivary glands, at an early phase of Sjögren's syndrome, sialectasis (punctate 1 mm lesions representing cystic dilatation of the ducts within salivary glands) can be observed during sialography throughout the glandular tissue; the main ducts appear normal, and the intraglandular ducts may be narrowed. In advanced disease states, punctate lesions increase in size and have an irregular shape, and cavitary sialectasis throughout the gland can be apparent.

14. Which medical conditions except Sjögren's syndrome can present with major salivary gland enlargement?

Unilateral:

- Primary salivary gland neoplasms
- Obstruction (stones or plugs), bacterial infection
- Chronic sialadenitis

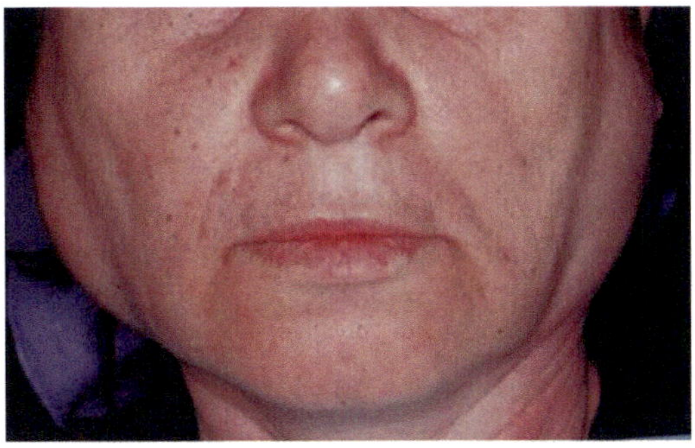

Fig. 6.4 Parotid gland enlargement: a 60-year-old lady with Sjögren's syndrome and persisting enlargement of both parotid glands. In this patient the possibility of lymphoma, sarcoidosis, and IgG4-related disease should be ruled out

Bilateral: (Fig. 6.4)

- Viral infection: Mumps, cytomegalovirus, influenza, and coxsackie A
- IgG4-related disease
- Granulomatous disease: Sarcoidosis, tuberculosis, and leprosy
- Acquired immunodeficiency (HIV)
- Alcoholism, malnutrition, hepatic cirrhosis, and chronic pancreatitis
- Diabetes mellitus
- Hyperlipoproteinemia types IV and V

15. Which are the clinical and laboratory similarities and differences between sicca syndrome caused by viral infection and Sjögren's syndrome?

Acquired immunodeficiency (HIV) and hepatitis C (HCV) viruses are epitheliotropic. They can infect the epithelial cells of the exocrine glands (lacrimal, salivary) leading to xerostomia and xerophthalmia. In that sense, viral sicca syndrome does not differ from sicca manifestations seen in patients with Sjögren's syndrome. However, viral sicca syndrome affects equally both sexes, while Sjögren's syndrome is predominantly a female disease. Furthermore, anti-Ro/SSA and anti-La/SSB reactivities which are found in the sera of two-thirds of Sjögren's syndrome patients are not present in the circulation of HIV-/HCV-induced sicca syndrome.

16. How are the extra-glandular manifestations of Sjögren's syndrome classified?

- Non-specific manifestations: Fatigability, arthralgias, myalgias, and Raynaud's phenomenon
- Manifestations due to peri-epithelial lymphocytic infiltrates (peri-bronchial, peri-cholangial, peri-renal tubular) leading to small-airway disease, biliary cirrhosis, and interstitial nephritis, respectively
- Manifestations due to immune complex-deposition: Raised purpura, peripheral neuritis, glomerulonephritis, and systemic vasculitis
- B-lymphocyte lymphoma [4]

17. What is the clinical picture of Raynaud's phenomenon in patients with Sjögren's syndrome?

Raynaud's phenomenon manifests in approximately one-third of Sjögren's syndrome patients. In around one out of four patients it precedes sicca manifestations. Its clinical course is pleomorphic since in a minority of patients it disappears during the clinical course of Sjögren's syndrome. In one-third of patients, the frequency of attacks decreases while in more than half of patients it remains stable. The local clinical findings of Raynaud's phenomenon in Sjögren's syndrome patients are swollen hands and on hand radiographs small, soft tissue calcifications are evident. However, in contrast to patients with scleroderma digital pulp ulcers, sclerodactyly or peri-ungual telangiectasias do not develop [5].

18. Which are the main skin rashes seen in patients with Sjögren's syndrome?

- Purpura (palpable or flat), red spots primarily on the lower extremities, 1–4 mm diameter (Fig. 6.5)
- Annular erythema (Fig. 6.6) consisting of wide erythematous plaques with elevated borders and central pallor located on the face, upper extremities, and back

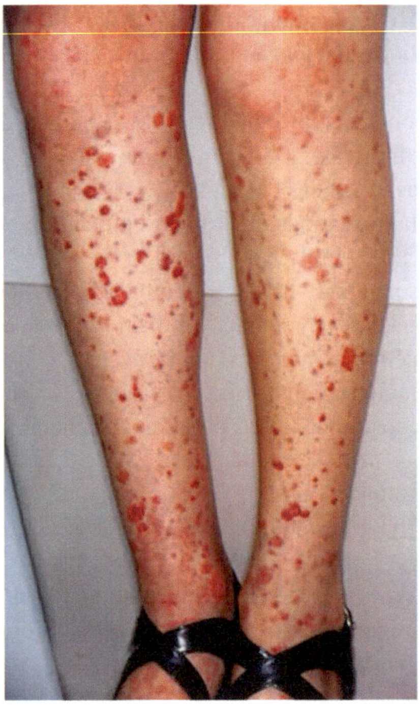

Fig. 6.5 Palpable purpura: of the lower extremities in a 50-year-old female patient with Sjögren's syndrome

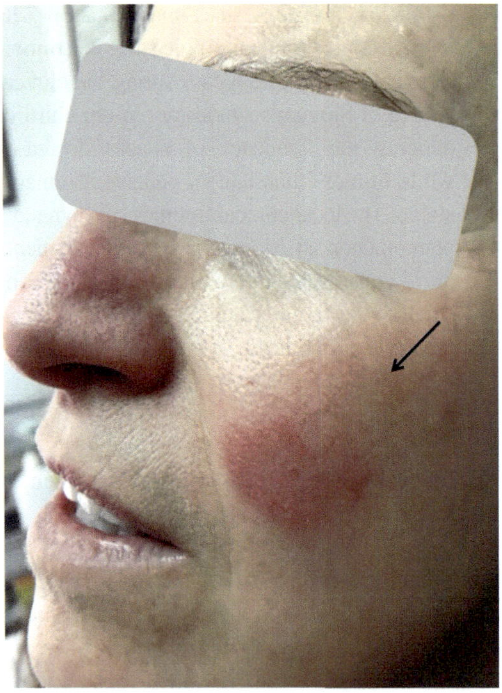

Fig. 6.6 Annular erythema on the left cheek of a 45-year-old woman with a history of Hashimoto thyroiditis, and Sjögren's syndrome

- Lupus pernio-like lesions of the distal extremities

19. Which are the types of purpura that can be seen in Sjögren's syndrome patients and what is the pathogenetic mechanism for its development?

- Palpable purpura which is due to small vessel vasculitis
- Flat (not palpable) purpura which can be the result of hypergammaglobulinemia (increased serum viscosity) and less often of thrombocytopenia

20. What is the commonest type of lymphoma in primary Sjögren's syndrome patients?

Non-Hodgkin's lymphoma develops in 5–10% of Sjögren's syndrome patients. The majority of lymphomas are marginal zone, low grade, and without B symptoms. Extra-nodal lymphomas are often identified in the salivary glands.

21. Which are the clinical, laboratory, and immunologic parameters which can predict future lymphoma development in a Sjögren's syndrome patient?

Univariate and multivariate analyses have revealed that salivary gland enlargement, Raynaud's phenomenon, lymphadenopathy, anti-Ro/SSA or anti-La/SSB autoantibodies, rheumatoid factor positivity, monoclonal gammopathy, and low serum C4 levels are independent predictors for non-Hodgkin's lymphoma (NHL) development in patients with Sjögren's syndrome. Presence of all seven factors in a patient with Sjögren's syndrome has a probability to predict future lymphoma development by 100% [6]. An additional clinical sign that should be taken under consideration when evaluating Sjögren's syndrome patients at risk for NHL is the morphology of the tongue. SS patients with the mucosa-associated lymphoid tissue (MALT) subtype of NHL seem to have a more atrophic and fissured tongue (Fig. 6.7) that those without MALT [7].

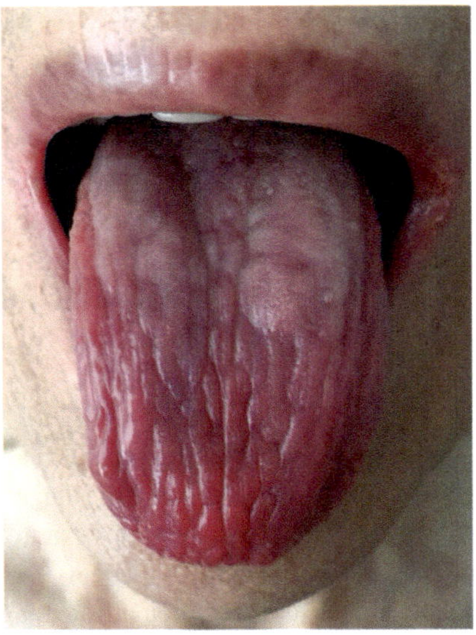

Fig. 6.7 Atrophic, sleek, and fissured tongue appearance in a female patient with Sjögren's syndrome and mucosa-associated lymphoid tissue (MALT) lymphoma

22. **Which manifestations of a Sjögren's syndrome patient will direct the physician to evaluate the patient for autoimmune liver disease?**

Elevated liver enzymes and antibodies against mitochondria or smooth muscle antigens.

23. **Which are the characteristics of Sjögren's syndrome patients with anti-centromere autoantibodies?**

Anti-centromere (ACA) autoantibody-positive Sjögren's patients are predominantly females as are Sjögren's patients without ACA. They present, however, higher incidence of Raynaud's phenomenon, dysphagia, and lower incidence of antibodies to Ro/SSA and La/SSB autoantigens. After a long follow-up period, a small fraction of these patients can evolve to scleroderma [8].

24. **Which is (according to incidence) the respiratory pathology seen in Sjögren's syndrome patients?**

The most common histopathological diagnoses in patients with primary Sjögren's syndrome and lung involvement are according to their incidence: xerotrachea, bronchitis sicca, bronchiolitis with small airway disease, lymphocytic and non-specific interstitial pneumonitis, and seldomly primary lymphoma. Pleurisy is more commonly seen in patients with Sjögren's syndrome associated with other connective tissue diseases.

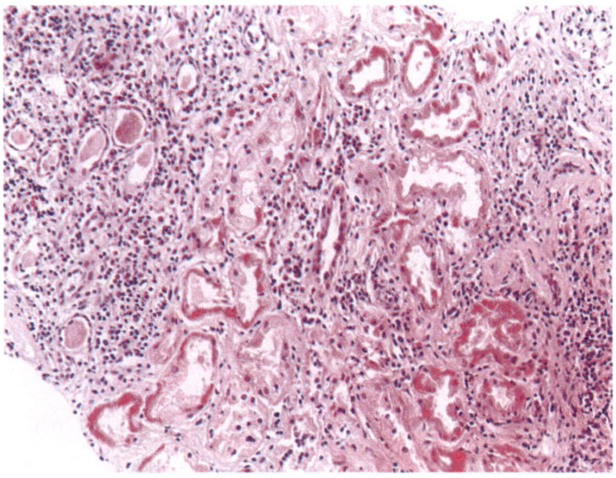

Fig. 6.8 Interstitial nephritis: a 26-year-old lady with Sjögren's syndrome with signs of distal tubular acidosis. Renal biopsy revealed heavy round cell interstitial infiltrates with tubular atrophy

25. **Which is the early and which is the late kidney disease in patients with Sjögren's syndrome? What is their clinical presentation?**

Clinically significant renal involvement in Sjögren's patients is infrequent (~5%). Approximately half of the patients with renal involvement develop interstitial nephritis (Fig. 6.8). Interstitial nephritis patients have an onset of Sjögren's syndrome at a younger age, and renal disease develops early in the disease course. Manifestations of the distal tubule malfunction prevail and include low blood pH (acidosis), high urine pH, hypokalemia, and hyperchloremia. Glomerulonephritis (GMN) develops seldomly in Sjögren's syndrome patients. It is usually membranoproliferative and rarely membranous glomerulonephritis. These patients have longer disease duration, present with hypertension, hematuria, and mild proteinuria. The majority of Sjögren's syndrome patients with GMN have circulating monoclonal cryoglobulins type II with rheumatoid factor activity and low serum complement C4 levels.

26. Which are the long-term sequelae of Sjögren's syndrome patients with renal disease?

After a 10-year follow-up, an equal percentage of interstitial nephritis- and glomerulonephritis-Sjögren's syndrome patients develop chronic renal disease and 20% of those require hemodialysis. Overall, the 5-year survival of Sjögren's syndrome patients with renal involvement is reduced compared to survival of patients without renal disease. Major causes of death among Sjögren's syndrome patients with renal involvement include lymphoma, cerebrovascular accidents, cardiovascular events, and infection. Sjögren's syndrome patients with glomerulonephritis have a higher risk to develop lymphoma, and their survival is poor compared to Sjögren's patients with interstitial nephritis [9].

27. Which are the main peripheral nervous system syndromes observed in Sjögren's syndrome patients?

Trigeminal neuropathy is not uncommon in Sjögren's syndrome patients as is carpal tunnel syndrome. Peripheral neuropathy is seen in Sjögren's syndrome patients with extra-glandular manifestations and is usually axonal. Sensory neuropathy and sensorimotor neuropathy are seen with the same frequency. Small fiber and autonomic neuropathy can also affect Sjögren's syndrome patients.

28. What is the psychopathologic profile of Sjögren's syndrome patients?

A high percentage of Sjögren's syndrome patients express neuroticism, psychoticism, obsessiveness, and psychological distress compared with age and sex-matched controls. After adjustment for personality characteristics and demographics, hypochondriasis was the main psychopathology feature associated with Sjögren's syndrome, suggesting that psychopathological manifestations of Sjögren's syndrome are primarily dependent on premorbid personality characteristics. Finally, the majority of Sjögren's syndrome patients experience stressful events in their lives and inability to handle them.

29. Which are the clinical, laboratory, and immunogenetic similarities and differences of patients with Sjögren's syndrome alone, patients with rheumatoid arthritis and Sjögren's syndrome, and patients with systemic lupus erythematosus and Sjögren's syndrome?

Sjögren's syndrome in rheumatoid arthritis patients develops many years after the diagnosis of rheumatoid arthritis, while Sjögren's syndrome in systemic lupus erythematosus patients can precede the systemic lupus erythematosus diagnosis or the two entities can appear at the same time. Clinically, parotid gland enlargement (transient or persistent) occurs more often in patients with Sjögren's syndrome alone called primary Sjögren's syndrome as well as in patients with Sjögren's syndrome/systemic lupus erythematosus. Antibodies to Ro-60 and La autoantigens appear in the circulation of patients with primary Sjögren's syndrome and Sjögren's syndrome/systemic lupus erythematosus, while their presence in the sera of patients with rheumatoid arthritis and Sjögren's syndrome can be found very infrequently.

In primary Sjögren's syndrome and Sjögren's syndrome/systemic lupus erythematosus patients, there is an association with the HLA-DR3 alloantigen, while in Sjögren's syndrome/rheumatoid arthritis patients there is an association with the HLA-DR4 alloantigen.

30. Which are the common clinical, serologic, histologic features, and therapeutic responses that patients with IgG4-related diseases share?

IgG4-related diseases (IgG4-RD) are immune-mediated fibroinflammatory disorders that affect multiple organs, generating varied manifestations. IgG4-RD are capable of mimicking—and being mimicked by—many other conditions, which should be considered and excluded before setting the diagnosis of IgG4-RD. Nonetheless, IgG4-RD share some common features [10]:

Clinical: Characteristic (at times tumor-like) clinical or radiological involvement of a typical organ (e.g., pancreas, salivary glands, bile ducts, orbits, kidney, lung, aorta, retroperitoneum, pachymeninges, pituitary or thyroid gland).

Histological: Pathological evidence of an inflammatory process accompanied by a lymphoplasmacytic infiltrate of uncertain etiology in one of these same organs containing more than 30–50 IgG4+ plasmacytes per high-power field or an IgG4+/IgG+ ratio greater than 40%, a peculiar pattern of fibrosis (known as storiform fibrosis), a tendency to affect veins by vascular inflammation that leads to obliterative phlebitis, and a mild-to-moderate tissue eosinophilia.

Serologic: Serum IgG4 concentration >135 mg/dL and elevated serum IgG2 and IgE levels.

Therapeutic response: Prompt response to glucocorticoids.

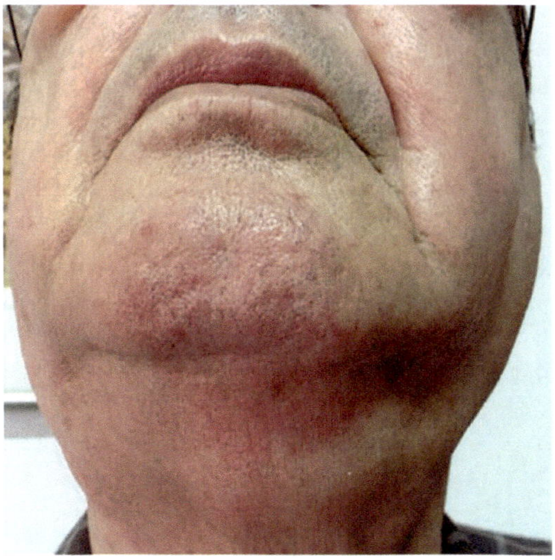

Fig. 6.9 Sclerosing sialadenitis (Mikulicz's disease): enlargement of submandibular and parotid glands is evident in a 60-year-old man who fulfilled diagnostic criteria of IgG4-related sialadenitis (*Reproduced from Fragoulis GE et al. 2017*) [12]

31. Which IgG4-related disease patients have the highest probability of having elevated serum IgG4 levels?

Patients older than 65 years of age with active disease, a greater number of involved organs, lower levels of complement proteins, higher absolute number of peripheral blood eosinophils, and higher serum IgE levels [11].

32. Which are the similarities and differences of sclerosing sialadenitis (Mikulicz's disease) and Sjögren's syndrome?

Similarities: Glandular enlargement, sicca symptoms, arthralgias, hypergammaglobulinemia, hypocomplementemia, and presence of ANA.

Differences: Sclerosing sialadenitis affects more often men, while Sjögren's syndrome is mostly a disease of females. Anti-Ro/SSA and anti-La/SSB autoantibodies are infrequently found in the sera of patients with sclerosing sialadenitis, the numbers of IgG4+ plasma cells in the salivary gland infiltrates of patients with sclerosing sialadenitis are increased, and sclerosing sialadenitis patients can benefit from corticosteroid therapy [12].

33. Which previously recognized conditions are now acknowledged to fall within the spectrum of IgG4-related disease?

- Mikulicz's syndrome (affecting the salivary and lacrimal glands) (Fig. 6.9)
- Küttner's tumor (affecting the submandibular glands)
- Sclerosing dacryoadenitis/orbital pseudotumor (Fig. 6.10a, b) [13]
- Riedel thyroiditis
- Sclerosing cholangitis
- Autoimmune pancreatitis (type I)
- Mediastinal fibrosis
- Retroperitoneal fibrosis (Ormond's disease)/periaortitis (Fig. 6.11)
- Inflammatory aortic aneurysm
- Idiopathic hypocomplementemic tubulointerstitial nephritis with extensive tubulointerstitial deposits
- Hypophysitis
- Inflammatory pseudotumor (affecting the orbits, lungs, kidneys, hypophysis, prostate, testicles, and other organs)

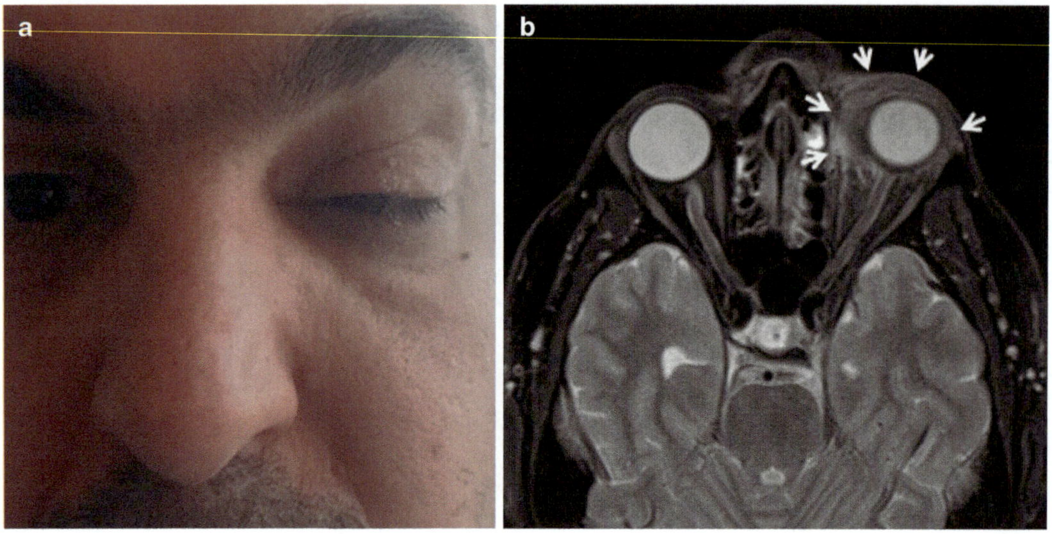

Fig. 6.10 Orbital mass: in a 41-year-old man who fulfilled diagnostic criteria of IgG4-related orbital pseudotumor. (**a**) Magnetic resonance imaging showed diffuse soft tissue swelling surrounding the left orbit, exhibiting hypointensity on T2-weighted images (**b**, arrows) (*Reproduced from Zampeli E et al. 2016*) [13]

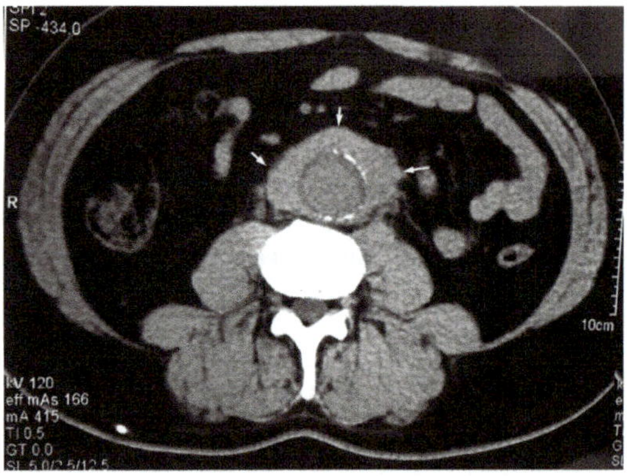

Fig. 6.11 Periaortitis: abdominal CT scanning revealing a soft tissue mass surrounding the aorta (arrows) in a 60-year-old man fulfilling the diagnostic criteria of IgG4-related disease

34. What is the clinical picture of IgG4-related lung disease (IgG4-RLD)?

Around 10% of patients with IgG4-related disease have pulmonary involvement. It may manifest as solid nodules or round-shaped mass (Fig. 6.12), diffuse ground-glass opacities, interlobular septal thickening, pleural nodules, effusion, or fibrosing (sclerosing) mediastinitis. The clinical manifestations of IgG4-RLD are diverse and non-specific. Cough, exertional dyspnea, and chest pain are presenting symptoms in half of IgG4-RLD patients, whereas the remaining present with findings on thoracic imaging in the absence of respiratory symptoms. Constitutional symptoms, such as fever and weight loss, are uncommon [14].

35. What is the incidence and prognosis of malignancy in patients with IgG4-related diseases (IgG4-RD)?

It is not clear if IgG4-RD patients have an increased risk for development of malignancies. In a prospective Chinese study, IgG4-RD patients were followed from January 2011 to August 2018. In the 587 Chinese patients with IgG4-RD, 17 malignancies were identified. Ten developed malignancy after the diagnosis of IgG4-RD (standard incidence ratio (SIR) of 2.78 (95%CI [1.33–5.12]). Multivariate logistic analysis revealed that autoimmune pancreatitis was positively associated with malignancy, whereas eosinophilia was negatively associated with malignancy. During the follow-up period (61.4 ± 26.4 months) all patients with malignancies and IgG4-RD survived. It appears from this study that IgG4-RD patients have a higher risk for development of malignancies [15].

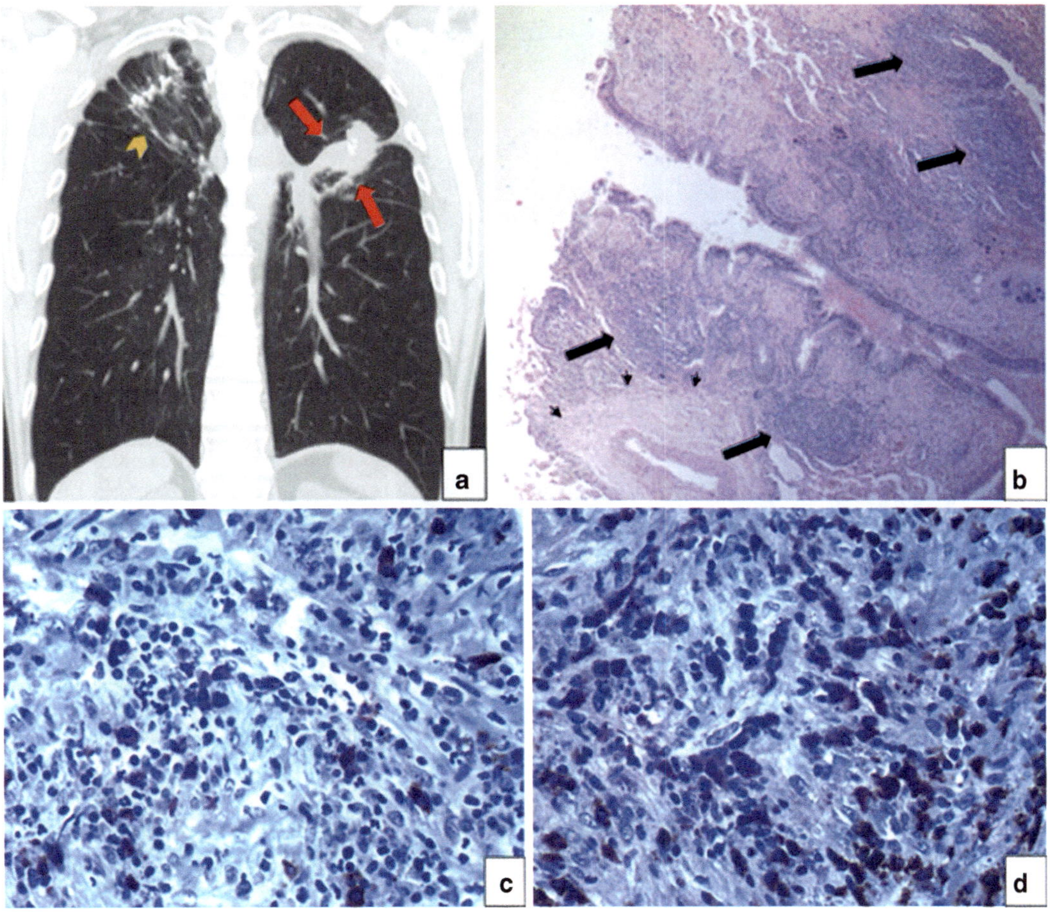

Fig. 6.12 A 50-year-old man, non-smoker, with a history of pulmonary tuberculosis (TB) 10 years ago, presented with cough producing dark-yellowish sputum. Chest computed tomography showed old fibrotic changes on the right lung apex (**a**, yellow arrowhead) and a new mass-like lesion (diameter >3 cm) on the left upper lobe (**a**, red arrows). Histopathology of nodular tissue revealed areas of intense fibrosis (**b**, arrowheads) and areas of round cell infiltrates (**b**, arrows). Tissue cultures did not grow any microbes. Tissue immunohistochemistry showed that the IgG4+ plasma cells constituted >35% (**c**) of the total plasma cells suggesting the diagnosis of IgG4-RLD. *(Reproduced from Skopouli FN, et al. 2017)* [14]

36. Which parts of the aorta can be affected in patients with IgG4-related diseases (IgG4-RD)?

In a study of 37 patients with IgG4-RD less than half had IgG4-related aortitis, which was detected with PET/CT revealing vessel wall thickening (6.3 ± 2.9 mm) and increased radioactive uptake. Almost 30% of the patients had involvement of the laryngeal arteries and the abdominal aorta (below the renal arteries), while 10% presented with involvement of the thoracic aorta and its branches and 6% had involvement of the abdominal aorta bifurcation (above the renal arteries) (Fig. 6.13) [16, 17].

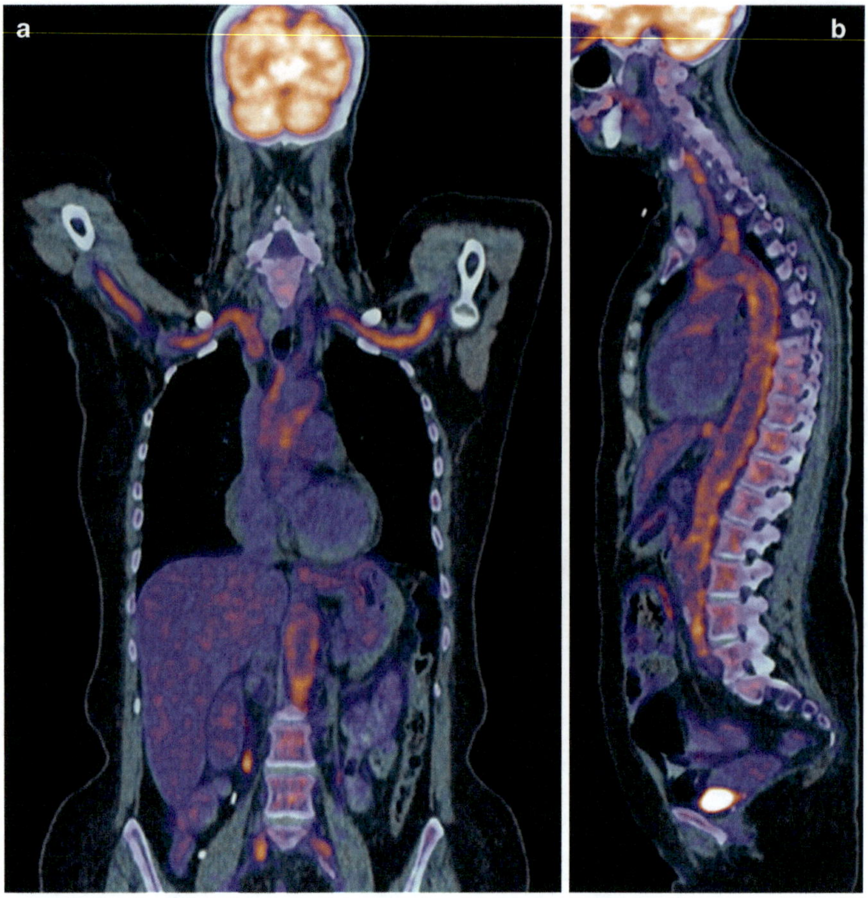

Fig 6.13 18F-Fluorodeoxyglucose Positron Emission Tomography/Computed Tomography (PET/CT), in a middle-aged woman with fever and systemic inflammatory findings such as chronic disease anemia, thrombocytosis and elevated acute phase proteins, revealed increased uptake of the radioactive material in the walls of the aorta and its main branches [(**a**) subclavian arteries, (**b**) thoracic, abdominal aorta and inguinal arteries] indicative of large vessel vasculitis. Serum IgG4 levels were highly elevated (530 mg/dL, normal value <140 mgdL) and bone marrow evaluation showed an increased number of IgG4+ plasma cells (25% of the plasma cells), findings suggesting that the patient suffered from IgG4 aortitis (*Reproduced from Serelis J, et al. 2019*) [17]

References

1. Christodoulou MI, Kapsogeorgou EK, Moutsopoulos HM. Characteristics of the minor salivary gland infiltrates in Sjögren's syndrome. J Autoimmun. 2010;34:400–7.
2. Moutsopoulos HM. Sjögren's syndrome: a forty-year scientific journey. J Autoimmun. 2014;51:1–9.
3. Shiboski CH, Shiboski SC, Seror R, Criswell LA, Labetoulle M, Lietman TM, et al. International Sjögren's Syndrome Criteria Working Group. American College of Rheumatology/European League Against Rheumatism classification criteria for primary Sjögren's syndrome: a consensus and data-driven methodology involving three international patient cohorts. Ann Rheum Dis. 2017;76:9–16.
4. Mavragani CP, Moutsopoulos HM. Sjögren syndrome. CMAJ. 2014;186:E579–86.
5. Skopouli FN, Talal A, Galanopoulou V, et al. Raynaud's phenomenon in primary Sjögren's syndrome. J Rheumatol. 1990;17:618–20.
6. Fragkioudaki S, Mavragani CP, Moutsopoulos HM. Predicting the risk for lymphoma development in Sjogren syndrome: an easy tool for clinical use. Medicine (Baltimore). 2016;95:e3766.
7. Zampeli E, Kalogirou EM, Piperi E, Mavragani CP, Moutsopoulos HM. Tongue atrophy in Sjögren syndrome patients with mucosa-associated lymphoid tissue lymphoma: autoimmune epithelitis beyond the epithelial cells of salivary glands? J Rheumatol. 2018;45:1565–71.
8. Vlachoyiannopoulos PG, Moutsopoulos HM. Anticentromere (ACA)-positive Sjögren's syndrome: a disease entity? Clin Exp Rheumatol. 2013;31:163–4.

9. Goules AV, Tatouli IP, Moutsopoulos HM, Tzioufas AG. Clinically significant renal involvement in primary Sjögren's syndrome: clinical presentation and outcome. Arthritis Rheum. 2013;65:2945–53.
10. Wallace ZS, Naden RP, Chari S, et al. The 2019 American College of Rheumatology/European League Against Rheumatism classification criteria for IgG4-related disease. Ann Rheum Dis. 2020;79:77–87.
11. Wallace ZS, Deshpande V, Mattoo H, Mahajan VS, Kulikova M, et al. IgG4-related disease: clinical and laboratory features in one hundred twenty-five patients. Arthritis Rheumatol. 2015;67:2466–75.
12. Fragoulis GE, Zampeli E, Moutsopoulos HM. IgG4-related sialadenitis and Sjögren's syndrome. Oral Dis. 2017;23:152–6.
13. Zampeli E, Moutsopoulos HM. IgG4-related orbital disease presenting with unilateral eyelid swelling. Arthritis Rheumatol. 2016;68:2824.
14. Skopouli FN, Panayotopoulos P, Moutsopoulos HM. IgG4-related nodular lung lesion. Arthritis Rheumatol. 2017;69:438.
15. Tang H, Yang H, Zhang P, et al. Malignancy and IgG4-related disease: the incidence, related factors and prognosis from a prospective cohort study in China. Sci Rep. 2020;10:4910.
16. Aguirre V, Connolly C, Stuklis R. IgG4-aortopathy: an underappreciated cause of non-infectious thoracic aortitis. Lung Circul. 2017:e79–e8.
17. Serelis J, Skopouli FN, Ioakimidou C, Moutsopoulos HM. Immunoglobulin G4 aortitis. Rheumatology. 2019;58:2077.

Systemic Sclerosis

7

Haralampos M. Moutsopoulos
and Evangelia Zampeli

Abstract

Systemic sclerosis (SSc) is an autoimmune systemic disease characterized by autoimmune reactivity (autoreactive B and T cells), which induces endothelial cell and fibroblast activation as well as overproduction of collagen leading to diffuse vascular pathology and widespread collagen accumulation. The vascular pathology is expressed by Raynaud's phenomenon, telangiectasias, ischemic digital ulcers, and pulmonary arterial hypertension (PAH). SSc can have three distinct clinical presentations: (a) limited cutaneous systemic sclerosis characterized by skin thickening on the face, neck, and distal aspects of the extremities, long-standing Raynaud's phenomenon, esophageal hypomotility, anti-centromere antibodies, and a tendency for developing PAH; (b) diffuse cutaneous systemic sclerosis characterized by extensive and rapidly progressive skin thickening, acute development of Raynaud's phenomenon and arthritis, presence of anti-topoisomerase I and anti-RNA polymerase III antibodies, a higher risk for interstitial lung disease, and scleroderma renal crisis development; and (c) systemic sclerosis sine scleroderma which refers to patients who develop internal organ involvement without skin involvement. Scleroderma can also present as a localized disease type which involves only the skin, and then it is termed morphea (single or multiple painless, discolored patches of the skin) or linear scleroderma (bands of skin thickening affecting a unilateral limb or the scalp and face, which may extend deeper into fascia, muscle, and bone and cause tissue atrophy). Diffuse fasciitis with eosinophilia, scleredema, and scleromyxedema are some of the scleroderma mimickers, and differential diagnosis can be challenging, especially early in the disease course.

H. M. Moutsopoulos (✉)
Athens Academy, Athens, Greece
e-mail: hmoutsop@med.uoa.gr

E. Zampeli
Bioclinic General Hospital of Athens and Institute for Autoimmune Systemic and Neurological Disorders, Athens, Greece
e-mail: ezampeli@bioclinic.gr

1. **Which are the main clinical characteristics of localized scleroderma?**

In localized scleroderma, skin changes consist of cutaneous fibrosis without involvement of internal organs. The two types of localized scleroderma are:

- *Morphea*: Single or multiple painless, discolored patches of the skin (Fig. 7.1a). Typically, the skin changes appear on the trunk, can

H. M. Moutsopoulos, E. Zampeli (eds.), *Immunology and Rheumatology in Questions*,
https://doi.org/10.1007/978-3-030-56670-8_7

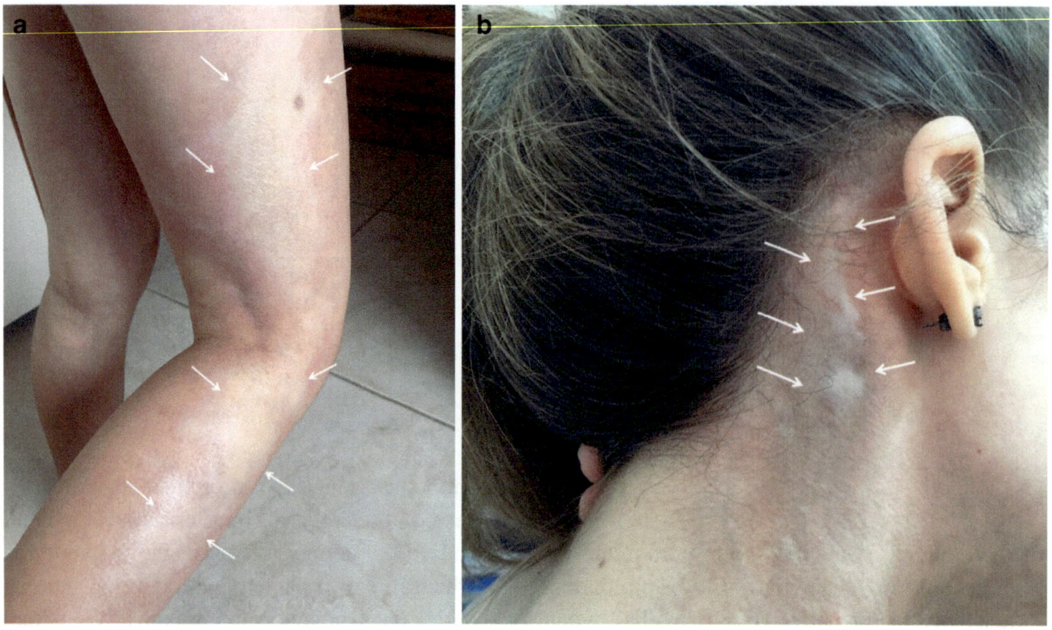

Fig. 7.1 Localized scleroderma (morphea): (**a**) multiple painless, discolored sclerotic skin lesions which become confluent in the lateral aspect of the right thigh in a 24-year-old female patient (**b**) ivory-colored band of thickened skin and atrophic changes in the right retroauricular area in a patient with linear localized scleroderma (linear morphea)

occur on the extremities, but spare the hands and the fingers. Patients with morphea do not suffer from Raynaud's phenomenon, and internal organs of the patients are not affected. The skin lesions can be circumscribed (focal skin and subcutaneous fibrosis), generalized (defined as four or more lesions >3 cm in size that become confluent in two or more anatomical sites), and pansclerotic (generalized involvement including the face, trunk, and extremities; these patients are at greater risk for squamous cell carcinoma development)

- *Linear scleroderma* (*linear morphea*): Bands of skin thickening affecting a unilateral limb or sometimes the scalp (Fig. 7.1b) and face (*en coup de sabre*). It can extend beyond the skin to fascia, muscle, and bone leading to tissue atrophy. Patients with linear scleroderma do not suffer from Raynaud's phenomenon; arthritis can be a manifestation in a minority (10–15%) of these patients, while internal organs are not affected

2. Which are the main clinical characteristics of limited cutaneous systemic sclerosis?

Patients with limited cutaneous systemic sclerosis (lcSSc) have skin thickening restricted to the face, neck, or distal aspects of upper and lower extremities (below the elbows and knees). These patients often have a history of longstanding Raynaud's phenomenon and gastroesophageal reflux disease and may develop telangiectasias (Fig. 7.2), skin calcifications (calcinosis), puffy hands and fingers, and sclerodactyly (Fig. 7.3a). In the past, the term CREST (calcinosis, Raynaud's, esophageal dysmotility, sclerodactyly, and telangiectasia) was used to refer to a subgroup of patients with lcSSc, but nowadays this term has been abandoned, as it describes only a narrow part of the spectrum of clinical manifestations. In patients with lcSSc, the presence of anti-Scl70 (anti-topoisomerase) antibody is associated with high risk for the development of interstitial lung disease (ILD), and the presence of anti-centromere antibodies is associated with a particularly high risk of pulmonary arterial hypertension (PAH). Scleroderma renal crisis very rarely affects patients with lcSSc.

3. Which are the main clinical characteristics of diffuse cutaneous systemic sclerosis?

Patients present with skin thickening proximal to the elbows and knees, or trunk. Symptoms including puffy hands, Raynaud's phenomenon, rapidly progressive skin thickening, and arthritis appear relatively acutely. Patients with diffuse cutaneous systemic sclerosis (dcSSc) are at higher risk to develop scleroderma renal crisis (even higher if positive for anti-RNA polymerase III antibodies) and progressive interstitial lung disease (particularly within the first 5 years of disease onset).

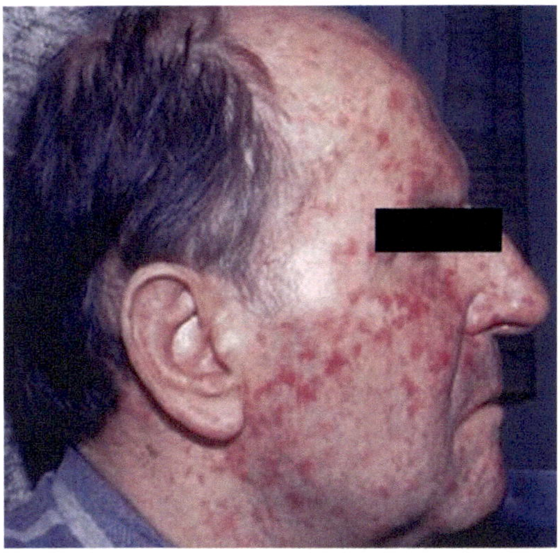

Fig. 7.2 Telangiectasias: multiple small dilated blood vessels close to the surface of the skin in a 70-year-old man with limited scleroderma

4. Which are the main clinical characteristics of systemic sclerosis sine scleroderma?

Systemic sclerosis sine scleroderma refers to patients with systemic sclerosis manifestations from internal organ, such as esophageal involvement and interstitial lung disease (ILD), along with scleroderma-specific autoantibodies (anti-Scl-70, anti-centromere, anti-RNA polymerase III) without evidence of skin fibrosis.

5. Which environmental agents have been implicated in the development of scleroderma?

Exposure to silica, solvents, epoxy resins, silicone breast implants, pesticides, and welding fumes have been implicated in the pathogenesis of scleroderma.

6. Which are the pathogenetic steps that lead to scleroderma development?

An environmental agent in a genetically predisposed individual leads to activation of innate/adaptive immune system abnormalities, which result to (1) the production of autoantibodies and

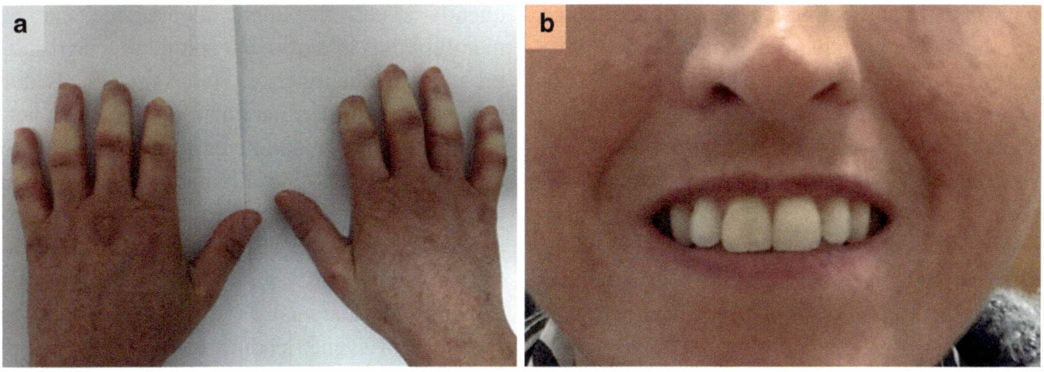

Fig. 7.3 A 33-year-old lady with systemic sclerosis: thickened skin of the face neck, trunk, and extremities with (**a**) sclerodactyly resulting in claw deformity of the fingers and (**b**) microstomia

cell-mediated autoimmunity, (2) microvascular endothelial cell/small vessel fibroproliferative vasculopathy, and (3) fibroblast hyperactivity leading to excessive accumulation of collagen and other matrix components in skin and internal organs.

7. What is microchimerism? Does it play any role in the pathogenesis of autoimmune diseases?

Fetal cells, including stem cells, cross the placenta during normal pregnancy, and enter maternal blood. They reside in maternal tissues during and after pregnancy and remain for decades in the bone marrow and other organs. This small number of fetal cells, being genetically distinct, constitutes an allogeneic cell population within the host, the mother in this case. This is called microchimerism. Although persistent fetal cells were first implicated in autoimmune disease, and particularly in the pathogenesis of systemic sclerosis, subsequent studies have shown that microchimeric cells can be found in healthy as well as in tissues from individuals with non-autoimmune disease [1].

8. Which are the characteristics of the "scleroderma pattern" seen in nailfold capillaroscopy?

In nailfold capillaroscopy the "scleroderma pattern" is characterized by giant capillaries (especially in the early and active stages of the disease) or the combination of abnormal shapes with an extremely lowered number of capillaries. Capillaries with a "hairpin" shape, crossing, or tortuous shapes are defined as being "normal," on the condition that their tip is convex. All other shapes are defined as being "abnormal" [2]. In contrast to scleroderma, in Sjögren's syndrome patients who present with Raynaud's phenomenon, capillaroscopic findings range from nonspecific findings (crossed capillaries) to more specific findings such as confluent and pericapillary hemorrhages. However, patients with Sjögren's syndrome and anti-centromere autoantibodies manifest capillaroscopic findings similar to those seen in patients with scleroderma [3].

9. Which are the oral manifestations of scleroderma?

- Microstomia (tightening of the face skin around the mouth resulting in reduction in the size of the oral aperture) (Fig. 7.3b)
- Xerostomia
- Loosening of periodontal tooth ligament and tooth mobility
- Accelerated tooth decay
- Shortening of the frenulum linguae
- Temporomandibular joint disease
- Telangiectasias of the mucosal lining of the lips
- Mandible resorption

10. In which body areas of patients with scleroderma telangiectasias can be seen?

Telangiectasias in scleroderma patients can occur on the face (Fig. 7.2), neck, anterior and posterior chest wall, hands, mucous membranes (inner lining of the lips), tongue, and mucosa of gastrointestinal tract, particularly in the antrum or the last part of the stomach giving the appearance of "watermelon" (streaky long red arches).

11. Which are the symptoms and findings of large intestine involvement in patients with scleroderma?

According to different series, the large intestine is involved in 10–50% of scleroderma patients. Involvement of the large bowel frequently affects the anorectal area and can be manifested as loss of rectal sphincter tone resulting in fecal incontinence. This is most likely due to neuropathy (arteriolar changes of the vasa nervorum) and not to sphincter atrophy/fibrosis. In the colon, atrophy and thinning of the muscular wall can lead to formation of wide mouth diverticula. Scleroderma patients have poor gastrointestinal tract motility with abdominal distension causing pain and malabsorption. The proposed sequence of events leading to malabsorption in scleroderma patients is diminished peristalsis leading to stasis, which results in colonic bacterial overgrowth and finally to diarrhea.

12. Which are the characteristics of interstitial lung disease in scleroderma patients?

The most common interstitial lung disease (ILD) patterns seen in scleroderma (SSc) patients are fibrotic non-specific interstitial pneumonia (F-NSIP) (Fig. 7.4) seen in 75% of cases, followed by usual interstitial pneumonia (UIP) (Fig. 7.5) in 25% of cases. In the sera of SSc patients with NISP antinuclear autoantibodies (ANA) with nucleolar pattern, anti-SCL70, anti-Th/To, anti-U3RNP, and anti-Pm/Scl antibodies are present [4].

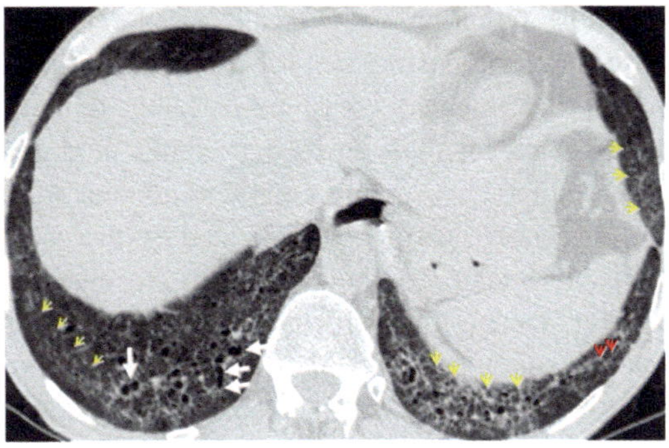

Fig. 7.4 *Non-specific interstitial pneumonia* in a 57-year-old male patient with diffuse systemic sclerosis. Chest computed tomography (CT) scan shows predominantly ground-glass opacities (yellow arrows), irregular reticular opacities (red arrows) with or without traction bronchiectasis (white arrows), minimal honeycomb changes, and subpleural sparing, which are some of the radiographic characteristics that differentiate non-specific from usual interstitial pneumonia (*Figure courtesy of Christos Kampolis, MD*)

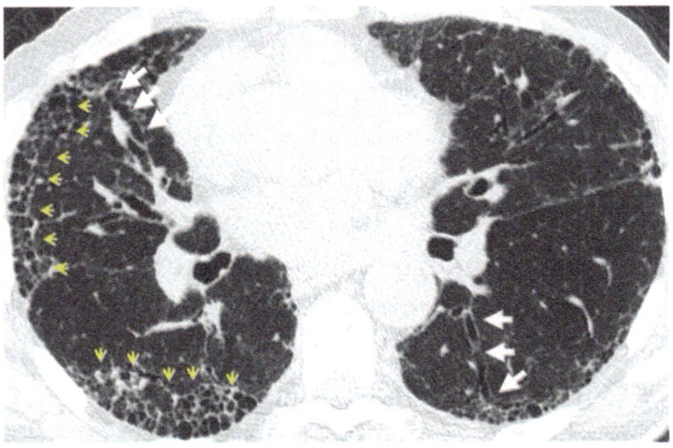

Fig. 7.5 Usual interstitial pneumonia in a 46-year-old female patient with diffuse systemic sclerosis. Chest computed tomography (CT) scan in usual interstitial pneumonia shows a pattern characterized by reticular septal thickening and honeycombing (yellow arrows) with or without traction bronchiectasis (white arrows) with a predominantly subpleural-basal distribution (*Figure courtesy of Christos Kampolis, MD*)

13. Which clinical and laboratory manifestations are indicative of scleroderma renal crisis?

Scleroderma renal crisis is the abrupt onset of arterial hypertension (>150/90 mmHg; however, 10% are normotensive and have a worse prognosis), hypertensive retinopathy, and rapid deterioration of renal function. Pericardial effusion and myocardial involvement can be present. Abnormal laboratory tests include elevated serum creatinine levels, consumptive thrombocytopenia, microangiopathic hemolysis (schistocytes on peripheral blood smears), mild proteinuria, and elevated renin levels.

14. Which scleroderma patients are more at risk to develop scleroderma renal crisis?

Those scleroderma patients with the following characteristics:

- Females with clinical features of diffuse cutaneous SSc
- Short disease duration (<4 years)
- Rapid skin thickening
- Tendon friction rubs
- New-onset microangiopathic hemolytic anemia
- New cardiac events (pericarditis, myocarditis, and congestive heart failure)
- High doses of corticosteroids
- Cyclosporine-A use
- Anti-RNA polymerase III antibody positivity

15. Which are the renal histopathologic findings in patients with scleroderma renal crisis?

The primary renal histopathologic changes are localized in the small arcuate and interlobular arteries and the glomeruli. The characteristic finding is intimal proliferation and thickening that leads to narrowing and obliteration of the vascular lumen, with concentric "onion skin-like" hypertrophy. These histopathologic findings are similar to systemic sclerosis-associated vascular lesions found in other organs. Scleroderma renal crisis is thrombotic microangiopathy similar to malignant nephrosclerosis, thrombotic thrombocytopenic purpura, hemolytic uremic syndrome, and antiphospholipid syndrome.

16. Which scleroderma patients are prone to develop pulmonary arterial hypertension (PAH)?

Those scleroderma patients with:

- Clinical features of lcSSc
- Duration of Raynaud's phenomenon more than 8 years
- Anti-centromere antibody positivity
- Anti-nucleolar antibodies
- Extensive telangiectasias
- Diffusing capacity of the lungs for carbon monoxide (DLCO) <60% in the absence of extensive interstitial lung disease
- Forced vital capacity (FVC%)/DLCO% ratio >1.6

17. Which autoantibody specificity predicts cancer development in scleroderma patients?

Scleroderma patients have an increased risk of cancer in comparison to the risk of cancer in the general population. Those patients with autoantibodies to RNA polymerase III are more likely to be diagnosed with cancer synchronously (−6 months to +12 months) or within 3 years of scleroderma onset. Patients with these autoantibodies and diffuse scleroderma seem to have an increased risk for breast cancer while patients with anti-RNA polymerase III antibodies and limited scleroderma have a high risk for lung cancer. On the contrary, scleroderma patients with anti-centromere antibodies show a lower risk for cancer development. On the basis of these findings, it is of paramount clinical importance, the scleroderma patients with RNA polymerase III autoantibodies to be closely followed, at least during the first 5 years after scleroderma development, in order to detect the possible malignancy at its early stages [5].

18. Does radiation therapy in patients with scleroderma and breast cancer have an impact on cancer and on scleroderma?

Scleroderma has been considered as an absolute contraindication for radiation therapy (RT) by most radiation oncologists, based on short case series suggesting that RT exaggerates fibrosis of the affected breast, underlying skin, or lungs. A recent study sheds light in this field. RT seems not to have an impact on scleroderma or on breast cancer outcome as indicated by the comparison of scleroderma patients who received or not RT. During follow up, there were no differences observed in modified Rodnan skin score (mRSS) and in forced vital capacity (FVC), nor in the proportion of patients who remain cancer free. Additionally, local RT toxicity was not different among scleroderma and non-scleroderma patients [6].

19. Is it possible for a patient with localized scleroderma (morphea or linear scleroderma) to evolve to systemic sclerosis?

The possibility that a patient with localized scleroderma evolves to systemic sclerosis is very low (<1%), and it has been described very infrequently in morphea patients who have positive anti-centromere antibodies (ACA) (2% of morphea patients).

20. Which organ in addition to the skin can be affected in limited scleroderma?

Other organs that can be affected in limited scleroderma besides the skin (skin thickening, telangiectasia, calcinosis, Raynaud's) include the joints (arthralgias-arthritis), the esophagus (esophageal dysmotility), and the lungs (pulmonary arterial hypertension, pulmonary fibrosis).

21. Which are the early electrocardiographic findings in patients with scleroderma cardiomyopathy?

The heart is one of the major organs which can be involved in systemic sclerosis. Cardiac involvement can be manifested as myocardial disease, conduction system abnormalities, arrhythmias, or pericardial disease. The most frequent abnormalities on the resting electrocardiogram of scleroderma patients are left anterior fascicular block (16%) and first-degree atrioventricular heart block (8%). Supraventricular arrhythmias are considered to be more common in scleroderma patients, occurring in approximately two-thirds of the cases, and much more frequent than ventricular tachyarrhythmias.

22. Which are the magnetic resonance imaging findings in patients with scleroderma cardiomyopathy?

Cardiac magnetic resonance imaging (MRI) can detect heart pathologies in up to 75% of affected scleroderma patients, including:

- Increased intensity signal of the myocardium (T2-weighted images)
- Thinning of the left ventricle
- Pericardial effusion
- Reduced left and right ventricle ejection fractions
- Left ventricle diastolic dysfunction and kinetic abnormalities
- Myocardial delayed contrast enhancement (Fig. 7.6a–c)
- In addition, cardiac MRI can be used to differentiate structural from functional pathologies, such as myocardial inflammation and fibrosis (the extent of fibrosis and viable tissue is properly measured after contrast enhancement). The method gives an opportunity for quantitative assessment of myocardial perfusion and the effect of vasodilators [7]

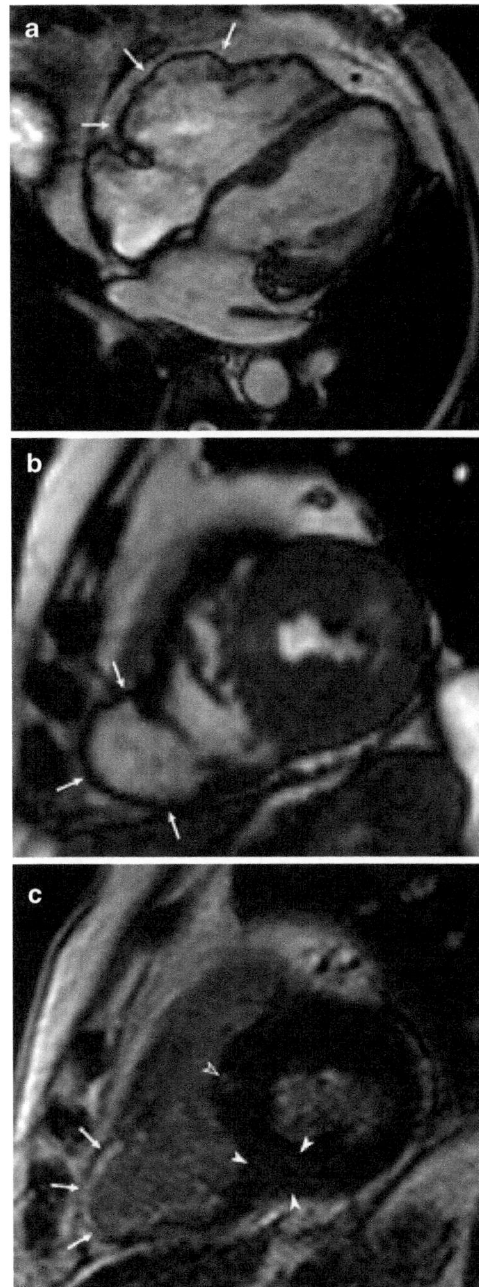

Fig. 7.6 Myocardial involvement in a 60-year-old female with systemic sclerosis. Cardiac magnetic resonance imaging (MRI) revealed thinning of the right ventricular (RV) myocardium with aneurysm formation (**a**, **b**, arrows) in the subtricuspid area. An abnormal linear enhancement (**c**, arrows) of the aneurysmal myocardium, as well as a patchy subtle enhancement (**c**, arrowheads) of the lower RV insertion point, and a somewhat more intense focal enhancement (**c**, open arrowhead) at the anteroseptal medial segment of the left ventricular myocardium are seen (*Figure courtesy of Sotiris C. Plastiras, MD*)

23. What is the pregnancy outcome in patients with systemic sclerosis?

Different studies have shown that women with systemic sclerosis (SSc) with meticulous obstetric monitoring have similar pregnancy outcomes (fetal morbidity and mortality) compared to those of women with rheumatoid arthritis (RA) and healthy age-matched controls. Infertility is not a frequent problem in this patient group. Preterm births and small full-term babies, however, may occur slightly more frequently in both SSc and RA patients compared to control subjects. Nevertheless, patients with early, rapidly progressive SSc and diffuse skin thickening and presence of autoantibodies to Scl-70 should be advised to avoid pregnancy until the disease is stabilized.

24. What is calcinosis cutis?

Calcinosis cutis refers to cutaneous deposits of basic calcium phosphate that typically occur in the hands (especially over proximal interphalangeal joints and fingertips), periarticular areas, and over bony prominences (especially the extensor surface of the elbows Fig. 7.7, and the knees) but can occur virtually anywhere on the body. The deposits of calcium are firm and irregular and can become inflamed, infected, or ulcerated and discharge a chalky white material.

25. What are the clinical differences between scleroderma and diffuse fasciitis with eosinophilia?

Diffuse fasciitis with eosinophilia is a disorder of unknown cause. In 50% of the cases, it has been reported to develop after strenuous exercise and mostly during spring and autumn. In contrast to systemic sclerosis, it does not involve the skin and subcutaneous tissues of the face or the hands and feet of the affected individuals. Raynaud's phenomenon, fingertip ulcerations, and telangiectasias are not present. Internal organ involvement (esophagus, lungs, and kidneys) is exceedingly rare [8].

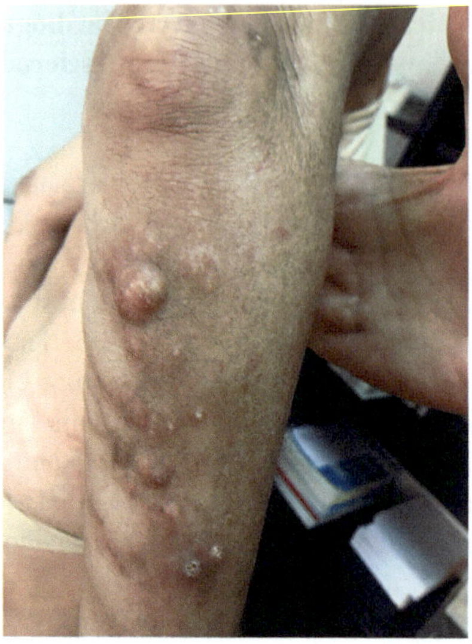

Fig. 7.7 Calcinosis cutis on the extensor surface of the elbows in a female patient with scleroderma and positive anti-centromere antibodies

26. What is the clinical picture of diffuse fasciitis with eosinophilia?

It may have a rapid onset with generalized manifestations like low-grade fever, muscle aches, cramps, and fatigability. Initially pitting edema, usually on both arms and legs simultaneously, becomes apparent, and typically the face, hands, and feet are spared. Carpal tunnel syndrome can be an early symptom in many patients. As the disease progresses, the skin becomes stiff, having a woody texture and an "orange peel" appearance (*peau d' orange*) (Fig. 7.8). At later stages, the fascia is involved and flexion contractures as well as muscle atrophy, yet without muscle weakness, can occur.

27. Which are the laboratory and histopathologic differences among scleroderma and diffuse fasciitis with eosinophilia?

The major laboratory finding in the initial phase of diffuse fasciitis with eosinophilia is peripheral eosinophilia (85%), while hypergammaglobulinemia and increased erythrocyte sedimentation rate are present in all phases of

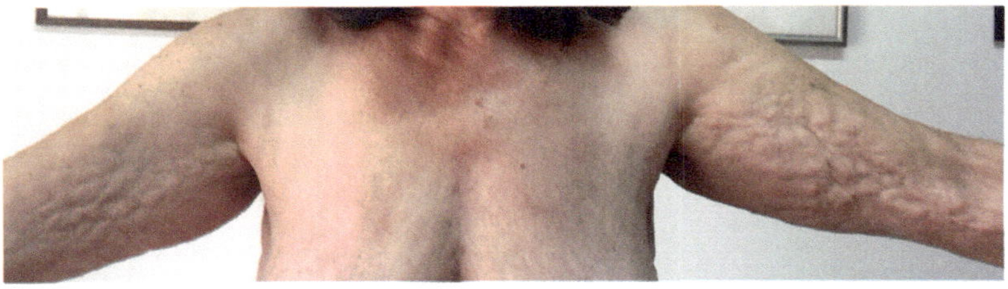

Fig. 7.8 Diffuse fasciitis with eosinophilia: a hard lumpy dimpling of the skin (*peau d'orange*) and subcutaneous tissue of the brachial areas of the arms in a 51-year-old woman, following unusual exercise

diffuse fasciitis with eosinophilia. A small number of patients may show a transient positivity of rheumatoid factor and antinuclear autoantibodies.

Histologically the diagnosis of diffuse fasciitis with eosinophilia is confirmed by a deep wedge en bloc full-thickness biopsy of the involved area. The most typical histological finding is thickening of the deep fascia due to inflammation, edema, and fibrosis. The inflammatory cells are predominantly lymphocytes, histiocytes, and plasma cells with scattered clusters of eosinophils. The dermis is not thickened and does not show condensation of fibrous tissue. In contrast, in scleroderma, the deep fascia shows no significant abnormality, whereas the dermis appears thickened.

28. What are the entities scleredema and scleromyxedema?

Scleredema is a sclerotic skin disease. It is characterized by firm, non-pitting skin edema that begins in the neck and upper back and spreads to the shoulders and trunk. The face and extremities are less commonly involved, while the hands and feet are typically spared. Scleredema generally occurs in association with poorly controlled diabetes mellitus, following streptococcal infection or in association with a paraproteinemia (usually IgG or IgA). Skin biopsy shows normal epidermis but thickened dermis with deposition of excessive collagen and mucin between collagen bundles.

Scleromyxedema is characterized by multiple flesh-colored papules of 2–3 mm in diameter on the face, posterior auricular area, glabella, neck, upper trunk, distal forearms, and hands but sparing the palms. Over 80% of individuals have an IgG mini-monoclonal protein (usually IgGλ) while 10% develop multiple myeloma. Systemic involvement has been reported with the occurrence of dysphagia, myopathies, and cardiopulmonary involvement. Skin biopsy shows normal epidermis, mucin deposition in the dermis, fibroblast proliferation, and fibrosis [9].

References

1. Nelson JL. The otherness of self: microchimerism in health and disease. Trends Immunol. 2012;33:421–7 .
2. Smith V, Herrick AL, Ingegnoli F, et al. Standardisation of nailfold capillaroscopy for the assessment of patients with Raynaud's phenomenon and systemic sclerosis. Autoimmun Rev. 2020;19:102458.
3. Tektonidou M, Kaskani E, Skopouli FN, Moutsopoulos HM. Microvascular abnormalities in Sjögren's syndrome: nailfold capillaroscopy. Rheumatology (Oxford). 1999;38:826–30.
4. Chartrand S, Lee JS, Swigris JJ, et al. Clinical characteristics and natural history of autoimmune forms of interstitial lung disease: a single-center experience. Lung. 2019;197:709–13.
5. Igusa T, Hummers LK, Visvanathan K, et al. Autoantibodies and scleroderma phenotype define subgroups at high-risk and low-risk for cancer. Ann Rheum Dis. 2018;77:1179–86.
6. Shah DJ, Hirpara R, Poelman CL, et al. Impact of radiation therapy on scleroderma and cancer outcomes in scleroderma patients with breast cancer. Arthritis Care Res (Hoboken). 2018;70:1517–24.
7. Tzelepis GE, Kelekis NL, Plastiras SC, Mitseas P, Economopoulos N, Kampolis C, Gialafos EJ, Moyssakis I, Moutsopoulos HM. Pattern and distribution of myocardial fibrosis in systemic sclerosis: a delayed enhanced magnetic resonance imaging study. Arthritis Rheum. 2007;56:3827–36.
8. Tyndall A, Fistarol S. The differential diagnosis of systemic sclerosis. Curr Opin Rheumatol. 2013;25: 692–9.
9. Sharma A. Scleroderma-like Disorders. Curr Rheumatol Rev. 2018;14:22–7.

Vasculitides and Related Diseases

8

Haralampos M. Moutsopoulos
and Evangelia Zampeli

Abstract

The term "vasculitis" stands for a spectrum of diseases characterized by an inflammatory injury of the vascular wall which may affect arteries and veins; it may lead to necrosis or to granulomatous inflammation of the vascular wall, occlusion of the vascular lumen, and ischemic injury of the affected tissues. Depending on the size of vessels affected, vasculitides are categorized into large-vessel vasculitis—affecting the aorta and its direct branches—such as giant cell arteritis (GCA) and Takayasu arteritis (TA); medium-vessel vasculitis, such as polyarteritis nodosa (PAN) and Kawasaki disease (KD); as well as small-vessel vasculitis. The small-vessel vasculitides comprise the ANCA-associated vasculitides (AAV), which are associated with the presence of circulating antineutrophil cytoplasmic antibodies (ANCA), and the ones without autoantibodies. The AAV are granulomatosis with polyangiitis (GPA, formerly known as Wegener's granulomatosis), microscopic polyangiitis (MPA), and eosinophilic granulomatosis with polyangiitis (EGPA, formerly known as Churg-Strauss syndrome). Other non-ANCA-associated small-vessel vasculitides are typically characterized by either the presence of immune complex deposition (cryoglobulinemic and IgA vasculitis/Henoch-Schönlein purpura) or are the result of neoplasia (paraneoplastic phenomenon).

GCA is diagnosed by temporal artery biopsy, while for TA, gadolinium-enhanced magnetic resonance angiography (MRA) and positron emission tomography associated with computed tomography (PET/CT) are both used for diagnosis and assessment of disease activity. Medium- and small-sized vasculitides should be diagnosed by biopsy of affected tissues. Microaneurysms seen with conventional angiography in the tripod of Haller support the diagnosis of PAN.

H. M. Moutsopoulos (✉)
Athens Academy, Athens, Greece
e-mail: hmoutsop@med.uoa.gr

E. Zampeli
Bioclinic General Hospital of Athens and Institute for Autoimmune Systemic and Neurological Disorders, Athens, Greece
e-mail: ezampeli@bioclinic.gr

1. Which are the clinical and histological characteristics of giant cell arteritis?

Giant cell arteritis (GCA) occurs primarily in patients over 50 years of age (female: male = 2–3:1) and affects mostly the extracranial branches of carotid arteries. Clinically detectable

H. M. Moutsopoulos, E. Zampeli (eds.), *Immunology and Rheumatology in Questions*,
https://doi.org/10.1007/978-3-030-56670-8_8

involvement of the aorta and its branches occurs in 15% of the cases. Symptoms of GCA include low-grade fever, polymyalgia rheumatica (PMR)-related symptoms, anorexia, new headache, scalp tenderness, jaw claudication, and weight loss. Enlarged/difficult to compress/pulseless temporal arteries, visual symptoms (diplopia, amaurosis fugax, unilateral loss of vision), and limb claudication are additional disease findings. Rare manifestations include hypertension, cough, tongue pain/ulcers, mononeuritis multiplex (affects the shoulder producing sudden weakness and pain mimicking a C5 radiculopathy), and large artery disease (aorta and major branches). Diagnosis of GCA can be set by Doppler ultrasound of temporal arteries (Fig. 8.1a, b). In case that the results of Doppler ultrasound are dubious, temporal artery biopsy is necessary for GCA diagnosis. Histologically, inflammation of the arterial wall is evident, especially at arterial bifurcations, with fragmentation and disruption of the internal elastic lamina being a classic finding. Multinucleated giant cells are found in 50% of the cases [1].

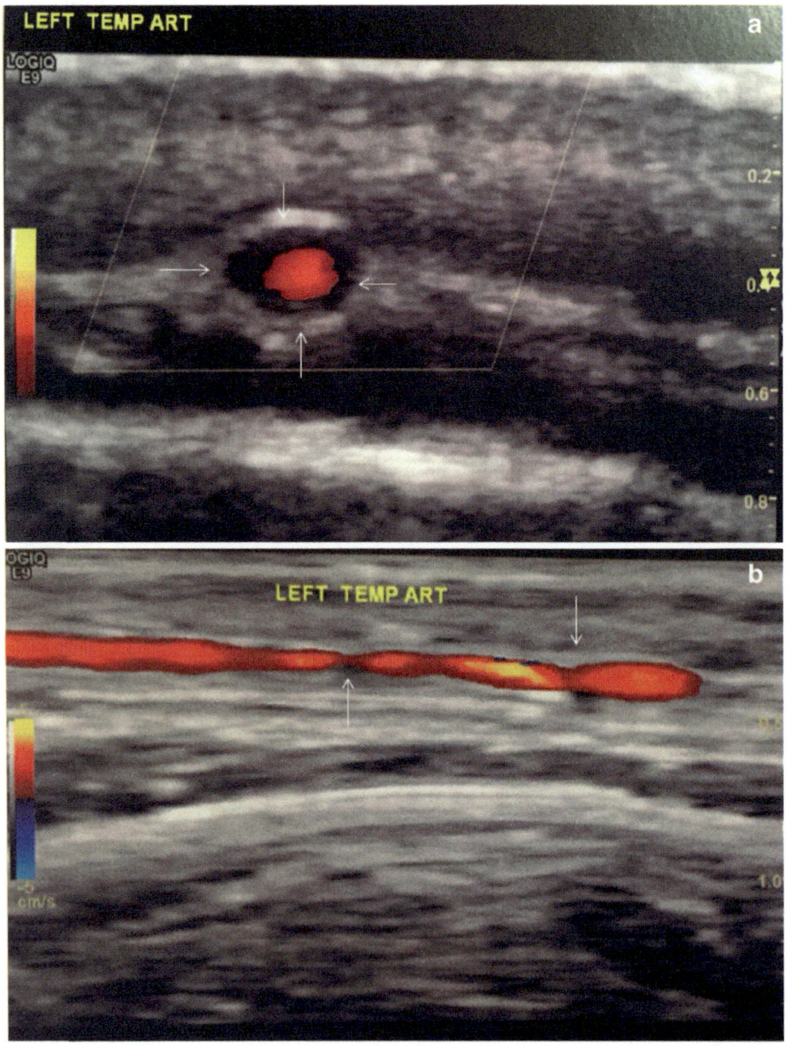

Fig. 8.1 Giant cell (Temporal) arteritis-temporal artery ultrasound findings: (**a**) a hypoechogenic ring area is apparent around the lumen of the temporal artery (*halo sign*), and (**b**) segmental artery stenosis is seen on sagittal sections in a 72-year-old man whose temporal artery biopsy confirmed the diagnosis of giant cell arteritis

2. Which large vessels (LV) can be affected by giant cell arteritis (GCA)?

Estimated incidence of LV-GCA varies greatly between studies due to various radiological modalities used. Based on recent studies, aorta involvement is seen in 10% and overall LV involvement in 15% of GCA patients. The most frequently involved LV are common carotid arteries, subclavian arteries, axillary arteries, thoracic aorta, renal arteries, celiac trunk, and superior mesenteric artery (Fig. 8.2a, b) [2, 3]. Stenoses are overall more frequent. Occlusive lesions are mostly seen in the inferior mesenteric artery while aneurysms are common in the thoracic and abdominal aorta or the renal arteries. In LV-GCA patients signs or symptoms of polymyalgia rheumatica with a lower initial systemic inflammatory response are more common [4]. Involvement of coronary arteries in GCA patients is rare [5].

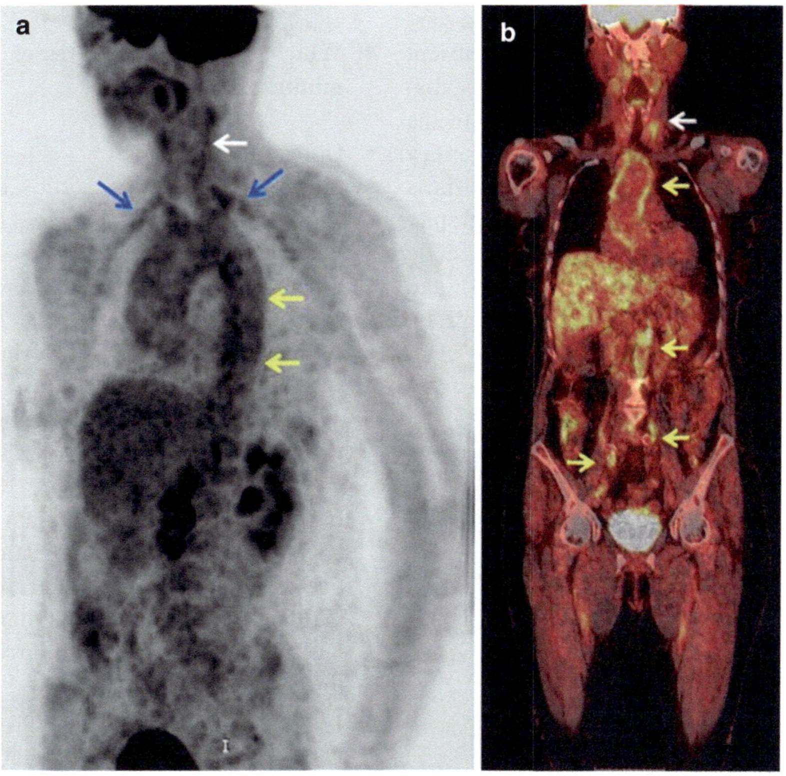

Fig. 8.2 A 56-year-old female presented with progressively deteriorating left arm weakness, normocytic anemia (Hb: 9.6 g/dl, MCV: 86 fL), thrombocytosis (platelets: 525000/μL), high erythrocyte sedimentation rate (ESR, 130 mm/h) and C-reactive-protein (CRP: 154 mg/l, normal value <5 mg/l). Temporal artery biopsy confirmed the diagnosis of giant cell arteritis. (**a**) Coronal 18Fluorodeoxyglucose positron emission tomography (PET) and (**b**) PET-CT showed involvement of large vessels with intense uptake throughout carotid (white arrows) and subclavian arteries (blue arrows), the thoracic and abdominal aorta, the superior mesenteric artery and the inguinal arteries (yellow arrows)

3. **Which are the clinical and histologic characteristics of Takayasu arteritis?**

Takayasu arteritis (TA) occurs most commonly in young women (female:male = 8:1), of young age (median age of 25 years; in 15% it occurs after the age of 40). TA affects primarily the aorta and its branches and more commonly the aortic arch and the abdominal aorta. Initial manifestations can be non-specific, including constitutional symptoms such as low-grade fever, fatigue, arthralgias, anorexia, and weight loss. Later on, typical manifestations and findings include claudication of upper extremities, bruits on large-vessel auscultation, decreased or even absent pulses (therefore also called "pulseless disease"), and asymmetric blood pressure in the extremities. Pulmonary and coronary artery involvement is less frequent. TA diagnosis is nowadays based on computer tomography angiography, gadolinium-enhanced magnetic resonance angiography (MRA) (Fig. 8.3), and positron emission tomography (PET). Thickening of the arterial wall and narrowing of the arterial lumen with subsequent aneurysmal dilatations are characteristic TA imaging findings.

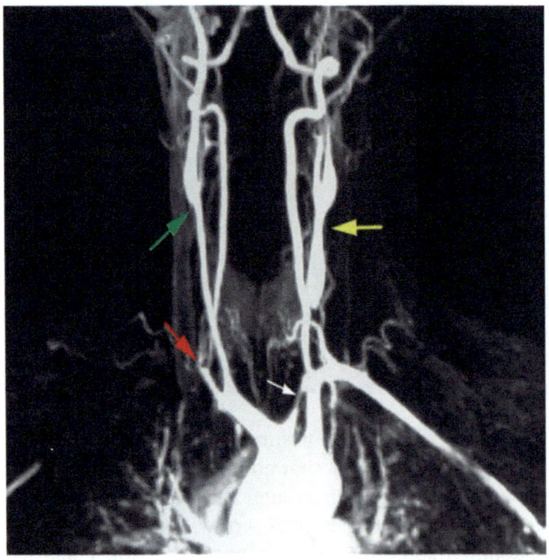

Fig. 8.3 Takayasu arteritis: Magnetic resonance angiography of the major aortic arch branches revealing complete obstruction of the right subclavian artery (red arrow) obstruction and post-stenotic dilatation of the right common carotid artery (green arrow), severe stenosis of the left subclavian artery (white arrow), and stenosis of the left common carotid artery with post-stenotic dilatation in a 30-year-old female diagnosed with Takayasu arteritis

The histologic appearance of TA is a focal panarteritis that can be very similar to giant cell arteritis (GCA). Like GCA, focal "skip lesions" are common, and lesions can be active, chronic, or healed. Mononuclear cell infiltrates (CD4 and CD8 lymphocytes, plasma cells, and macrophages) in the outer parts of the media and adventitia are prominent, in contrast to GCA where inflammatory infiltrates concentrate around the inner half of the media.

4. **Which are large-vessel vasculitis mimickers**?

- Diffuse atherosclerosis
- Infections: Tuberculous aortitis, and syphilitic aortitis
- Inherited connective tissue diseases, such as Ehlers-Danlos type IV, Marfan syndrome, Neurofibromatosis type 1
- Aortitis associated with ankylosing spondylitis

5. **Which imaging tests are recommended for the diagnosis of large vessel vasculitis?**

- In patients with suspected giant cell arteritis (GCA), predominantly cranial, an early positive imaging test (ultrasound of temporal ± axillary arteries) can set the diagnosis, without an additional test (biopsy or further imaging)
- If ultrasound is not available or inconclusive, magnetic resonance angiography (MRA) of cranial arteries may be used alternatively
- CT angiography (CTA) and PET-CT are not recommended for the assessment of inflammation of cranial arteries
- Ultrasound, PET, MRA, and/or CTA may be used to support the diagnosis of large vessel-GCA, as mural inflammation and/or luminal changes in extracranial arteries can be detected
- In patients with suspected Takayasu arteritis (TA), MRA should be used as the first imaging test to set the diagnosis

- Conventional angiography is not recommended for the diagnosis of GCA or TA
- Imaging is not routinely recommended for GCA or TA patients in clinical and biochemical remission. It should only be used when a flare is suspected [6]

6. **Which are the clinical and laboratory features of polymyalgia rheumatica?**

Polymyalgia rheumatica (PMR) is an inflammatory syndrome affecting older individuals (>50 years of age) and women more often than men (2:1). PMR is about two to three times more common than giant cell arteritis (GCA). Cardinal features include abrupt onset of pain and morning stiffness, especially in the neck and shoulder/pelvic girdles, which can be so severe that patients may be unable to lift their arms to comb their hair, rise from a chair, or even get out of bed without assistance. At times patients with PMR may present with peripheral arthritis (knees, wrists, and sternoclavicular joints) which is non-erosive and asymmetrical. These symptoms are accompanied by constitutional symptoms, including low-grade fever and weight loss, in more than 50% of patients and are particularly common in patients aged 70 years or older.

Elevated acute-phase reactants (ESR, CRP), as well as absence of rheumatoid factor and anti-citrullinated protein antibodies is characteristic for patients with PMR. A remarkable response to corticosteroid administration is not diagnostic, yet poor or unsustained response to this therapy may indicate another diagnosis, including GCA, cancer-related muscle pain, fibromyalgia, chronic infection, or endocrinopathy (such as hypothyroidism). In all cases of PMR, concurrence of GCA should be considered, as GCA may occur in 30% of patients with PMR and PMR may be the initial symptom in 20–40% of patients with GCA.

7. **What other diseases should be considered before setting the diagnosis of polymyalgia rheumatica?**

The diagnosis of polymyalgia rheumatica is a clinical one and is made after excluding other possible disease entities, such as:

- Occult infection
- Giant cell arteritis
- Malignancy
- Rheumatoid arthritis
- Polymyositis
- Fibromyalgia

8. **Which are the main clinical manifestations of patients with microscopic polyangiitis?**

Microscopic polyarteritis (MPA) is one of the ANCA-associated vasculitides affecting small vessels (capillaries, arterioles, or venules). Its main clinical characteristics are:

- Nonspecific constitutional symptoms, such as fever, malaise, myalgias, and weight loss, are common
- Kidney involvement is typical, and rapidly progressive glomerulonephritis (GMN) (focal segmental necrotizing, pauci-immune) is detected in more than 80% of MPA patients
- Lung involvement is not uncommon, and it can manifest with symptoms ranging from pulmonary effusions and infiltrates to diffuse alveolar hemorrhage with hemoptysis and even pulmonary fibrosis
- Mononeuritis multiplex occurs in almost 60% of MPA patients
- Cutaneous vasculitis (palpable purpura, ulcers, and vesiculobullous lesions)
- Migratory arthralgias or arthritis, which is pauciarticular or polyarticular, yet non-destructive
- Gastrointestinal tract involvement with mesenteric vasculitis

9. Which are the main laboratory findings in patients with microscopic polyangiitis?

- Mild-to-moderate leukocytosis and thrombocytosis
- Elevated acute-phase reactants (ESR and CRP)
- Positive rheumatoid factor in 40–50% of MPA patients
- Microscopic hematuria and proteinuria
- Perinuclear antineutrophil cytoplasmic antibodies (pANCAs) directed against myeloperoxidase (MPO) are detected in the serum of the majority of MPA patients and support the diagnosis; yet a few MPA patients may have cytoplasmic antineutrophil cytoplasmic antibodies (cANCAs), directed against proteinase 3 (PR3)

10. Which are poor prognostic factors in patients with microscopic polyangiitis and renal involvement?

In patients with microscopic polyangiitis and renal involvement age $\geq$ 65 years at the time of diagnosis, serum creatinine level $\geq$ 500 μmol/L, and interstitial lung disease or pulmonary fibrosis, at the time of diagnosis, seem to be associated with increased mortality [7, 8].

11. Which are the main clinical manifestations of patients with eosinophilic granulomatosis with polyangiitis (formerly Churg-Strauss syndrome)?

Eosinophilic granulomatosis with polyangiitis (EGPA) is an ANCA-associated granulomatous vasculitis affecting small- and medium-sized vessels. Its main clinical characteristics are:

- The majority of patients have a history of allergic manifestations such as allergic rhinitis, nasal polyposis, and adult-onset asthma
- It affects the lungs, the heart, the peripheral nerves, the skin, and the gastrointestinal tract and is associated with peripheral blood and tissue eosinophilia
- Lung involvement presents with patchy transient pulmonary infiltrates without cavitation
- Heart involvement can manifest as pericarditis, pericardial effusion, valvular heart disease, cardiomyopathy, acute myocardial infarction, myocarditis, and acute heart failure
- Although uncommon, cardiac involvement represents a major cause of morbidity and mortality
- Mononeuritis multiplex and asymmetric sensorimotor polyneuropathy (glove/stocking distribution) are frequent (65–75%) manifestations
- Subcutaneous nodules, petechiae, palpable purpura, and ulcers due to skin infarction are manifestations of skin involvement
- Eosinophilic gastroenteritis with abdominal pain and bloody diarrhea occurs in some EGPA patients
- Kidney involvement is uncommon, and acute kidney injury may be caused by eosinophil-mediated interstitial nephritis

12. Which are the main laboratory findings in patients with eosinophilic granulomatosis with polyangiitis?

- Peripheral blood eosinophilia (often >3000/mm^3)
- Elevated acute-phase proteins (CRP/ESR) and serum IgE levels
- ANCAs directed against myeloperoxidase (MPO) (30–40%)
- Patients who are MPO positive tend to have a higher prevalence of arthritis and glomerulonephritis than those who are MPO negative

13. Which are common lung radiological and computerized tomography (CT) findings in patients with eosinophilic granulomatosis with polyangiitis (EGPA)?

The most frequently observed X-ray findings in patients with EGPA are transient and often migrant opacities with bilateral, mostly peripheral distribution, without predilection for any lung zone. These findings are similar to eosinophilic pneumonia and organizing pneumonia. The most common abnormality on chest CT, seen in up to 90% of EGPA patients, is bilateral ground-glass opacities or consolidations with a symmetric and peripheral distribution. Other relatively common findings are the presence of airway involvement consisting of bronchial dilatation, bronchial wall thickening, and small peribronchial and centrilobular nodules related to eosinophilic infiltration of the bronchial wall and asthma. Smooth interlobular septal thickening, which may reflect the presence of edema secondary to cardiac involvement or eosinophilic septal infiltration, can be seen in 50% of patients.

14. Which hypereosinophilic conditions should be considered in the differential diagnosis of eosinophilic granulomatosis with polyangiitis?

- Strongyloidiasis: Infection from the nematode *Strongyloides stercoralis*
- Löffler syndrome
- Chronic eosinophilic pneumonia
- Eosinophilic gastroenteritis
- Hypereosinophilic syndrome
- Eosinophilic fasciitis
- IgG4-related disease
- Eosinophilic leukemia [9]

15. Which are the main clinical manifestations of patients with granulomatosis with polyangiitis (formerly Wegener's granulomatosis)?

Granulomatosis with polyangiitis (GPA) is a systemic ANCA-associated vasculitis affecting small- to medium-sized vessels (both arterial and venous). Its main clinical characteristics are:

- GPA presents usually in a subacute way. Chronic sinusitis and inflammation of the nasal mucosa and purulent/hemorrhagic nasal discharge, nasal mucosa crusts, and/or ulcerations are common initial manifestations
- Patients are frequently *Staphylococcus aureus* carriers, which can lead to GPA relapses
- Oral manifestations include typically painful ulcers on the lateral sides of the tongue (Fig. 8.4) and gum inflammation giving the appearance of "strawberry gums"
- Acute suppurative otitis media or chronic serous otitis media as well as mixed-type conductive and sensorineural hearing loss
- Scleritis, episcleritis, retinal artery occlusion, and orbital pseudotumors
- Chronic inflammation of the laryngeal and tracheal mucosa can lead to hoarseness and subglottic stenosis
- Lung involvement is the presenting symptom in 50% of GPA patients, while more than 80% will present clinical evidence of lower respiratory tract involvement during their disease course. The typical appearance of lung involvement consists of multiple nodules or masses that may demonstrate cavitation. Diffuse multifocal air-space opacities with or without cavitation may also be seen. Pulmonary hemorrhage due to pulmonary capillaritis is another well-known presenting manifestation of GPA
- Pulmonary fibrosis may result from healing of acute or chronic inflammation
- Kidney involvement is very frequent (80% of GPA patients). It can manifest as microscopic hematuria, proteinuria, cellular casts, and variable degree of renal function compromise

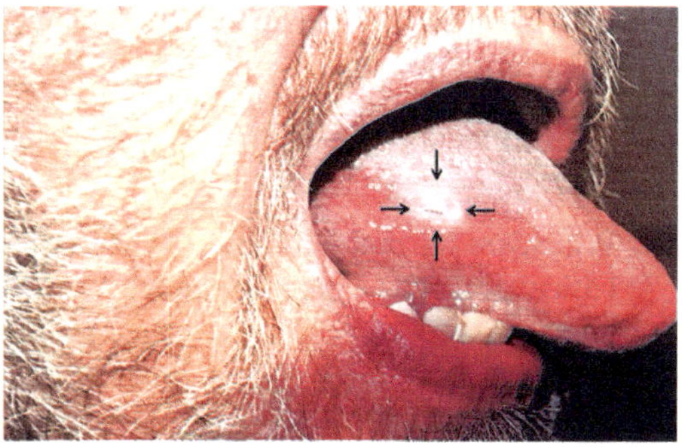

Fig. 8.4 Deep painful tongue ulcer in a 62-year-old male with granulomatous polyangiitis (Wegener's granulomatosis)

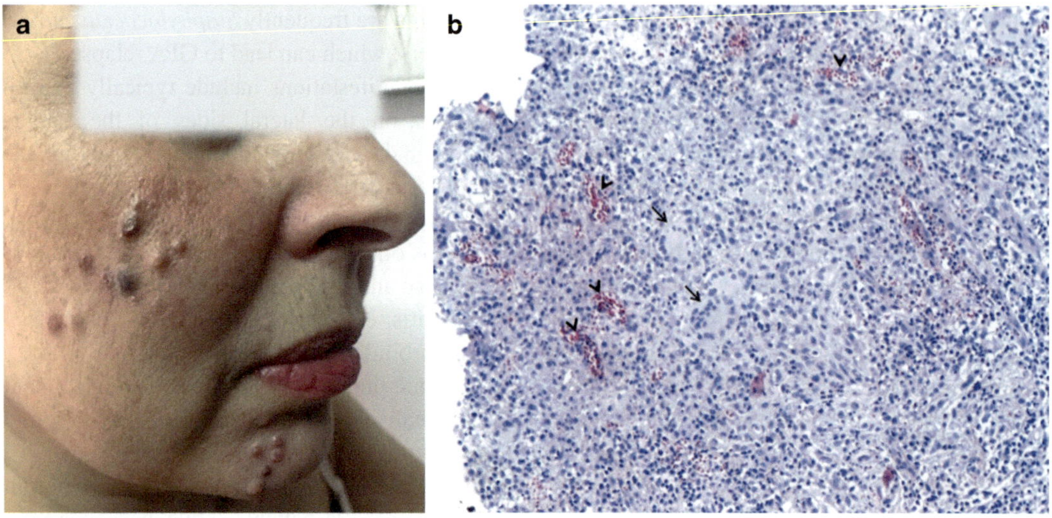

Fig. 8.5 (**a**) A 39-year-old woman, with limited pulmonary granulomatosis with polyangiitis on exacerbation developed red-brown-black, painless, non-pruritic papular lesions on her right cheek and chin areas. (**b**) Biopsy of the lesions revealed granulomatous dermal inflammation with multinuclear histiocytic giant cells in the dermis (arrows) without vasculitis cells and extravasated red blood cells (arrowheads) (H&E × 100). Acid-fast and periodic acid-Schiff stains and cultures did not uncover any organisms. (*Reproduced by Zampeli E* et al. *2020*) [10]

The histopathologic renal lesion is pauci-immune focal segmental necrotizing glomerulonephritis

- Deep vein thrombosis can occur in GPA patients as a result of venous circulation involvement
- Skin manifestations include a wide range of cutaneous vasculitis signs: palpable purpura, subcutaneous nodules, facial papules (Fig. 8.5), ulcers, and vesicles
- Peripheral and central nervous system involvement in the form of mononeuritis multiplex, meningeal inflammation, and central nervous system vasculitis

16. Which are the main laboratory findings in patients with granulomatosis with polyangiitis?

- Anemia and elevated acute-phase reactants (ESR and CRP) are common
- Microscopic hematuria and proteinuria occur with renal involvement
- Rheumatoid factor may be positive in 30–40%
- Cytoplasmic ANCAs directed against proteinase 3 (PR3) are found in 90%

17. Which are the common lung computerized tomography (CT) findings in patients with granulomatosis with polyangiitis?

The most common CT findings are cavitating pulmonary nodules, (2–4 cm) usually multiple, bilateral, and well defined (Fig. 8.6), which tend to increase with disease activity and progression. Cavities are usually thick walled with an irregular inner margin. The nodular lesions are often related to the vessels, and they tend to involve mainly the subpleural regions but have no predilection for the upper or lower lung zones. The presence of a rim of ground-glass opacity around the nodules (halo sign) is frequent and denotes alveolar hemorrhage. An air bronchogram within the pulmonary nodules can often be seen. After treatment, the lesions usually show a slow regression characterized by a marked wall thinning. In cases of diffuse alveolar hemorrhage bilateral ground-glass opacities and consolidations are prominent in the perihilar areas.

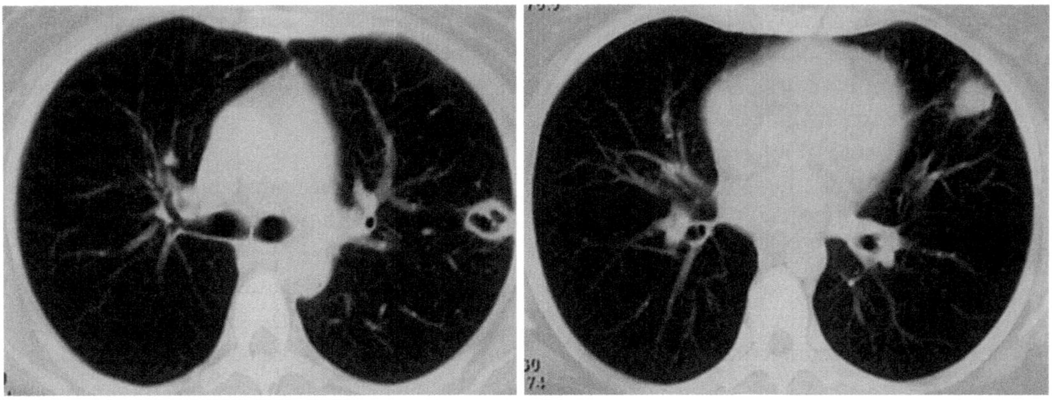

Fig. 8.6 Granulomatous polyangiitis (Wegener's granulomatosis) lung lesions: Chest computerized tomography (CT) showing bilateral round opacities with and without cavitation in a 36-year-old male patient with granulomatosis with polyangiitis (*Figure courtesy of Christos Kampolis, MD*)

18. Which drugs have been implicated in drug-induced ANCA-associated vasculitis?

Propylthiouracil, minocycline, clozapine, levamisole, allopurinol, hydralazine, montelukast, and anti-tumor necrosis factor agents have been reported to be possibly implicated in drug-induced ANCA vasculitis. Constitutional symptoms, skin vasculitis, and arthralgias are common manifestations, while lung and kidney involvement occurs less frequently. Timely withdrawal of the offending drug usually leads to recovery, while late withdrawal of the drug and more advanced disease may require administration of immunosuppressive therapy. In these patients multiple antigens can be responsible for ANCA positivity.

19. With which group of diseases could ANCA-associated vasculitis possibly overlap?

In patients with a confirmed diagnosis of ANCA-associated vasculitis (AAV), mainly granulomatosis with polyangiitis, atypical manifestations such as pachymeningitis, orbital mass, chronic periaortitis or other inflammatory pseudo-tumors have been described. Since these manifestations are included in the spectrum of IgG4-related diseases (IgG4-RD), a recently emerging entity is the IgG4-RD/AAV overlap syndrome, in which tumoral lesions could be related to IgG4-RD rather than refractory granulomatous lesions [11]. It has been postulated that class switching of ANCA toward IgG4 may also contribute to AAV pathogenesis, since IgG4 ANCA exhibit stimulatory properties on oxidative burst. Furthermore, IgG subclasses are produced in a temporal manner (IgG3 < IgG1 < IgG2 < IgG4) during an immune response, which could implicate that affinity maturation and class switching are potentially concomitant influential events in the ANCA production and consequently in the development of both AAV and IGG4-RD/AAV overlap [12]. Therefore, clinicians should bear in mind that atypical manifestations during AAV could be related to IgG4RD rather than to refractory granulomatous or vasculitis lesions.

20. Which are ANCA-associated small-vessel vasculitis mimickers?

- Infective endocarditis, disseminated intravascular coagulation, and sepsis
- Antiphospholipid syndrome
- Idiopathic diffuse alveolar hemorrhage/pulmonary alveolar proteinosis
- Emboli (cholesterol, cardiac myxomas, cardiac thrombus, endocarditis, mycotic aneurysm, and others)
- Asthma and eosinophilia (EGPA mimics): Toxocariasis, HIV, *Aspergillus* infection, hypereosinophilic syndrome, aspirin-

exacerbated respiratory disease, idiopathic eosinophilic pneumonia
- Midline destructive lesions (GPA mimics): Cocaine-induced midline destructive lesions, necrotizing sinonasal infections (tuberculosis, syphilis), NK/T cell lymphoma, Sarcoidosis, IgG4-related disease

21. Which are immune complex-associated small-vessel vasculitis mimickers?

- Purpuric lesions: Infectious emboli (endocarditis), scurvy, antiphospholipid syndrome, heparin-induced thrombocytopenia, thrombotic thrombocytopenic purpura, paroxysmal nocturnal hemoglobinuria, intravascular lymphoma
- Urticarial lesions: serum sickness-like eruption, autoinflammatory diseases, Sweet's syndrome, viral exanthems, Schnitzler's syndrome (Fig. 9.2a, b)
- Nodular lesions: Panniculitis (Weber-Christian disease), granulomatous diseases
- Ulcers: Peripheral venous/arterial disease, pyoderma gangrenosum, calciphylaxis, livedoid vasculopathy (Fig. 10.6a, b), malignant atrophic papulosis (Degos disease)

22. Which are the main clinical manifestations of patients with polyarteritis nodosa?

Polyarteritis nodosa (PAN) is a necrotizing inflammation of medium-sized arteries and muscular arterioles. The main clinical features suggestive of PAN are:

Anorexia, weight loss, myalgias, and low-grade fever.
Skin lesions: Livedo reticularis, palpable purpura, nodules, papules, ulcers, and digital ischemia/gangrene.
Peripheral neuropathy, most frequently mononeuritis multiplex.
Testicular pain.
Mesenteric vasculitis presenting with abdominal pain/intestinal angina.
Hypertension due to renal artery involvement.
Glomerulonephritis, lung involvement, and ANCA positivity are not PAN manifestations.

23. Which are the main laboratory findings in patients with polyarteritis nodosa?

- Elevated acute-phase proteins (CRP and serum complement)
- Leukocytosis, normochromic anemia, or thrombocytosis
- Presence of hepatitis B or C viral infection in around 30% of patients
- Elevated creatinine levels and mild proteinuria
- Elevated levels of liver enzymes
- Hypergammaglobulinemia (in 30% of patients with PAN)
- To confirm the diagnosis of PAN, biopsy of an accessible affected tissue, and/or visceral angiography should be performed

24. Which are the angiographic and histopathology findings of polyarteritis nodosa?

The typical angiographic findings in PAN are microaneurysms (small saccular aneurysms), occlusions, abrupt vessel cutoffs, irregularities of the vessel lumen, and stenosis of the small and medium vessels of the viscera. To confirm the diagnosis of PAN, biopsy of an accessible affected tissue should be performed. Skin, nerve, or muscle biopsies are preferred since they yield high diagnostic value with the lowest morbidity. The characteristic pathologic picture shows focal transmural necrotizing inflammation of small- and medium-sized arteries, disrupting the normal architecture of the vessel wall and leading to aneurysmal dilatations. The inflammatory process is pleomorphic with predominance of round (lymphocytes/macrophages) cells. The elastic lamina is disrupted and the vessel wall is destroyed. Proliferation of fibrous tissues and endothelial cells can lead to vessel lumen occlusion.

25. What is cutaneous polyarteritis nodosa?

Cutaneous PAN is a distinct subset of the systemic disease, where skin is the sole organ affected. Patients present with firm, painful subcutaneous nodules, which may ulcerate, most often found on the legs and feet. A deep skin biopsy, including subcutaneous tissue, is necessary for the accurate diagnosis of cutaneous PAN. Necrotizing inflammation of small- to medium-sized arterioles of the deep dermis and/or hypodermis with or without fibrinoid necrosis is the characteristic histopathologic finding (Fig. 8.7). Cutaneous PAN runs a chronic but relatively benign course.

26. Which are medium-vessel vasculitis mimickers?

- Infectious endocarditis and mycotic aneurysms
- Fibromuscular dysplasia (Fig. 8.8a, b)
- Thromboangiitis obliterans (Buerger's disease)
- Segmental arterial mediolysis
- Livedoid vasculopathy (Fig. 10.6a, b)

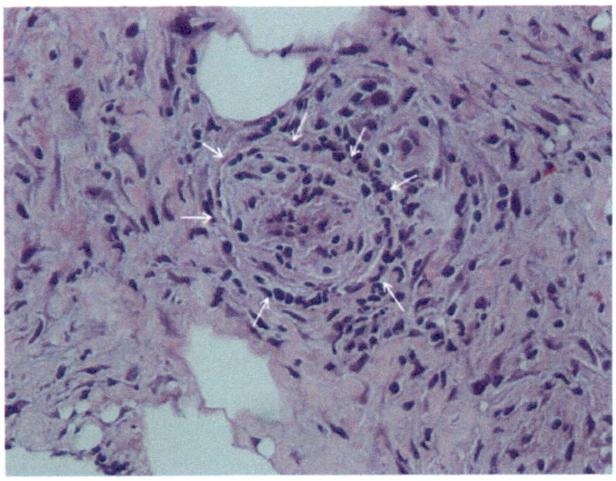

Fig. 8.7 Cutaneous polyarteritis nodosa: Deep skin biopsy (HE × 200) revealing focal fibrinoid necrosis, a mixed inflammatory infiltrate, as well as occlusion of the arteriole's lumen in the medium-sized arterioles of hypodermis in a 56-year-old female patient with recurrent painful, indurated subcutaneous nodules on the lower extremities

27. Which collagen disorders fibromuscular dysplasia can mimic?

Fibromuscular dysplasia is due to noninflammatory and non-atherosclerotic hypoplasia of the medial vessel wall. It affects more often young women but also men of all ages. The etiology is unknown, but a small percentage of patients have a family history. The affected arteries show stenotic areas alternating with dilatation resembling "string of beads" (Fig. 8.8a, b). Renal arteries and carotid arteries are more often affected, but all arteries can be affected. Other conditions producing arterial microaneurysms, such as atherosclerosis, hereditary collagen diseases, polyarteritis nodosa, Takayasu's arteritis, coronary vasospasm, and myocardial bridging, should be ruled out [13, 14].

28. Which conditions can present as pulmonary-renal syndrome?

Pulmonary-renal syndrome is defined as the combination of alveolar hemorrhage and glomerulonephritis. It can be caused by a variety of diseases, such as:

- Primary systemic vasculitis (especially microscopic polyangiitis and granulomatosis with polyangiitis)
- Goodpasture syndrome (associated with autoantibodies against type IV collagen, the major component of alveolar and glomerular basement membranes)
- Systemic lupus erythematosus
- Antiphospholipid syndrome

29. What is middle line lethal granuloma? Which autoimmune condition resembles it?

It is a natural killer/T-cell non-Hodgkin's lymphoma causing destruction of the nasal septum, the hard palate, the nasopharynx, and the orbit. It can resemble the clinical picture of granulomatosis with polyangiitis (Wegener's granulomatosis) when the latter affects the upper airways.

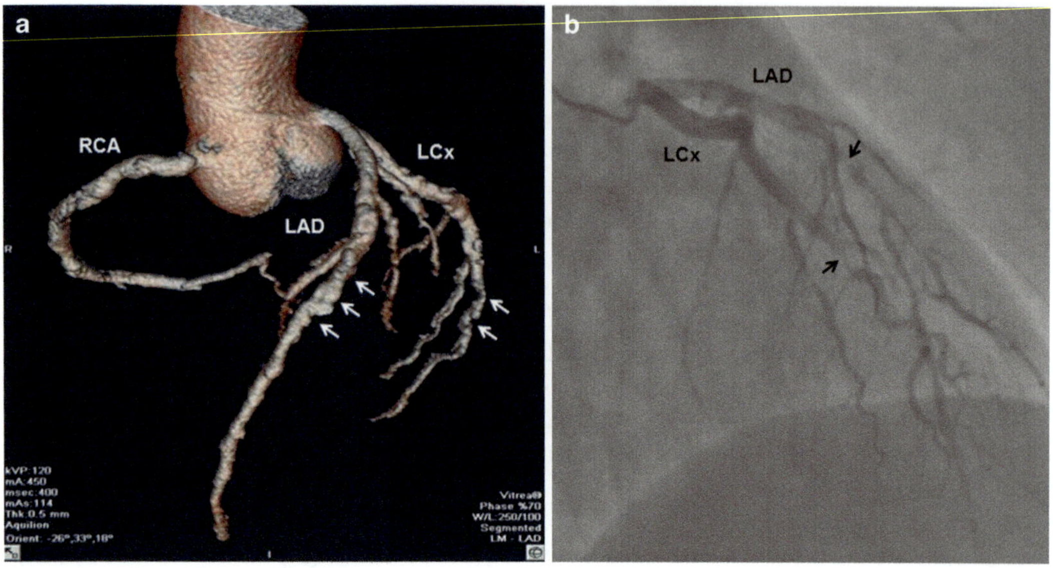

Fig. 8.8 CT coronary artery angiogram of a 39-year-old salesman with well-controlled hypertension on angiotensin converting enzyme inhibitor and a family history of coronary heart disease who suddenly experienced retrosternal chest pain radiating to the anterior part of the neck revealed in the coronary arteries areas of stenosis alternating with dilatation resembling "string of beads" (**a**, **b** arrows) findings characteristic of coronary artery fibromuscular dysplasia. (*Reproduced by Plastiras C et al. 2016)* [14]

30. Which clinical manifestations should be considered for the diagnosis of Behçet's disease?

- Oral aphthosis: Recurrent oral ulcerations (Fig. 8.9)
- Genital aphthosis: Recurrent oral ulcerations
- Ocular lesions: Anterior/posterior uveitis, or cells in vitreous on slit-lamp examination or retinal vasculitis
- Neurological manifestations
- Skin lesions: Erythema nodosum (Fig. 8.10), pseudofolliculitis or papulopustular lesions, or acneiform nodules in post-adolescent patients (Fig. 8.11)
- Vascular manifestations: Arterial thrombosis, large vein thrombosis, phlebitis, or superficial phlebitis
- Positive pathergy test (Fig. 8.12)

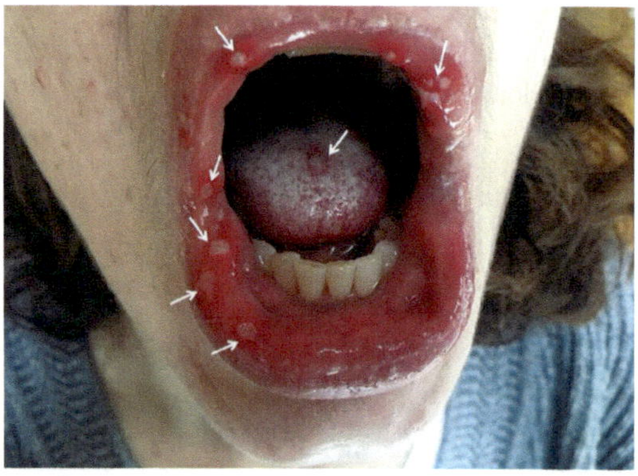

Fig. 8.9 Painful aphthous oral ulcers: in a 52-year-old woman with Behçet's syndrome

Based on the latest diagnostic criteria [15] oral aphthosis, genital aphthosis, and ocular lesions are each given 2 points, whereas 1 point is given to skin lesions, vascular manifestations, and neurological manifestations. A patient scoring 4 points or above is classified as having Behçet's disease. If pathergy testing is conducted one extra point may be assigned for a positive result.

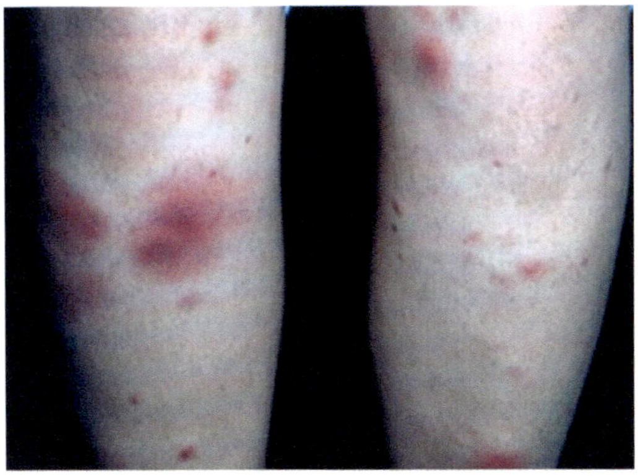

Fig. 8.10 Erythema nodosum: in a 29-year-old male patient with Behçet's syndrome

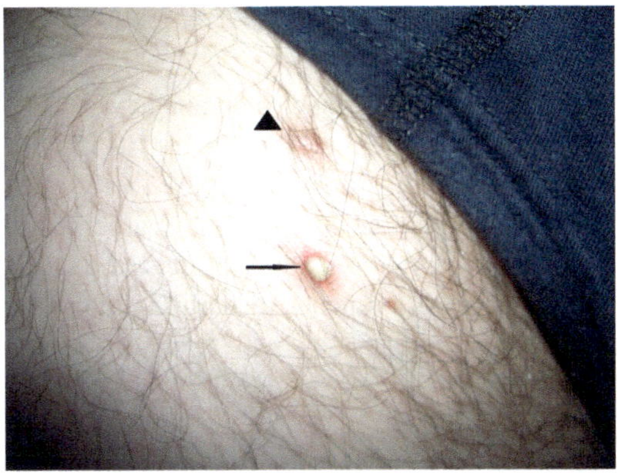

Fig. 8.11 Folliculitis in active phase (arrow) and in healing phase (arrowhead) in a 43-year-old male with Behçet's syndrome

31. What is pathergy test? In which patient population is it more often positive?

Pathergy is skin hyper-reactivity to any cutaneous injection or needle stick. Pathergy test (Fig. 8.12) is the development of a ≥ 2 mm erythema 24–48 h after a 20 or 21 gauge needle prick subcutaneously to a depth of 5 mm. This reaction is believed to be pathognomonic of Behçet's disease. The mechanism of pathergy is thought to be related to increased neutrophil chemotaxis. The rate of a positive reaction varies in different populations, being more common in Japan and Turkey.

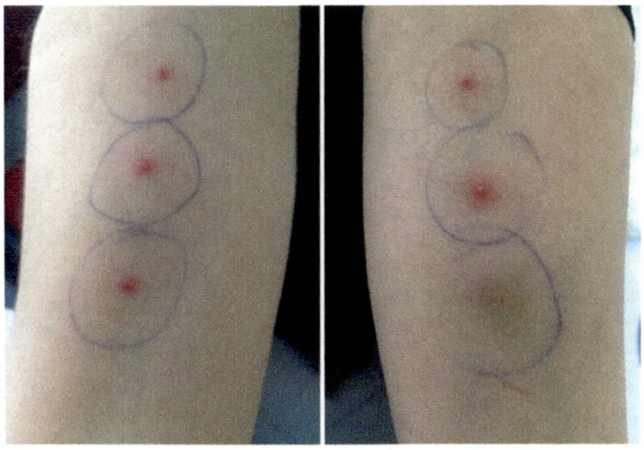

Fig. 8.12 Pathergy test: in a young male with Behçet's syndrome. Pustule formation could be seen in 5/6 needle insertion sites on the antecubital area (*Figure courtesy of Professor Emire Seyahi, MD*)

32. In which autoinflammatory diseases pulmonary artery aneurysms can manifest?

Behçet's disease (Fig. 8.13) and Takayasu arteritis.

33. Which are the commonest clinical manifestations of Cogan syndrome?

Cogan syndrome is a rare inflammatory disorder presenting with:

- Interstitial keratitis (non-syphilitic): manifests as an acute onset of unilateral or bilateral redness, pain, photophobia, and increased lacrimation. Uveitis, choroiditis, and retinal artery occlusion can occur with or without concomitant keratitis. Episcleritis/scleritis and uveitis are not uncommon in these patients
- Vestibulo-auditory dysfunction: is usually acute in onset and manifests with episodes of tinnitus, vertigo, and sensorineural (Ménière-like) hearing loss which might be initially fluctuating but progressively leads to deafness in more than 50% of cases. Unilateral involvement is typical

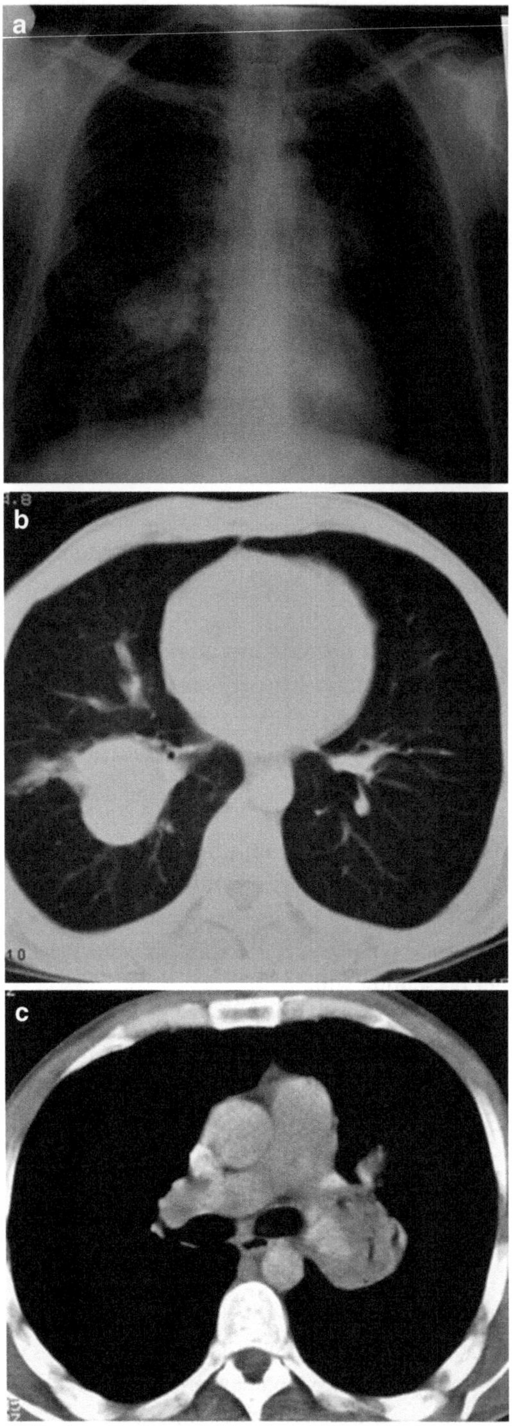

Fig. 8.13 Pulmonary artery aneurysms: (**a**) chest plain radiography and (**b**, **c**) computed tomography (CT) scans of a young male patient with Behçet's syndrome: multiple aneurysms completely thrombosed can be observed. Aneurysms are located on the right descendant artery (5 cm), distal portion of the left main artery (5 cm), and on the left descendant artery (1.5 cm) (*Figure courtesy of Professor Emire Seyahi, MD*)

34. Which are the systemic manifestations of Cogan syndrome?

The most common systemic manifestations in patients with Cogan syndrome are:

- Musculoskeletal complaints: Arthralgias, myalgias, and inflammatory arthritis
- Constitutional symptoms: Mostly in systemic disease
- Gastrointestinal involvement: Abdominal pain, bleeding, and hepatomegaly
- Cardiac involvement: Pericarditis and aortic insufficiency
- Neurologic manifestations: Headache, peripheral neuropathy, mononeuritis multiplex, and meningitis
- Skin: Nodules and rash
- Lymphadenopathy and splenomegaly
- Systemic vasculitis: Occurs in 10–15% of cases, usually affecting large- more often than medium-sized vessels. Large-vessel vasculitis predominantly affects the aorta and its major branches resembling Takayasu arteritis

35. What is the clinical picture of cryoglobulinemic vasculitis, and which are poor prognostic factors?

Cryoglobulinemic vasculitis is an immune-complex mediated small-vessel vasculitis associated with chronic infections (hepatitis C, hepatitis B virus, CMV, EBV, parvovirus B19, HIV, leishmaniasis, and Q fever caused by *Coxiella burnetii*), autoimmune disorders (systemic lupus erythematosus, Sjögren's syndrome) and B-cell lymphoproliferative disorders (diffuse large B cell lymphoma and Non-Hodgkin lymphoma). Patients with type I cryoglobulinemia have frequent manifestations from the skin (Raynaud's phenomenon, ulcers, gangrene), but rarely renal involvement. In patients with mixed cryoglobulinemia (type II and III), the skin, musculoskeletal system, and the kidneys are frequently affected. Skin manifestations include palpable purpura in dependent areas, digital ulcers, and gangrene. Arthralgias in hands and knees are frequent, yet without overt arthritis. Neurological symptoms present as distal sensory or sensorimotor polyneuropathy, mostly bilateral and symmetric. Male sex, age over 60 years old, type II cryoglobulinemia, renal and gastrointestinal tract involvement, as well as chronic hepatitis C infection are poor prognostic factors in patients with cryoglobulinemic vasculitis.

36. Which are the clinical and histopathologic findings of IgA vasculitis (formerly called Henoch-Schönlein purpura)?

This type of small-vessel vasculitis is more common than granulomatous polyangiitis. It is usually triggered either by an infection or a medication. It occurs more frequently in children than in adults. In adults, it presents with palpable purpura (Fig. 8.14a), arthritis of the lower extremities large joints, while gastrointestinal and kidney involvement is seen in two-thirds of the patients. In the majority of patients, it is self-limited. Direct immunofluorescence of the skin biopsy specimens reveals selective IgA deposition on the vessel wall of the dermis (Fig. 8.14b).

37. What is the etiopathogenesis and the clinical manifestations of Goodpasture syndrome?

Goodpasture syndrome is also termed anti-glomerular basement membrane (anti-GBM) disease. It involves both the lungs and kidneys, often presenting as pulmonary hemorrhage and glomerulonephritis (pulmonary-renal syndrome), in the presence of anti-glomerular basement membrane antibodies. Renal involvement presents as rapidly progressing glomerulonephritis. The pulmonary symptoms are typically present at disease initiation, or shortly after that. Hemoptysis of varying degrees is typical when there is pulmonary involvement. Mostly younger patients present simultaneously renal and pulmonary symptoms. Patients over 50 years of age tend to present with glomerulonephritis alone and follow a less severe

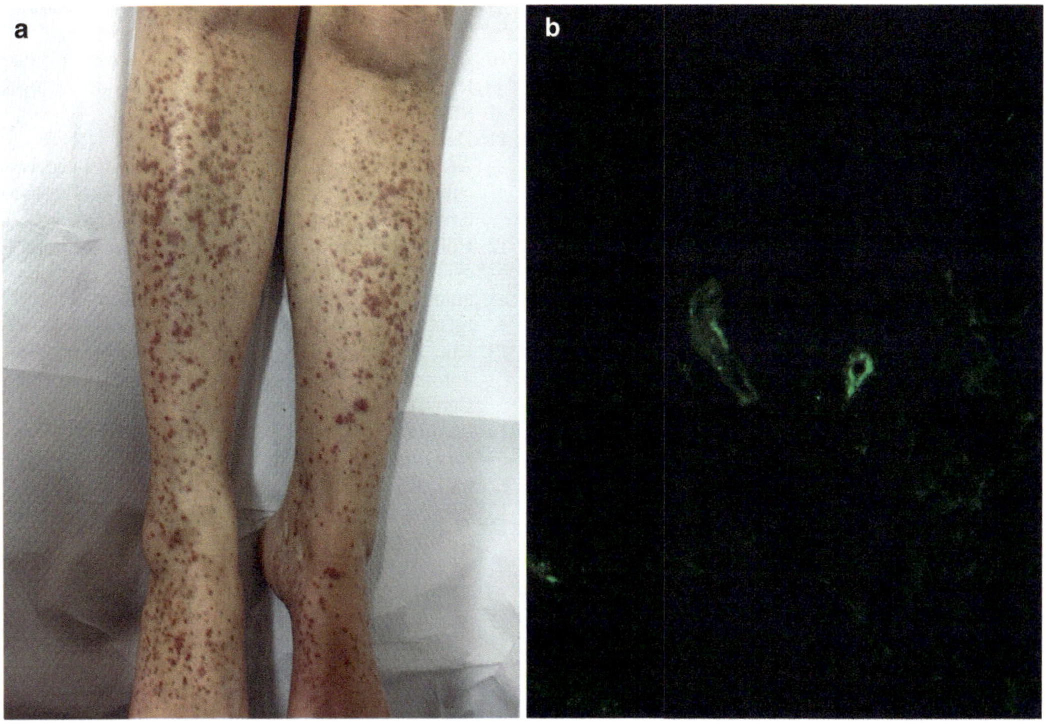

Fig. 8.14 IgA vasculitis (Henoch-Schönlein): (**a**) palpable purpura on the lower extremities, at sites coalescing to ecchymoses, in a 55-year-old lady. Skin biopsy of the lesions revealed leukocytoclastic vasculitis and (**b**) direct immunofluorescence showed selective IgA deposition on the vessel wall of the dermis

course. Besides the detection of serum anti-GBM antibodies, kidney biopsy is the gold standard for diagnosis. Immunofluorescence histology will show the linear deposition of IgG and C3 complement along the basement membrane.

38. What is Moya-Moya disease and which are its prominent clinical manifestations?

Moya-Moya disease is a rare cerebrovasculopathy characterized by progressive stenosis of the circle of Willis arteries (internal carotid, anterior, and middle cerebral arteries) and their branches. The term Moya-Moya (Japanese for "puff of smoke") refers to the appearance on angiography of abnormal vascular collateral networks that develop adjacent to the stenotic vessels. The steno-occlusive areas are usually bilateral.

The disease can present as transient ischemic attack or stroke in children, while adults usually present hemorrhagic stroke [16].

39. What is Sweet's syndrome?

Sweet's syndrome is also known as acute febrile neutrophilic dermatosis. Sweet's syndrome can present as a vasculitis mimicker. Its characteristic manifestations are acute presentation of raised painful papules on the extremities, face, neck, and trunk, accompanied by fever and polyarthritis in 20% of cases. Neutrophilic leukocytosis is common, and skin biopsy reveals dense dermal neutrophilic infiltrates without evidence of vasculitis. It is associated with underlying malignancy in 10–15% of patients (mostly with acute myelogenous leukemia). Other conditions associated with acute neutrophilic dermatosis are sun exposure, upper respiratory tract infection, inflammatory bowel disease, rheumatoid arthritis, lupus erythematosus, relapsing polychondritis, pregnancy, and drugs (oral contraceptives, trimethoprim-sulfamethoxazole, and minocycline).

References

1. Monti S, Floris A, Ponte C, Schmidt WA, Diamantopoulos AP, Pereira C, et al. The use of ultrasound to assess giant cell arteritis: review of the current evidence and practical guide for the rheumatologist. Rheumatology (Oxford). 2017;57(2):227–35.
2. Naderi N, Mohammad AJ, Turesson C. Large vessel involvement in biopsy-proven giant cell arteritis: incidence, distribution, and predictors. Scand J Rheumatol. 2017;46:215–21.
3. Kermani TA, Diab S, Sreih AG, et al. Arterial lesions in giant cell arteritis: a longitudinal study. Semin Arthritis Rheum. 2019;48:707–13.
4. Nuenninghoff DM, Hunder GG, Christianson TJH, et al. Incidence and predictors of large-artery complication (aortic aneurysm, aortic dissection, and/or large-artery stenosis) in patients with giant cell arteritis: a population-based study over 50 years. Arthritis Rheum. 2003;48:3522–31.
5. Ungprasert P, Koster MJ, Warrington KJ. Coronary artery disease in giant cell arteritis: a systematic review and meta-analysis. Semin Arthritis Rheum. 2015;44:586–91.
6. Dejaco C, Ramiro S, Duftner C, et al. EULAR recommendations for the use of imaging in large vessel vasculitis in clinical practice. Ann Rheum Dis. 2018;77:636–43.
7. Tzelepis GE, Kokosi M, Tzioufas A, Toya SP, Boki KA, Zormpala A, et al. Prevalence and outcome of pulmonary fibrosis in microscopic polyangiitis. Eur Respir J. 2010;36:116–21.
8. Shi J, Shen Q, Chen X, et al. Clinical characteristics and outcomes in microscopic polyangiitis patients with renal involvement: a study of 124 Chinese patients. BMC Nephrol. 2019;20:339.
9. Curtis C, Ogbogu P. Hypereosinophilic syndrome. Clin Rev Allergy Immunol. 2016;50:240–51.
10. Zampeli E, Moutsopoulos HM. Facial papular lesions in granulomatosis with polyangiitis. Arthritis Rheumatol. 2020;72:864.
11. Danlos F-X, Rossi GM, Blockmans D, et al. Antineutrophil cytoplasmic antibody-associated vasculitides and IgG4-related disease: a new overlap syndrome. Autoimmun Rev. 2017;16:1036–43.
12. Holland M, Hewins P, Goodall M, et al. Antineutrophil cytoplasm antibody IgG subclasses in Wegener's granulomatosis: a possible pathogenic role for the IgG4 subclass. Clin Exp Immunol. 2004;138:183–92.
13. Kim ES, Serhal M. The diagnosis and treatment of fibromuscular dysplasia: an update for cardiologists. Curr Treat Options Cardiovasc Med. 2016;18:37.
14. Plastiras C, Zampeli E, Moutsopoulos HM. Chest pain in a 39-year-old man: what could be the underlying cause? Am J Med. 2016;129:e329–30.
15. International Team for the Revision of the International Criteria for Behçet's Disease (ITR-ICBD). The international criteria for Behçet's disease (ICBD): a collaborative study of 27 countries on the sensitivity and specificity of the new criteria. J Eur Acad Dermatol Venereol. 2014;28:338–47.
16. Fujimura M, Bang OY, Kim JS. Moyamoya disease. Front Neurol Neurosci. 2016;40:204–20.

9 Autoinflammatory Syndromes

Haralampos M. Moutsopoulos
and Evangelia Zampeli

Abstract

Autoinflammatory syndromes constitute a group of genetic disorders, in which gene mutations coding for significant inhibitory inflammatory molecules have been identified. These disorders can manifest with inflammatory signs and symptoms of one or many organs without an apparent exogenous or endogenous insult. The mutated genes responsible for the main clinical syndromes are the MEFV gene on chromosome 16 in patients with Mediterranean fever; the type I TNF-α receptor (TNFRSF1A) gene on chromosome 12 in patients with TNF receptor-associated periodic syndrome (TRAPS); the mevalonate kinase (MVK) gene on chromosome 12 in patients with hyperimmunoglobulin D syndrome (HIDS); the CIAS1 gene on chromosome 1 in patients with cryopyrin-associated periodic syndrome (CAPS); the PSTPIP1 gene on chromosome 15q in patients with pyogenic arthritis, pyoderma gangrenosum, and acne (PAPA) syndrome; the IL1RN gene, which encodes interleukin-1 receptor antagonist, in patients with deficiency of the interleukin-1 receptor antagonist (DIRA) and the TMEM173 gene, encoding the stimulator of interferon genes (STING) in patients with STING-associated vasculopathy with onset in infancy (SAVI), a recently described autoinflammatory syndrome. The age onset of the different syndromes is variable. The clinical picture of these syndromes usually manifests with recurrent fevers, skin rashes, mucosal lesions, thoracic or abdominal pains (due to serositis), arthritis, and elevated acute-phase proteins. Cornerstone therapy of these disorders includes colchicine and anti-interleukin-1 receptor antagonist.

H. M. Moutsopoulos (✉)
Athens Academy, Athens, Greece
e-mail: hmoutsop@med.uoa.gr

E. Zampeli
Bioclinic General Hospital of Athens and Institute for Autoimmune Systemic and Neurological Disorders, Athens, Greece
e-mail: ezampeli@bioclinic.gr

1. **What is the role of the inflammasome in the pathogenesis of familial autoinflammatory syndromes?**

NALP3 is also known as cryopyrin, and it is encoded by the NLRP3 gene, located on chromosome 1. This protein is primarily found on neutrophils and monocytes and serves as an intracellular sensor of pathogens and danger signals. NALP3 consists of a pyrin domain (PYD), a nucleotide-binding oligomerization domain (NOD, also called NACHT), and a leucine-rich repeat (LRR) domain. Upon stimulation, NLRP3 interacts with

H. M. Moutsopoulos, E. Zampeli (eds.), *Immunology and Rheumatology in Questions*,
https://doi.org/10.1007/978-3-030-56670-8_9

adaptor proteins (ASC and cardinal), forming a multiprotein complex known as NLRP3 inflammasome. A cascade of interactions between the different protein parts of this complex leads to the activation of procaspase 1 to caspase 1. Caspase 1, in turn, activates pro-IL-1β to be released as the pro-inflammatory cytokine IL-1β. Genetic mutations of any of these protein parts can contribute to the development of familial autoinflammatory syndromes [1].

2. **Which are the main familial autoinflammatory syndromes?**

The main periodic fever syndromes are:

- Familial Mediterranean fever (FMF)
- Tumor necrosis factor (TNF) receptor-associated periodic Syndrome (TRAPS)
- Hyper-immunoglobulin D Syndrome (HIDS) also known as Mevalonate Kinase Deficiency (MKD)

The main cryopyrinopathies (cryopyrin-associated periodic syndromes, CAPS) are:

- Familial Cold Autoinflammatory Syndrome (FCAS)
- Muckle-Wells Syndrome (MWS)
- Neonatal-Onset Multisystem Inflammatory Disease (NOMID) (also called Chronic Infantile Neurologic Cutaneous Articular, or CINCA syndrome)

The main pyogenic disorders are:

- Pyogenic arthritis, pyoderma gangrenosum, and acne (PAPA) syndrome
- Deficiency of IL-1 receptor antagonist (DIRA) syndrome [2]

3. **Which are the major characteristics of familial Mediterranean fever?**

Familial Mediterranean fever (FMF) is associated with mutations in the MEFV gene on the short arm of chromosome 16 that encodes the pyrin protein. It is inherited in an autosomal recessive way. The diagnosis of FMF requires the presence of a pathogenic or likely pathogenic MEFV genotype along with at least one of the following clinical manifestations: recurrent episodes of fever lasting 12–72 h, non-destructive large joint arthritis (hip, knee, ankle, and wrist) typically non-responsive to prednisone, chest pain, or abdominal pain. In case of a non-confirmatory MEFV genotype at least two of the clinical manifestations are required to set the diagnosis [3]. FMF can present in two distinct ways: either as recurrent episodes of inflammation (patients, if untreated, can develop amyloidosis (AA) and subsequent renal failure) or it can present with AA amyloidosis (especially renal) as the first manifestation, without previous history of inflammatory episodes. FMF affects mainly children (<20 years) of Eastern Mediterranean ancestry (Armenian, Jewish, Arabian, and Turkish origin). Recurrence of attacks is usually every 2–4 weeks. Attacks respond to colchicine therapy.

4. **Which are the major characteristics of TNF receptor-associated periodic syndrome?**

TNF receptor-associated periodic syndrome (TRAPS) is due to mutations (mostly single-nucleotide missense) in the gene of type I TNF-α receptor (TNFRSF1A) on the short arm of chromosome 12. It is inherited in an autosomal dominant way. It can manifest in children as well as in middle-aged adults. Presents with high spiking fever of varying duration (yet always more than 5 days of duration); myalgias that can become migratory; migratory erythematous patches, or urticarial plaques over the areas of myalgias; ocular inflammation (conjunctivitis, periorbital edema); peritonitis; pleurisy; and arthralgias (rarely synovitis), all responding to glucocorticoids. A familial distribution with relatives affected can often be noted. These patients do not respond to colchicine. The attacks reoccur two to six times per year [3].

5. Which are the major characteristics of hyperimmunoglobulin D syndrome?

Hyperimmunoglobulin D syndrome (HIDS) is due to a mutation of the mevalonate kinase (MVK) gene on chromosome 12 that encodes the MVK enzyme. It is inherited in an autosomal recessive way. The symptomatology starts in infancy (younger than 1-year old). Infants present with fever (lasting 1–10 days) which is associated with cervical adenopathy, abdominal pain and vomiting, aphthous stomatitis, splenomegaly, maculopapular skin rash (on face, palms, and soles), genital ulcers, large joint arthritis, and myalgias. Elevated serum IgD levels and during flares increased urinary mevalonic acid can be detected [3].

6. Which are the major characteristics of cryopyrin-associated periodic syndromes (CAPS)?

Cryopirin-associated periodic syndromes (CAPS) are due to mutations in CIAS1 gene found on the long arm of chromosome 1, which encodes for cryopyrin (NALP3). They are inherited in an autosomal dominant way or are due to sporadic mutations. Their diagnosis requires the presence of a confirmatory or not confirmatory NLRP3 genotype and at least one or two clinical manifestations among the following respectively: cold/stress-triggered episodes, urticarial rash, red eye (conjunctivitis, episcleritis, and uveitis), and neurosensorial hearing loss [3]. More precisely:

(a) Familial cold autoinflammatory syndrome (FCAS): is the mildest form of CAPS. Symptoms develop within the first year of life and get less severe with aging. Fever, chills, rash (Fig. 9.1), arthralgias, and conjunctivitis, within 1–3 h after cold exposure, are typical
(b) Muckle-Wells syndrome: starts in adolescence, and the episodes can be triggered by fatigue, hunger, or cold exposure. Attacks last 24–48 h and are characterized by fever, chills, abdominal pain, myalgia, urticarial rash, and conjunctivitis. Late onset of sensorineural hearing loss is common and renal AA amyloidosis can occur

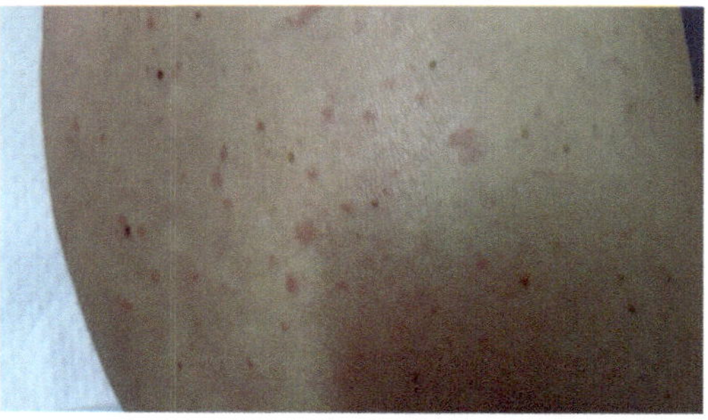

Fig. 9.1 Urticaria-like rash in a 65-year-old woman with cryopyrin-associated periodic syndrome (CAPS) triggered by exposure to cold (*Figure courtesy of Professor Fotini N.Skopouli, MD*)

(c) Chronic infantile neurologic, cutaneous, and articular syndrome (CINCA)/neonatal-onset multisystem inflammatory disease (NOMID): it is the most severe form of CAPS. It is characterized by the triad of chronic aseptic meningitis, neonatal-onset skin lesions, and arthropathy. Prognosis is poor with 20% mortality in childhood

7. Which are the major characteristics of pyogenic arthritis, pyoderma gangrenosum, and acne syndrome?

Pyogenic arthritis, pyoderma gangrenosum, and acne (PAPA) syndrome is inherited in an autosomal dominant way. It is due to a mutation in the proline-serine-threonine phosphatase-interacting protein 1 (PSTPIP1) gene on chromosome 15q. Clinical features of PAPA syndrome include early-onset, painful flares of recurrent sterile arthritis involving a prominent neutrophilic infiltrate along with skin ulcerations, frank pyoderma gangrenosum, or severe cystic acne. Symptoms persist into adulthood, leading to severe joint destruction.

8. What is the clinical picture of deficiency of the interleukin-1 receptor antagonist syndrome?

Deficiency of the interleukin-1 receptor antagonist (DIRA) is an autosomal recessive autoinflammatory syndrome, which is due to mutations in the gene encoding interleukin

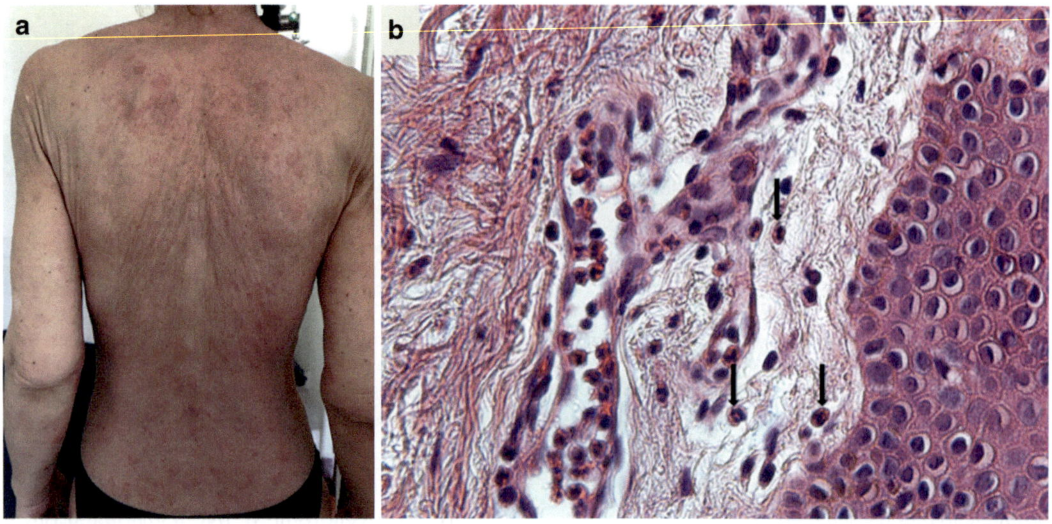

Fig. 9.2 Maculopapular urticarial rash on the back (**a**) of a 55-year-old woman with high-grade fever and generalized bone pain, who was diagnosed with Schnitzler's syndrome. Skin biopsy (H&E × 100) (**b**) showed edema of the dermis, vascular dilatation, presence of scattered polymorphs (neutrophils and eosinophils) and a slight perivascular T-cell (CD3$^+$) lymphocytic infiltrate, findings indicative of urticarial neutrophilic dermatosis

(IL)-1 receptor antagonist. This genetic defect has as a result the production of an abnormal non-secretory protein, which exposes the cells to a continuous IL-1 activity. The syndrome is clinically expressed with a wide range of symptoms from very serious (i.e., respiratory distress syndrome and cerebral vasculitis) to arthritis, hepatomegaly/splenomegaly, osteomyelitis, and oral ulcers/stomatitis.

9. What is the clinical picture of Schnitzler syndrome?

Schnitzler syndrome is a rare, acquired, late-onset auto-inflammatory disease sharing similar symptoms with periodic fever syndromes, in particular the cryopyrin-associated periodic syndromes, nonetheless there are controversial reports on Schnitzler patients baring mutation variations of the NLRP3 gene. It is characterized by recurrent fever in association with non-pruritic urticarial rash (Fig. 9.2a), histologically shown to be a neutrophilic dermatosis (Fig. 9.2b), arthralgia, bone pain, fatigue, weight loss, and systemic inflammation, while the presence of a monoclonal IgM is the hallmark of the syndrome. Interleukin-1-receptor antagonist (anakinra) is the only treatment that has proved efficient for the treatment of this syndrome. In fact, a rapid and immediate amelioration of all signs and symptoms after a single anakinra injection is supportive of the diagnosis. In cases of unresponsiveness to anakinra, the diagnosis should be reconsidered [4–6].

10. What is STING-associated vasculopathy with onset in infancy?

STING-associated vasculopathy with onset in infancy (SAVI) is a recently identified autoinflammatory disease caused by sporadic or inherited gain-of-function mutations in TMEM173 gene. This gene encodes for a protein called STING (stimulator of interferon gene), which is involved in the production of beta-interferon (IFN-β). Overproduction of IFN-β causes excessive inflammation which results in tissue damage, leading to the signs and symptoms of SAVI.

The signs and symptoms of SAVI begin in the first few months of life. Recurrent low-grade fever, lymphadenopathy, livedo reticularis, and Raynaud's phenomenon may be the presenting symptoms. Affected infants present extended vasculopathy with areas of severely damaged

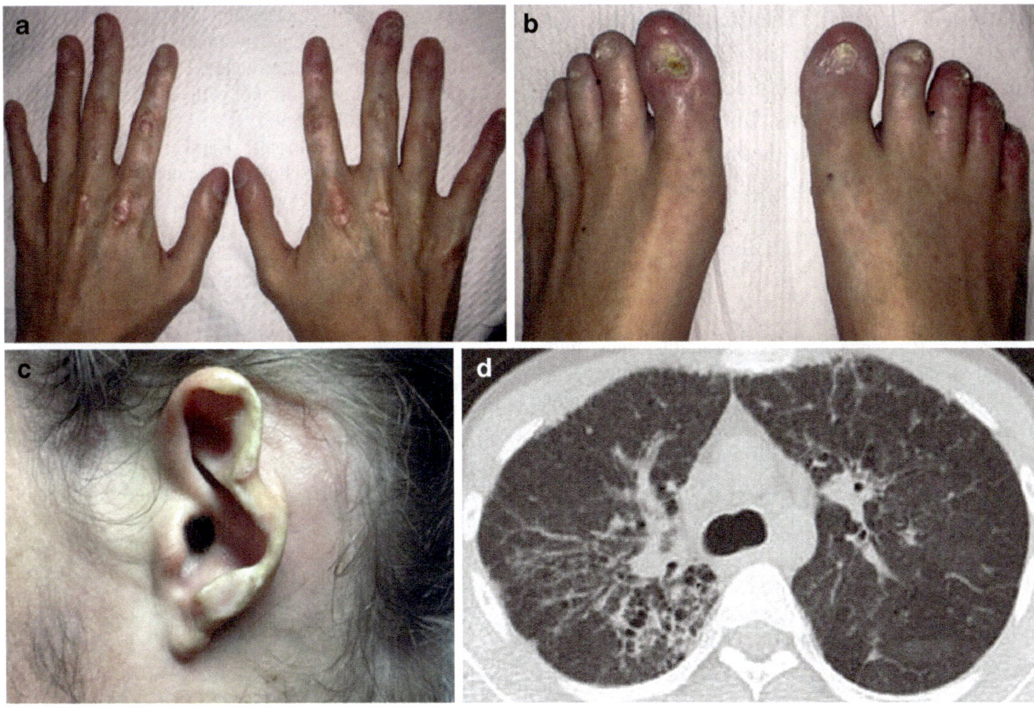

Fig. 9.3 STING-associated vasculopathy with onset in infancy (SAVI): recurrent vasculitic skin lesions of the fingers, the toes, the ears, and the nose, unresponsive to immunosuppression, which led to resorption of distal phalanges, nail dystrophy (**a**, **b**), scarred ears (**c**), and interstitial lung disease with areas of honeycombing, reticular opacities, and patchy ground glass (**d**) in an 18-year-old male in whom genetic analysis revealed a mutation in exon 6 of TMEM173 gene (encoding STING—stimulator of interferon genes) (*Reproduced from Manoussakis MN et al. 2017*)

skin, particularly the face, ears, nose, fingers, and toes. These lesions begin as rashes and can progress to become ulcerated and necrotic. The skin lesions are worse upon exposure to cold and stress and may lead to scarring of the ears, nasal septum perforation, and absorption of the distal phalanges (Fig. 9.3a–c). The most severe and potentially lethal complication in SAVI patients is rapidly progressive interstitial lung disease (Fig. 9.3d). Options for treating patients with SAVI are currently limited, but the blockade of interferon signaling with a Janus kinase (JAK) inhibitor could offer a therapeutic strategy [7, 8].

11. What is haploinsufficiency of A20 (HA20)?

Tumor necrosis factor alpha-induced protein 3 gene (TNFAIP3) encodes the tumor necrosis factor alpha-induced protein 3 (TNFAIP3, also known as A20), which is a negative regulator of the nuclear factor kappa B (NF-κB) signaling pathway. Loss-of-function mutations in TNFAIP3 result in deficient suppression of NF-κB activity and inflammasome activation leading to overproduction of proinflammatory cytokines, (IL-1β, IL-6, IL-18, and TNF-α). Dysregulation of innate immunity is the major cause of the autoinflammatory disease-haploinsufficiency of A20 (HA20). The majority of HA20 patients is either Caucasian or Japanese and has a family history. Symptomatology of HA20 starts at a mean age of 14 years. Oral and/or genital ulcers appear to be the hallmark feature of the disease. Almost half of the reported cases present recurrent fever, skin rashes (ranging from non-specific to psoriasiform, folliculitis or malar rash), and gastrointestinal symptoms (abdominal pain, vomiting, and diarrhea). One-third of them present also musculoskeletal symptoms, such as arthralgia or arthritis. Few patients with HA20 have ocular involvement (uveitis). The main disorder that should be ruled out is Behçet's disease. Glucocorticoids and colchicine are used in treating most of these patients. Immunosuppressives such as cyclosporine-A, methotrexate, and azathioprine have also been widely used [9, 10].

References

1. Tsoukas P, Canna SW. No shortcuts: new findings reinforce why nuance is the rule in genetic autoinflammatory syndromes. Curr Opin Rheumatol. 2017;29:506–15.
2. Álvarez-Errico D, Vento-Tormo R, Ballestar E. Genetic and epigenetic determinants in autoinflammatory diseases. Front Immunol. 2017;8:318.
3. Gattorno M, Hofer M, Federici S, et al. Classification criteria for autoinflammatory recurrent fevers. Ann Rheum Dis. 2019;78:1025–32.
4. Vanderschueren S, Van der Veen A. The Schnitzler syndrome: chronic urticaria in disguise: a single-Centre report of 11 cases and a critical reappraisal of the literature. Clin Exp Rheumatol. 2017;35:69–73.
5. Gilson M, Abad S, Larroche C, Dhote R. Treatment of Schnitzler's syndrome with anakinra. Clin Exp Rheumatol. 2007;25:931.
6. Zampeli E, Marinos L, Karakatsanis SJ. Images of the month 1: Schnitzler syndrome: an acquired autoinflammatory syndrome. Clin Med (Lond). 2020;20:229–30.
7. Crow YJ, Casanova JL. STING-associated vasculopathy with onset in infancy—a new interferonopathy. N Engl J Med. 2014;371:568–71.
8. Manoussakis MN, Mavragani CP, Nezos A, Zampeli E, Germenis A, Moutsopoulos HM. Type I interferonopathy in a young adult. Rheumatology (Oxford). 2017;56:2241–23.
9. Zhou Q, Wang H, Schwartz DM, et al. Loss-of-function mutations in TNFAIP3 leading to A20 haploinsufficiency cause an early-onset autoinflammatory disease. Nat Genet. 2016;48:67–73.
10. Yu MP, Xu XS, Zhou Q, et al. Haploinsufficiency of A20 (HA20): updates on the genetics, phenotype, pathogenesis and treatment. World J Pediatr. 2019;10.1007/s12519-019-00288-6.

Part III

Rheumatic Disorders and Manifestations in Various Organs, Systems and Disciplines

The Skin, the Eyes, and the Ears in Rheumatic Diseases

10

Haralampos M. Moutsopoulos and Evangelia Zampeli

Abstract

The skin, the eyes, and the ears are sense organs, which are very frequently involved in rheumatic diseases. The skin is an easily accessible organ to physical examination and biopsy. Taking into account the morphology, location, distribution, and histological characteristics of cutaneous manifestations in patients with rheumatic disorders, particular skin rashes may aid the diagnosis (e.g., butterfly rash and systemic lupus erythematosus) and/or define disease activity and prognosis (e.g., raised purpura and risk factor for lymphoma development in patients with Sjögren's syndrome).

Ocular manifestations may serve as a guide to proper diagnosis of an autoimmune disorder or indicate necessity for intensified treatment of the underlying rheumatic disease. Keratoconjunctivitis sicca, keratitis, uveitis, scleritis, and retinal vasculitis are often diagnosed in patients with rheumatic diseases. Some ocular symptoms of rheumatic diseases (e.g., amaurosis fugax in giant cell arteritis) or of drugs used to treat the diseases (e.g., antimalarial agents causing maculopathy) are sight-threatening, and they should be recognized promptly to prevent permanent loss of vision.

Ear manifestations of rheumatic diseases can often be the initial symptom of an undiagnosed autoimmune disease. Hearing disturbances may be encountered in systemic lupus erythematosus, relapsing polychondritis, Sjögren's syndrome, granulomatosis with polyangiitis, eosinophilic granulomatosis with polyangiitis, Cogan syndrome, sarcoidosis, and Behçet's disease. They can manifest as otalgia, otitis, uni- or bilateral sensorineural or conductive hearing loss, as well as audiovestibular deficits.

The questions and answers of this chapter aim (a) to familiarize a rheumatologist and any related subspecialty physician with the vast variety of rashes associated with rheumatic diseases, (b) to depict the different ocular manifestations of autoimmune diseases, and (c) to raise the clinical awareness that hearing disturbances can be the initial manifestation of a rheumatic disease.

H. M. Moutsopoulos (✉)
Athens Academy, Athens, Greece
e-mail: hmoutsop@med.uoa.gr

E. Zampeli
Bioclinic General Hospital of Athens and Institute for Autoimmune Systemic and Neurological Disorders, Athens, Greece
e-mail: ezampeli@bioclinic.gr

H. M. Moutsopoulos, E. Zampeli (eds.), *Immunology and Rheumatology in Questions*,
https://doi.org/10.1007/978-3-030-56670-8_10

1. **With which autoimmune disorder(s) chronic autoimmune urticaria coexists?**

Chronic autoimmune urticaria is caused by autoantibody formation against the Fc portion of the immunoglobulin (Ig) E receptor and less frequently by an autoantibody against IgE. These autoantibodies activate blood basophils and cutaneous mast cells, which release histamine and other proinflammatory mediators. A high percentage of patients with autoimmune thyroid disease have chronic autoimmune urticaria. Female patients with chronic urticaria present a higher incidence of rheumatoid arthritis, Sjögren's syndrome, systemic lupus erythematosus, celiac disease, and type I diabetes mellitus [1].

2. **Which skin rashes are suggesting a diagnosis of a clinical entity?**

- *Heliotrope* (Fig. 5.2) on eyelids and *Gottron's papules* (Fig. 5.1) over the metacarpophalangeal and proximal interphalangeal joints = dermatomyositis
- *Butterfly rash* = systemic lupus erythematosus (Fig. 4.6)
- *Lupus pernio* = sarcoidosis (Fig. 10.1)
- *Erythema migrans* = Lyme disease (Fig. 10.2)
- *Salmon-rash* = adult-onset Still's disease (Fig. 10.3)
- *Annular-psoriasiform rash* on the trunk and upper extremities = subacute cutaneous lupus erythematosus (Fig. 4.8)
- *Erythema marginatum* = rheumatic fever

3. **Can you tell from the location of the rash on the dorsum of the hands which patient has dermatomyositis and which systemic lupus erythematosus?**

Erythematous lesions on the dorsum of the hands and fingers affecting the skin between the finger joints is a rash seen in systemic lupus erythematosus patients, while erythematous papules over the metacarpophalangeal and proximal interphalangeal joints is a character-

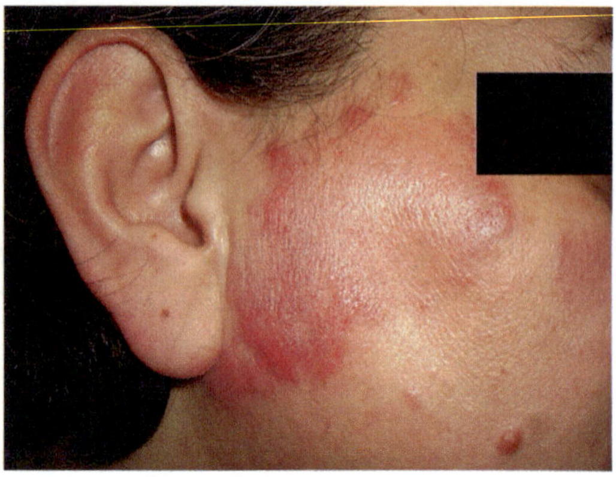

Fig. 10.1 Lupus pernio: a red-purple, swollen, shiny plaque on the cheek of a 30-year-old female with sarcoidosis

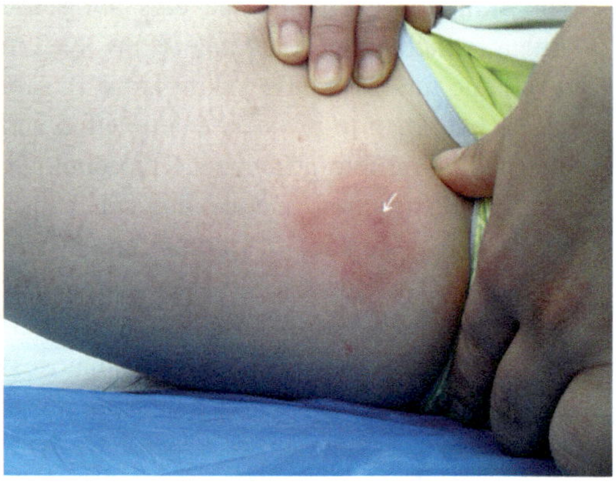

Fig. 10.2 Erythema migrans: A painless round skin rash, 5 cm in diameter, on the right inner thigh with a central spot (tick bite, arrow) ringed by an expanding red rash (like a bull's eye) in a 39-year-old female patient with IgM antibodies to *Borrelia burgdorferi*. *(Figure courtesy of Professor Alexandros A. Drosos, MD)*

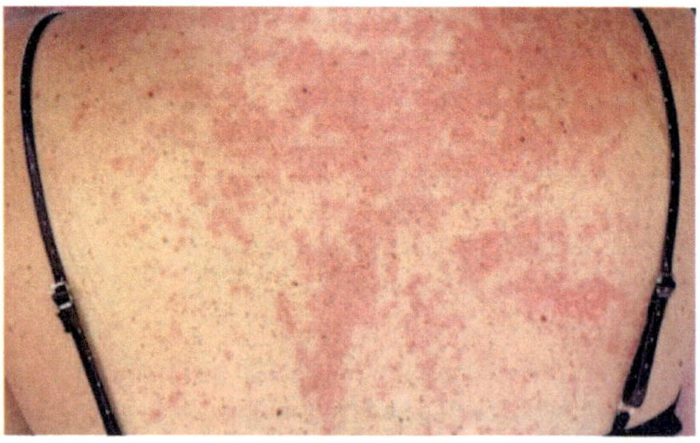

Fig. 10.3 Salmon-like rash in a 31-year-old female patient with adult-onset Still's disease

istic rash for dermatomyositis (Gottron's papules) (Fig. 5.1).

4. What is lupus pernio? What is its etiology?

Lupus pernio is truly a misnomer. It is a particularly disfiguring skin manifestation of sarcoidosis and not a skin manifestation of lupus. It is characterized by erupting violaceous plaques (Fig. 10.1) and nodules of the nose/nostrils, malar areas, and nasolabial folds, around the eyes, in the scalp, and along the hairline.

5. What are subungual splinter hemorrhages and in which diseases can they be seen?

Subungual splinter hemorrhages appear as tiny linear longitudinal, reddish-brown to black subungual streak lesions that do not blanch under pressure in the distal one-third of nails. The most common cause of subungual splinter hemorrhages is trauma. Nonetheless, they are recognized as a classical sign of subacute bacterial endocarditis in association with Osler nodes (tender lumps with pale center on fingers or toes) and Janeway lesions (non-tender, often haemorrhagic macular lesions on the palms and soles or on the thenar and hypothenar eminences), as a result of septic emboli in small capillary vessels. Other infective causes of subungual splinter hemorrhages include meningococcal disease, psittacosis, disseminated histoplasmosis, and *Trichinella spiralis* infections. Subungual splinter hemorrhages can also be observed in autoimmune diseases, such as psoriasis with psoriatic nail disease, primary or SLE-associated antiphospholipid syndrome, Bechet's disease, but also cutaneous vasculitis. The mechanism of subungual splinter hemorrhages in systemic autoimmune diseases is most probably due to formation of inflammatory microemboli. Finally, some drugs have been implicated in the development of subungual splinter hemorrhages, such as tyrosine kinase inhibitors, nitrofurantoin, ganciclovir, and tetracycline.

6. What are the causes of livedo reticularis?

Livedo reticularis (Fig. 4.5), a mottled reticular vascular pattern, seems to occur more in women than in men and usually in the third decade of life. It has many causes. Spasm of the blood vessels or an abnormality of the local circulation and disturbances of hormonal and autonomic regulatory mechanisms may account for its pathogenesis. More specifically livedo reticularis can be seen either without any underlying cause (idiopathic) or in patients with:

- Hypercoagulable states: Antiphospholipid syndrome, coagulopathies related to proteins C and S or antithrombin III deficiencies
- Hyperviscosity states: Cryoglobulinemias (type I), paraproteinemias/multiple myeloma
- Vessel wall pathology: Medium-size vessel vasculitis (i.e., polyarteritis nodosa, granulomatosis with polyangiitis, microscopic polyangiitis), calciphylaxis (deposition of calcium within the vessel walls usually in chronic renal failure)
- Autoimmune diseases: Systemic lupus erythematosus, systemic sclerosis, Sjögren's syndrome, dermatomyositis, adult-onset Still's disease
- Embolic diseases: Cholesterol emboli, atrial myxoma
- Infections: Syphilis, tuberculosis, mycoplasma pneumonia, brucellosis, streptococcemia, meningococcemia, hepatitis C, endocarditis, parvovirus B19
- Neurologic diseases: Reflex and sympathetic dystrophy, Sneddon's syndrome [2]

7. What is the etiology, clinical, and histopathologic manifestations of linear IgA vesiculobullous dermatosis?

Linear IgA vesiculobullous dermatosis is a rare autoimmune subepidermal vesiculo-bullous disease caused by IgA autoantibodies directed against different antigens of the basement membrane zone of the skin and/or mucosae. It is often idiopathic but also secondary to drugs (vancomycin is the most commonly implicated

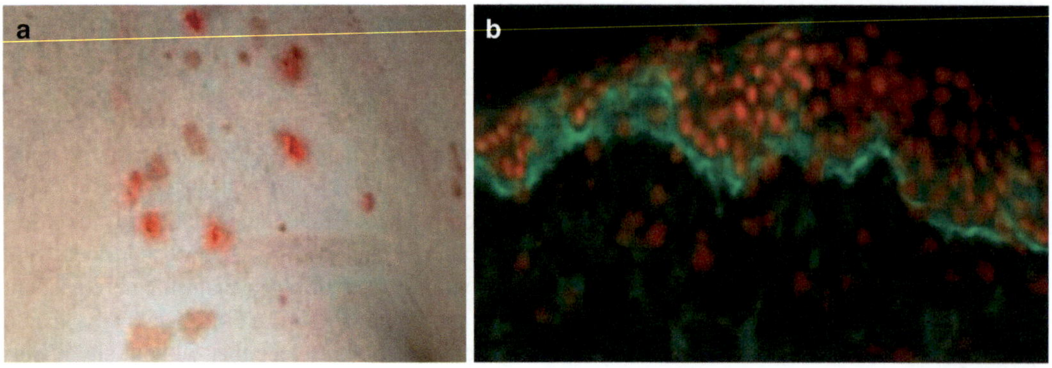

Fig. 10.4 (**a**) Blistering pruritic rash on an erythroid base over the extremities of a 42-year-old woman with Sjögren's syndrome. (**b**) Direct immunofluorescence microscopy of skin biopsy specimens demonstrates linear deposits of IgA along the basement membrane zone (*Reproduced from Mavragani CP et al. 2013*) [3]

drug), malignancy, infections, systemic autoimmune diseases, and inflammatory bowel diseases. It affects young children and adults with varying symptomatology. Papulovesicular lesions or larger bullae with an erythematous base develop in children, mostly in the lower abdomen, perineal area, and inner thighs while in adults the extensor surfaces (Fig. 10.4a), trunk, buttocks, and face are mainly affected. The hands, and feet are rarely involved, while mucous membranes may be involved with the oral cavity and the eyes being the most commonly affected. Direct immunofluorescence microscopy of skin biopsy specimens demonstrates linear deposits of IgA along the basement membrane (Fig. 10.4b) [3].

8. What are the causes of erythema nodosum? Name them according to their incidence

Erythema nodosum is a type of panniculitis, an inflammatory disorder affecting subcutaneous fat. It manifests as tender, erythematous, subcutaneous nodules that are typically located symmetrically on the anterior surface of the lower extremities. Causes of erythema nodosum according to incidence are: idiopathic (60–70%), streptococcal pharyngitis, drugs (penicillin, oral contraceptives, and sulfonamides), infectious diseases (hepatitis C, tuberculosis, leprosy, syphilis, yersinia, Epstein-Barr virus infection, and cat-scratch disease), inflammatory bowel disease, Behçet's disease, sarcoidosis, systemic lupus erythematosus, and malignancy (lymphoma, carcinoid, and pancreatic cancer) [4].

9. What are the clinicopathologic features and therapy of Weber-Christian panniculitis (WCP)?

WCP affects primarily women. The lesions appear as bilateral, symmetrical, painful subcutaneous nodules, and are more frequently seen on the lower legs (Fig 10.5a) but they can develop on the upper back, abdominal area, breasts, face, and buttocks. Very infrequently the nodules can develop on the mesentery of the small or large bowel, the lungs, the heart or other internal organs and produce a systemic disease with poor prognosis. There are usually associated constitutional symptoms like fever, malaise arthralgias, and myalgias. Clinical course is characterized by exacerbations and remissions. There are no specific laboratory tests to aim the diagnosis, but biopsy of the nodule will confirm the diagnosis (Fig 10.5b). A large and deep incisional biopsy of early lesions is preferred as late-stage lesions show non-specific findings. Treatment of WCP is empirical. Corticosteroids along with steroid-sparing agents like cyclosporine-A, methotrexate, leflunomide, azathioprine, mycophenolate mofetil,

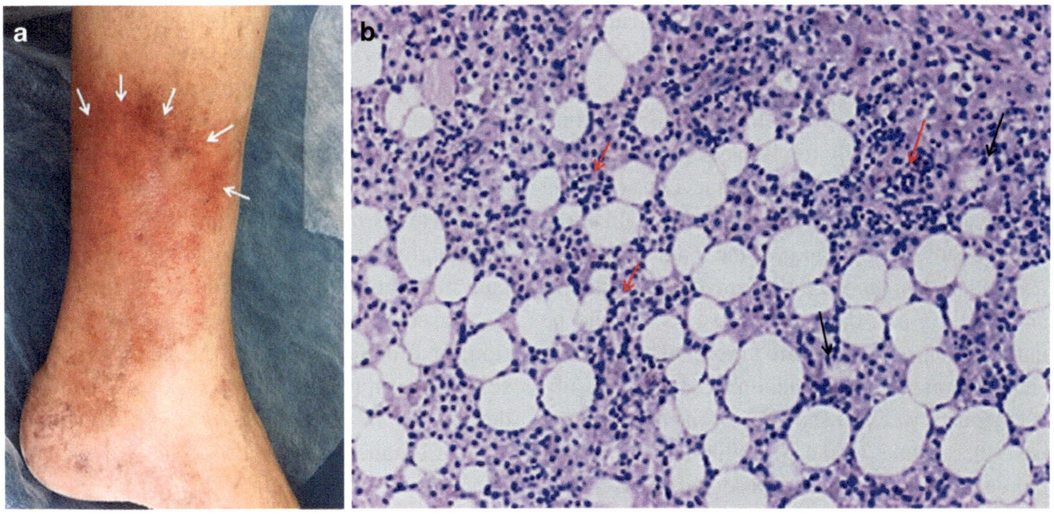

Fig. 10.5 (**a**) A 45-year-old woman with a well-demarcated brownish sunken skin area on the medial aspect of her left tibia. The upper part of the lesion was hot and indurated (arrows) while the rest was indented most probably due to fat necrosis. (**b**) Histology (H&E × 40) revealed panniculitis of the subcutis with a dense histio-lymphocytic infiltrate surrounding fat cells showing different stages of degeneration (red arrows) and scattered foamy cells (black arrows), in the absence of vasculitis, findings supporting the diagnosis of Weber-Christian disease (relapsing febrile nodular non-suppurative panniculitis)

or even cyclophosphamide have been successful in diminishing the disease relapses or even completely suppress the disease process [5].

10. What is the pancreatitis, panniculitis, and polyarthritis (PPP) syndrome?

PPP syndrome is a combination of extra-pancreatic manifestations occurring in some patients with pancreatitis. The pathogenesis is unknown; nevertheless, it is postulated to be due to augmented secretion of pancreatic enzymes in the circulation leading to systemic fat necrosis, especially in subcutaneous fat tissue (panniculitis) as well as in bones and joints (polyarthritis). Clinical manifestations include pancreatitis (most commonly due to pancreas carcinoma, usually with mild abdominal symptoms), arthritis (usually ankles and knees) with non-inflammatory and creamy synovial fluid (lipid droplets that give the creamy appearance stain with Sudan black), red and tender nodules on the extremities (lobular panniculitis with fat necrosis), eosinophilia, febrile pleuropericarditis, and osteolytic bone lesions. Amylase, lipase, and trypsin are elevated in the serum [6].

11. What is hidradenitis suppurativa?

Chronic recurrent hidradenitis (hidradenitis suppurativa) is an inflammatory skin disease affecting the apocrine glands of the skin mainly in the areas of the axillae, inframammary folds, groin, and perineum. It is characterized by painful groups of small skin abscesses which can persist for years, are difficult to heal, and often lead to sinus tracts and scar formation. Flares are triggered by sweating, stress, warm/humid environment, and hormonal changes. Genetic predisposition has been identified and autoimmune reactivity plays a significant role.

12. Is the risk of inflammatory arthritis increased in patients with newly diagnosed hidradenitis suppurativa?

A follow-up study of a large cohort of patients with hidradenitis suppurativa (HS) showed an increased risk of ankylosing spondylitis, psoriatic arthritis, and rheumatoid arthritis in patients with HS compared to those without HS. However, the incidence of any inflammatory arthritis was low (2 and 6 additional arthritis cases per 10,000 patients with HS per 1.5 years) [7].

13. What is the treatment of hidradenitis suppurativa?

For mild cases, topical clindamycin (1% solution or gel twice daily for 12 weeks) or resorcinol (15%) have proven effective. Tetracycline (500 mg p.o. twice daily for 10 weeks) is used in more widespread disease, and if the patient fails to respond, combination of clindamycin and rifampicin (600 mg p.o. daily for 12 weeks) should be initiated. In patients who are unresponsive or intolerant to oral antibiotics, adalimumab (40 mg subcutaneously weekly) should be considered as the next therapeutic modality. Infliximab (5 mg/kg intravenously) should be considered as a second-line option treatment, only after failure of adalimumab. Surgical intervention should be applied for particular cases. In addition to pharmaceutical treatment, all patients should be advised to lose weight, keep the skin clean to reduce odor and discontinue tobacco smoking [8].

14. Which pathologic conditions present with flat and which with raised purpura? Provide the pathogenic mechanisms

Purpura is caused by extravasation of blood into the skin or mucous membranes producing red-purple lesions. It can be palpable/raised or non-palpable/flat and typically non-blanching upon pressure. *Flat purpura* can be subdivided into petechiae (small lesions <3 mm) and ecchymoses (larger lesions >3 mm). It occurs either when the hydrostatic pressure inside the capillaries is increased as in the case of hypergammaglobulinemia (Waldenström's hypergammaglobulinemic purpura), because of decreased or altered platelet formation, destruction, or function, or when the integrity of vessels is disrupted as in the case of vitamin C deficiency. In contrast, *palpable purpura* is a sign of cutaneous vasculitis. The major causes of small-vessel vasculitis leading to palpable purpura are cryoglobulinemic purpura, IgA vasculitis, and leukocytoclastic vasculitis.

15. Which conditions can present with the clinical picture resembling livedoid vasculopathy (atrophie blanche)?

Livedoid vasculopathy (LV) is a vasculopathy of middle-aged women, presenting as an occlusive disorder of the capillary microcirculation leading to cutaneous ischemia and infarction (Fig. 10.6a). It can be idiopathic or secondary. The literature on LV presents a confusing picture

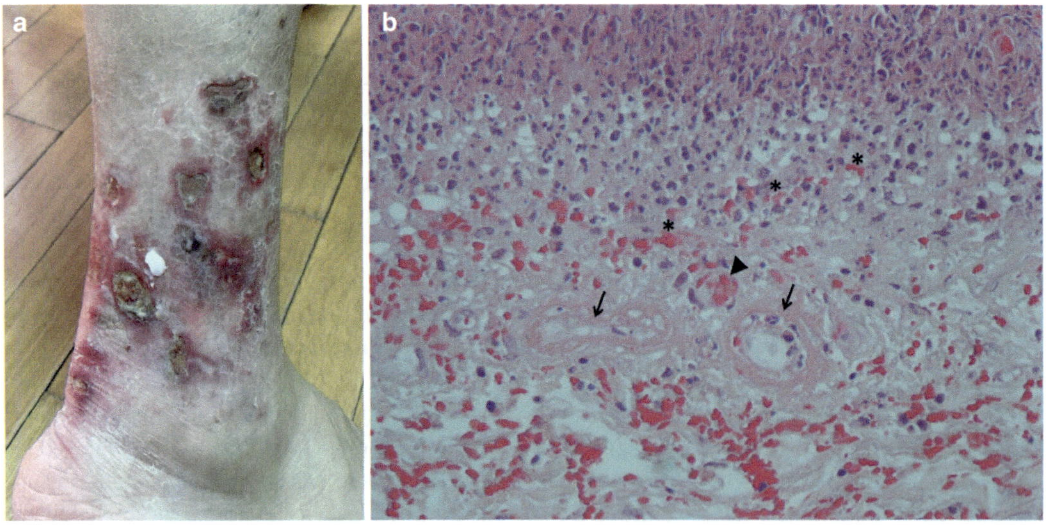

Fig. 10.6 Livedoid vasculopathy: (**a**) multiple, painful, deep, well-demarcated ulcers on a livedoid base, surrounded by atrophic white-ivory skin in the lower legs in a 55-year old. (**b**) Skin biopsy of the ulcers (HE × 400) showed in the mid-dermis segmental thickening of vessel wall containing fibrin material (black arrows), vessel occlusion with hyaline microthrombi (arrowhead), and extravasated erythrocytes (asterisks) without features of inflammation (*Reproduced from Zampeli E et al. 2017*) [9]

regarding its causes, pathogenesis, and treatment. Differential diagnosis should include cutaneous small-vessel vasculitis (leukocytoclastic vasculitis), cutaneous polyarteritis nodosa, antiphospholipid syndrome, chronic venous stasis, pyoderma gangrenosum, factitious dermatitis, pseudo-Kaposi sarcoma and malignant atrophic papulosis, inherited or acquired thrombophilias, chronic myelogenous leukemia, cryoglobulinemia, and heavy-chain disease [9].

16. Which are the cutaneous histopathologic lesions of livedoid vasculopathy?

Histology of livedoid vasculopathy (Fig. 10.6b) typically reveals occlusion by fibrin thrombi of capillary vessels in the upper and middle dermis as well as fibrinoid degeneration of the vessel walls in the sense of a vasculopathy. In contrast to primary vasculitis, only a slight or no perivascular inflammatory infiltrate is found initially, and later the secondary inflammation is less prominent. Hyalinization of the dermis and capillary walls characterizes livedoid vasculopathy [9].

17. What is the pathogenetic mechanism of relapsing polychondritis?

The main hypothesis on the pathophysiology of relapsing polychondritis (RP) is an autoimmune reaction initially directed against the cartilage, later on spreading to non-cartilaginous tissues. Autoantibodies against cartilage and collagen (mostly type II) have been found in patients with RP, yet their diagnostic value is extremely poor, since they are found in a limited number of RP patients and can also be found in patients with other autoimmune diseases.

18. Which are the clinical manifestations of relapsing polychondritis?

Relapsing polychondritis (RP) is an infrequent autoimmune systemic disease manifesting with relapsing inflammation of cartilaginous tissues which can result in their deformity. The typical clinical presentation of RP is a combination of chondritis (auricular, nasal, laryngeal, tracheal, and cartilaginous bronchi)—which is necessary for the diagnosis—with inflammation of other proteoglycan-rich tissues such as the eyes, heart valves, blood vessels, external or inner ears. The most common and suggestive feature of the disease is chondritis of the pinna of the ear (Fig. 10.7a), which presents in up to 90% of patients during the disease course. Chondritis can be acute, subacute, or chronic and unilateral or bilateral. In the acute presentation, the pinna of the ear (helix, antihelix, tragus, antitragus, and external auditory canal) is inflamed, swollen, painful, and red. Typically, the inflammation spares the ear lobe, which does not contain cartilage. The external auditory canal may be obstructed by the inflammatory infiltrate or collapsed, leading to conductive hearing loss and/or recurrent otitis externa. The inflammation may involve surrounding retroauricular soft tissues and could be sometimes associated with lymphadenopathy. Patients cannot press their ear on the telephone handset or the pillow. The inflammation lasts for a couple of days to a few weeks and often resolves spontaneously. Complications include loss of the auricular cartilage resulting in a floppy distorted pinna, giving the appearance of a "cauliflower ear" (Fig. 10.7b). On the other hand, the pinna can also become thickened with calcification and deformity of the cartilaginous structure. Arthritis (Fig. 10.7c) and constitutional symptoms, including fatigue, weight loss, and unexplained prolonged fever, may be the presenting symptoms of RP [10].

19. Which autoimmune or autoinflammatory conditions affect the sclera and produce episcleritis or scleritis?

Episcleritis: Rheumatoid arthritis, inflammatory bowel disease, ANCA-associated vasculitis

Scleritis: Rheumatoid arthritis, granulomatosis with polyangiitis (Wegener's granulomatosis), relapsing polychondritis, systemic lupus erythematosus, inflammatory bowel disease, seronegative spondyloarthritis

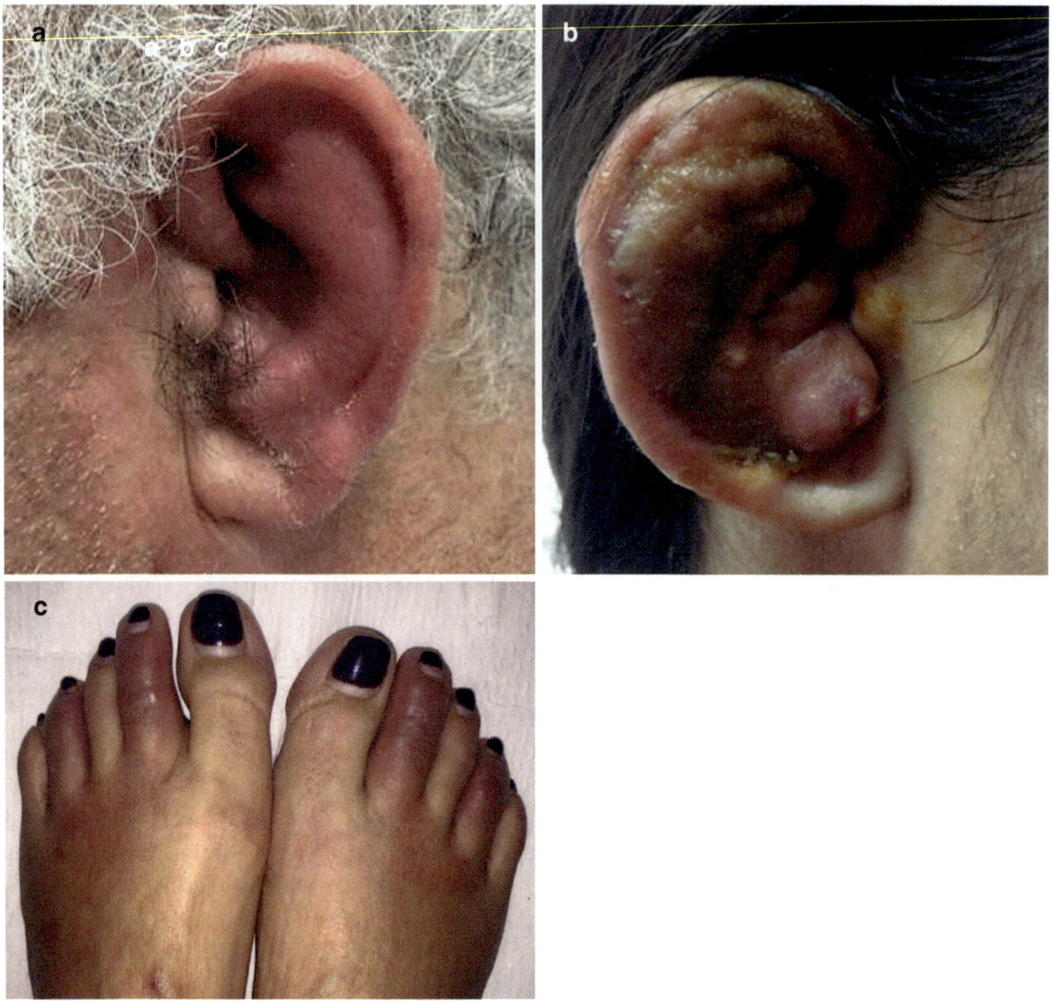

Fig. 10.7 (**a**) Relapsing polychondritis: Recurrent bouts of erythematous swelling of the ear pinna accompanied by hoarseness of voice and scleritis in a 65-year-old male with relapsing polychondritis. (**b**) A 33-year-old woman with relapsing polychondritis had a 5 months long history of untreated right ear auricle inflammation, which resulted in an inflamed and deformed, like a cauliflower, right ear auricle (**c**) at presentation erythematous, painful and swollen second and fourth toes of the left foot were evident. *(b and c reproduced from Zampeli E et al. 2018)* [10]

20. Which are the fundoscopic findings in a patient with Ehlers-Danlos?

Angioid streaks, retinal detachment, carotid-cavernous sinus fistula, lens subluxation, keratoconus, and macular degeneration.

21. In which medical conditions angioid streaks are seen in the funduscopic examination?

Angioid streaks are fine, irregular lines deep to the retina arranged in a radiating fashion resulting from pathological breaks in Bruch's membrane. Angioid streaks may be idiopathic or associated with underlying systemic illnesses, such as *pseudoxanthoma elasticum*, Paget's disease, sickle cell disease, and Ehlers-Danlos syndrome.

22. In which rheumatic disorders hypopyon can be seen?

Hypopyon is the presence of inflammatory cell exudate in the anterior eye chamber. Hypopyon is commonly seen in HLA-B27 positive patients who develop acute anterior uveitis. It is also seen in 20% of patients with Bechet's disease and is a poor prognostic sign, because it is frequently associated with retinal involvement.

23. Which ophthalmological manifestations can be induced from rheumatic disorders or from their therapeutic agents?

The most common ocular manifestations of rheumatic diseases include keratoconjunctivitis sicca, anterior uveitis, epi- and/or scleritis, diffuse vitritis, papillitis, and retinal vasculitis. Cystoid macular edema and epiretinal membrane are common causes of visual impairment. Another cause of sudden vision loss is involvement of the ophthalmic artery in giant cell arteritis, which can be its sole presenting clinical manifestation. The most serious ophthalmologic complications of the inherited connective tissue disorders are cataract or lens subluxation. The most significant ophthalmologic complications from drug side-effects used in the therapy of rheumatic disorders is maculopathy induced by antimalarial agents and cataract by corticosteroids.

24. Which conditions are responsible for Bulls' eye retinopathy?

Bull's eye retinopathy refers to a maculopathy. Bull's eye retinopathy can be seen in inherited retinal conditions, Alport syndrome, or due to hydroxychloroquine (HCQ) toxicity. HCQ acts by raising lysosomal pH. When this happens in the retinal pigment epithelium cells, the lysosomal activity slows down and lipofuscin builds up in the subretinal space. This eventually exerts cytotoxic effects on retinal pigmented epithelium causing destruction of macular rods and cones with sparing of foveal cones producing a pale ring-shaped, pattern of damage around the darker area of macula on retinal examination giving the typical bull's eye appearance. The patient may present blurred vision, central scotomas, photophobia, poor color vision, and diminished visual acuity. HCQ should be discontinued, but since it has a long half-life (about 1 month) maculopathy continues even after discontinuation of the medication.

25. What are the clinical symptoms of uveitis?

Uveitis can be anterior, intermediate, or posterior. Anterior uveitis is acute in onset. Pain, redness, and photophobia are the cardinal symptoms along with a variable degree of visual acuity loss. In intermediate uveitis patients usually complain of blurred vision with floaters and a distortion of central vision. There is no pain or photophobia. In posterior uveitis, the onset is usually subacute, with blurry vision, floaters, and scotomata being the main patient's complaints. The external eye has no signs of inflammation and pain and photophobia are absent [11].

26. Which rheumatic diseases can be associated with uveitis?

- Spondyloarthropathies: in around 40% of patients with ankylosing spondylitis, most commonly associated with unilateral anterior uveitis of acute onset and recurrent
- Psoriatic arthritis and inflammatory bowel disease-related inflammatory arthritis: most commonly associated with bilateral, chronic anterior uveitis of subacute onset
- Juvenile idiopathic arthritis: most commonly associated with bilateral anterior uveitis of subacute onset
- Reactive arthritis: usually mild conjunctivitis is the classical eye manifestation, but sudden-onset unilateral anterior uveitis is also well described
- Sarcoidosis: bilateral anterior, posterior or intermediate and in 90% chronic
- Behçet's disease: in 60–80% of patients with Behçet's disease, usually bilateral and recurrent, may present as panuveitis of acute onset, often severe with associated retinal vasculitis
- Systemic lupus erythematosus and Sjögren's syndrome: most commonly associated with mild anterior uveitis [11]

  Medications do not usually cause uveitis, but possible culprits include intravenous bisphosphonates [12], TNF inhibitors [13], checkpoint inhibitors [14], and several antibiotics [15]

27. What is the etiology and clinical manifestations of autoimmune inner ear disease (AIED)?

To date, the etiology of the AIED is still not well understood. Many antigens in the inner ear and possibly in the endolymphatic sac have been recognized as possible AIED targets. Among those, cochlin, an extracellular matrix protein specifically present in the inner ear, has been proposed as a possible cochlear antigen involved in the pathogenetic mechanism of AIED. The clinical expression of AIED is bilateral and mostly asymmetrical sensorineural hearing loss, characterized by a rapidly progressive onset over weeks or months (usually progressively developing between 3 and 90 days), which typically benefits from a steroid and immunosuppressive therapy. In about 50% of the AIED patients, hearing loss is also associated with vestibular symptoms, such as imbalance and motion intolerance, ataxia, and positional or episodic vertigo. In up to 30% of cases, AIED is secondary to systemic autoimmune disease [16].

28. In which autoimmune disorders the inner ear can be affected?

- Systemic lupus erythematosus
- Sjögren's syndrome
- Rheumatoid arthritis
- Seronegative spondyloarthritis
- Inflammatory bowel diseases
- Cogan syndrome
- Systemic vasculitis (ANCA-associated, polyarteritis nodosa)
- Behçet's disease
- Antiphospholipid syndrome
- Relapsing polychondritis [17]

References

1. Confino-Cohen R, Chodick G, Shalev V, Leshno M, Kimhi O, Goldberg A. Chronic urticaria and autoimmunity: associations found in a large population study. J Allergy Clin Immunol. 2012;129:1307–13.
2. Sangle SR, D'Cruz DP. Livedo reticularis: an enigma. Isr Med Assoc J. 2015;17:104–7.
3. Mavragani CP, Asvesti K, Moutsopoulos HM. Linear IgA dermatosis in a patient with primary Sjögren's syndrome. Rheumatology (Oxford). 2013;52:403–4 .
4. Psychos DN, Voulgari PV, Skopouli FN, Drosos AA, Moutsopoulos HM. Erythema nodosum: the underlying conditions. Clin Rheumatol. 2000;19:212–6.
5. Zheng W, Song W, Wu Q, et al. Analysis of the clinical characteristics of thirteen patients with Weber-Christian panniculitis. Clin Rheumatol. 2019;38:3635–41.
6. Arbeláez-Cortés A, Vanegas-García AL, Restrepo-Escobar M, Correa-Londoño LA, González-Naranjo LA. Polyarthritis and pancreatic panniculitis associated with pancreatic carcinoma: review of the literature. J Clin Rheumatol. 2014;20:433–6.
7. Schneeweiss MC, Kim SC, Schneeweiss S, et al. Risk of inflammatory arthritis after a new diagnosis of Hidradenitis Suppurativa. JAMA Dermatol. 2020;156:342–5.
8. Saunte DML, Jemec GBE. Hidradenitis Suppurativa: advances in diagnosis and treatment. JAMA. 2017;318:2019–32.
9. Zampeli E, Moutsopoulos HM. Livedoid vasculopathy. Arthritis Rheumatol. 2017;69:2096.
10. Zampeli E, Moutsopoulos HM. Relapsing polychondritis: a diagnosis not to be missed. Rheumatology (Oxford). 2018;57:1768.
11. Rosenbaum JT, Dick AD. The eyes have it: a Rheumatologist's view of uveitis. Arthritis Rheumatol. 2018;70:1533–43.
12. Patel DV, Horne A, House M, Reid IR, McGhee CN. The incidence of acute anterior uveitis after intravenous zoledronate. Ophthalmology. 2013;120:773–6.
13. Lim LL, Fraunfelder FW, Rosenbaum JT. Do tumor necrosis factor inhibitors cause uveitis? A registry-based study. Arthritis Rheum. 2007;56:3248–52.
14. Conrady CD, Larochelle M, Pecen P, Palestine A, Shakoor A, Singh A. Checkpoint inhibitor-induced uveitis: a case series. Graefes Arch Clin Exp Ophthalmol. 2018;256:187–91.

15. Eadie B, Etminan M, Mikelberg FS. Risk for uveitis with oral Moxifloxacin: a comparative safety study. JAMA Ophthalmol. 2015;133:81–4.
16. Strum D, Kim S, Shim T, Monfared A. An update on autoimmune inner ear disease: a systematic review of pharmacotherapy. Am J Otolaryngol. 2020;41:102310.
17. Stone JH, Francis HW. Immune-mediated inner ear disease. Curr Opin Rheumatol. 2000;12:32–40.

Suggested Reading

18. Agarwal A, Sepah YJ, Nguyen QD. Ocular manifestations of systemic autoimmune diseases. In: Ikezu T, Gendelman H, editors. Neuroimmune pharmacology. Cham: Springer; 2017.
19. Griffiths C, Barker J, Bleiker T, Chalmers R, Creamer D, editors. Rook's textbook of dermatology, vol. 4. 9th ed: Wiley-Blackwell; 2016.

Rheumatic Disorders Associated with Metabolic, Endocrine, and Hematological Diseases

11

Haralampos M. Moutsopoulos
and Evangelia Zampeli

Abstract

The interconnection of metabolic/endocrine disorders and autoimmune/rheumatic diseases is multifaceted. Metabolic and endocrine diseases can be autoimmune in nature (e.g., type I diabetes mellitus, Graves' disease, and Hashimoto's thyroiditis). On the other hand, many metabolic/endocrine disorders present with musculoskeletal manifestations that can mimic a rheumatic disease. Patients with hyperlipidemias and metabolic syndrome can present with gout, migratory arthritis, Achilles tendinitis, and rotator cuff syndrome. Hyperuricemia, gout, and calcium pyrophosphate crystal deposition disease (pseudogout) can be found in patients with primary hyperparathyroidism. A well-documented association between diabetes mellitus and several rheumatic syndromes exists, with severity of the former determining the extent of rheumatic manifestations. Carpal tunnel syndrome, trigger fingers, Dupuytren's contractures, diabetic cheiroarthropathy, diffuse idiopathic skeletal hyperostosis, shoulder bursitis, and neuropathic arthropathy are some of the musculoskeletal manifestations associated with diabetes. In patients with hyperthyroidism, rheumatic manifestations include osteoporosis, painless proximal muscle weakness, thyroid acropathy, and adhesive shoulder capsulitis. In patients with autoimmune thyroiditis, rheumatic manifestations (osteoarthritis, fibromyalgia, Raynaud's phenomenon, sicca symptoms, and arthritis) frequently occur even in the absence of overt thyroid dysfunction. On the other hand, patients with systemic autoimmune diseases such as rheumatoid arthritis, polymyalgia rheumatica, Sjögren's syndrome, systemic lupus erythematosus, and scleroderma present an increased prevalence of thyroid autoimmune disease. Finally, corticosteroids, which are commonly used in the treatment of various autoimmune disorders, can be an iatrogenic cause of endocrine disorders, such as diabetes mellitus, steroid myopathy, and Cushing's disease.

Hemochromatosis, hemophilia, sickle cell disease, thalassemia, leukemia, lymphoma, myelodysplastic syndromes, multiple myeloma, and cryoglobulinemia may all present with a great variety of autoimmune and rheumatic manifestations.

H. M. Moutsopoulos (✉)
Athens Academy, Athens, Greece
e-mail: hmoutsop@med.uoa.gr

E. Zampeli
Bioclinic General Hospital of Athens and Institute for Autoimmune Systemic and Neurological Disorders, Athens, Greece
e-mail: ezampeli@bioclinic.gr

H. M. Moutsopoulos, E. Zampeli (eds.), *Immunology and Rheumatology in Questions*,
https://doi.org/10.1007/978-3-030-56670-8_11

1. **Which are the risk factors associated with increased serum uric acid and gout ?**

- Genetic predisposition (family history)
- Gender and age (more common in men than in women, more common in adults than in children)
- Obesity
- Increased alcohol consumption
- Purine-rich diet (anchovies, sardines, scallops, herring, liver, kidneys, asparagus, mushrooms, dried beans, and peas)
- Comorbidities: hypertension, diabetes, hyperlipidemia, and metabolic syndrome
- Renal insufficiency
- Medications (diuretics, salicylate-containing drugs, cyclosporine-A, niacin, and levodopa)

2. **Which conditions predispose to acute gout attacks?**

Trauma, binge alcohol drinking, consumption of food containing high amounts of purines, intense-stressful life events.

3. **Which are the risk factors associated with calcium pyrophosphate deposition disease (CPPD, pseudogout)?**

- Older females, after 60 years old with:
- Hyperparathyroidism
- Gout, osteoarthritis, rheumatoid arthritis, and hemochromatosis
- Osteoporosis
- Hypomagnesemia and calcium supplementation
- Chronic kidney disease

4. **Which is the easiest and cheap test to diagnose gout and pseudogout?**

Synovial fluid aspiration and detection of monosodium urate (gout) and calcium pyrophosphate (pseudogout) crystals respectively remains the gold standard for diagnosis. In 30% of patients with pseudogout, knee X-ray can reveal chondrocalcinosis (calcification of articular fibrocartilage as punctate or linear densities in the fibrocartilaginous menisci of the knee) (Fig. 11.1).

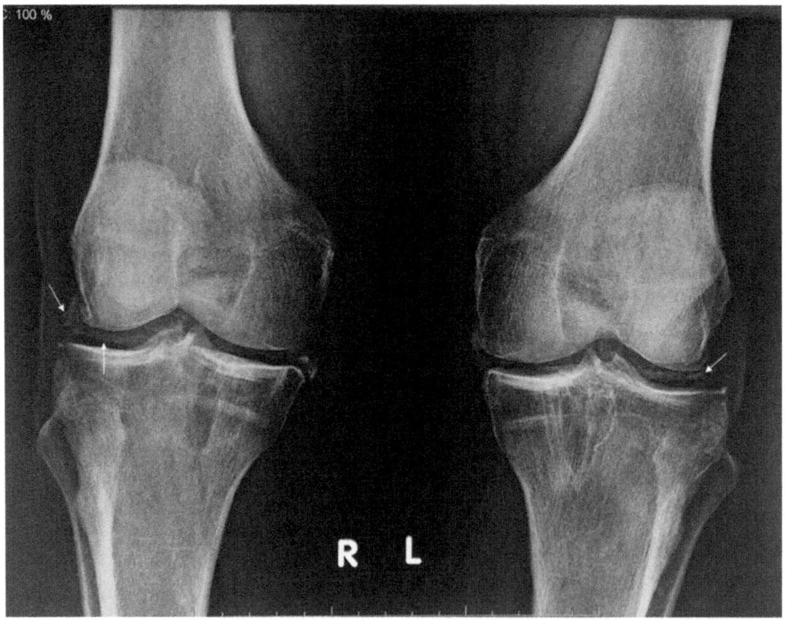

Fig. 11.1 Pseudogout (calcium pyrophosphate dihydrate crystal deposition disease): Knee X-ray showing degenerative changes and chondrocalcinosis (arrows) in a 60-year-old man with pseudogout

5. Which is the birefringence difference among monosodium urate and calcium pyrophosphate crystals?

Monosodium urate crystals are typically needle-shaped and negatively birefringent. On polarized microscopy, they appear yellow. Calcium pyrophosphate crystals are bright rhomboid-shaped crystals with weakly positive birefringence. They appear blue when viewed under polarized light.

6. Which are the commonly affected joints from gout and which from pseudogout?

Gout: Commonly affected joints are the first metatarsophalangeal joints (Fig. 11.2), the midfoot, ankle, heel, and the knee. In chronically untreated patients, the following joints can be also affected: the elbow, wrist, and finger joints. Any other joint, especially with underlying osteoarthritis can be affected. Besides the joints, other periarticular structures such as tendons and bursae may also be involved.

Pseudogout: Commonly affected joints are the knees (Fig. 11.1), wrists, and less often the hips, shoulders, elbows, finger joints, toes, and ankles. Jaccoud's arthropathy can occur in patients with pseudogout.

7. In which medical conditions cholesterol crystals can be seen and in which tissues can they be found?

Cholesterol crystals are often found in the synovial fluid of patients with rheumatoid arthritis (RA), systemic lupus erythematosus, osteoarthritis, hyperlipidemia, and chronic tophaceous gout. Defective synovial fluid drainage, local destruction, increased permeability of synovial membrane, and intraarticular bleeding are possible etiologies for their presence. They are also found in xanthomas, calcinosis cutis, rheumatoid nodules, and pleural and pericardial effusions due to RA, tuberculosis, or malignancy. Cholesterol crystals are best identified by polarized light microscopy but may also be seen with ordinary light microscopy.

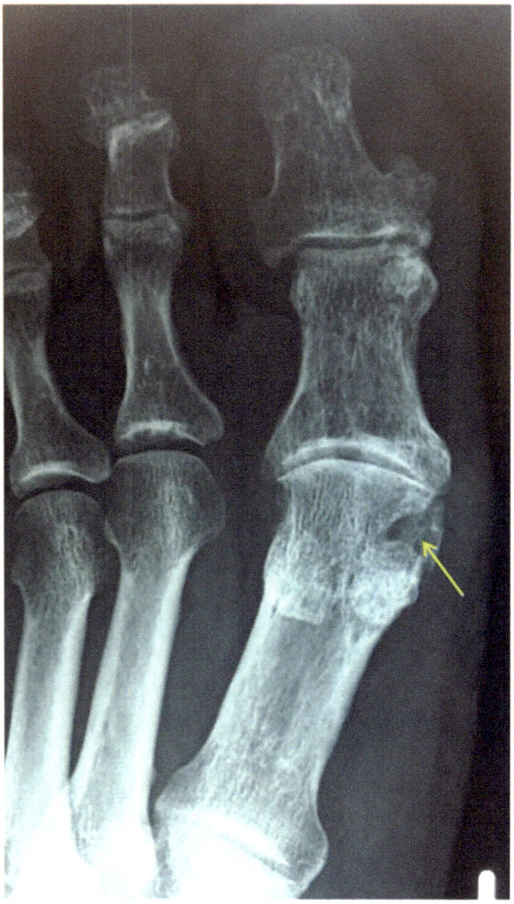

Fig. 11.2 Gout: Foot X-ray showing a major erosive, punched-out lesion on the first metatarsal bone (arrow) in a 56-year-old male with recurrent gout attacks (podagra)

8. Which are the musculoskeletal manifestations seen in diabetic patients?

- Pseudosclerodactyly: Thickened, waxy skin changes are most apparent in the fingers
- Flexor tenosynovitis of the hands (trigger fingers) is quite frequently seen in diabetic patients
- Dupuytren's contractures occur in around 15% of diabetics
- Carpal tunnel syndrome is seen in 20% of diabetics
- Diabetic stiff hand syndrome (diabetic cheiroarthropathy). The fingers are commonly affected, with stiffness, limited movement, and contractures. Flexion contractures of the proximal and distal interphalangeal joints

result in the "prayer sign," an inability to close the gap between opposed palms and fingers. It is associated with advanced disease and diabetic microvascular disease elsewhere
- Periarthritis: Adhesive capsulitis of the shoulder is commonly seen in diabetic patients
- Diffuse idiopathic skeletal hyperostosis (DISH) is seen in one out of ten diabetic patients
- Shoulder bursitis, usually bilateral, is more common in females with insulin-dependent diabetes
- Neuropathic arthropathy (Charcot joint) occurs in 1% of diabetics (both type I and type II) and is equally frequent in males and females. These patients have usually long-standing, poorly controlled diabetes complicated by diabetic peripheral neuropathy. It affects the feet, ankles, and knees
- Diabetic amyotrophy is an asymmetric ischemic myopathy presenting with pain and dysesthesia of the proximal muscles of the pelvis and lower limbs leading to muscle wasting and unsteady gait. The shoulder girdle muscles can also be involved. It usually appears in long-standing diabetes

9. Which rheumatic manifestations have been associated with hyperparathyroidism?

Rheumatic manifestations are rarely seen in patients with hyperparathyroidism. Hyperuricemia, gout, and calcium pyrophosphate crystal deposition disease (CPPD, pseudogout) have been described to be associated with primary hyperparathyroidism. Pseudogout, a result of calcium pyrophosphate crystal deposition in the cartilaginous tissues of the joints, has been reported after successful parathyroid surgery, though the mechanism of this association is unclear. In severe long-standing primary hyperparathyroidism osteitis fibrosa cystica is the characteristic sequelae. The excessive amount of circulating parathyroid hormone leads to increased osteoclast activity which in turn produces bone resorption. The bones are weakened as their calcified supporting structures are replaced with fibrous tissue. Radiolucent cystic-like lesions composed of fibrous tissue and decomposing blood, known as brown tumors, may form leading to spontaneous bone fractures which imitate malignancies. The key laboratory finding which differentiates osteitis fibrosa cystica from malignancies (metastatic carcinoma, bone cysts, osteosarcoma, and especially giant-cell tumor) are the elevated serum levels of parathyroid hormone. Diffuse osteopenia is common and the bones have a moth-eaten appearance. The softened bones which break easily release calcium from the bone into the circulation. Excess calcium in the blood leads to kidney stone formation and nonspecific manifestations such as anorexia and weight loss. Nevertheless, nowadays overt rheumatic manifestations associated with hyperparathyroidism are mainly of historical meaning and not part of the clinical spectrum of contemporary disease [1].

10. Which are the musculoskeletal manifestations of hyperthyroidism?

- Osteoporosis (most common musculoskeletal manifestation)
- Thyroid acropathy is a rare complication of Graves' disease. It usually occurs after the patient becomes euthyroid and presents with soft tissue swelling of the hands, digital clubbing, and periostitis particularly of the metacarpal and phalangeal bones. X-rays can reveal periosteal reaction along the shafts of these bones. Patients with Graves' disease complicated with acropathy usually present additionally with ophthalmopathy and pretibial myxedema
- Painless proximal muscle weakness
- Adhesive capsulitis of the shoulders [2, 3]

11. Which are the musculoskeletal manifestations of hypothyroidism?

- Hypothyroid arthropathy: Knees, hand joints, and wrists are more commonly involved; non-inflammatory effusions can occur in these joints
- Muscular pain and stiffness of extremities which can present as true myopathy in prolonged or severely hypothyroid patients

- Carpal tunnel syndrome
- Muscle cramps

12. Which musculoskeletal manifestations are associated with hyperlipidemias?

- Gout
- Tendon xanthomas
- Achilles tendinitis
- Transient Achilles tendon pain
- Oligoarthritis and migratory polyarthritis
- Osteoarthritis
- Rotator cuff syndrome
- Epicondylitis
- Meniscal tears

13. Which musculoskeletal manifestations are seen in patients with acromegaly?

Acromegaly results from the oversecretion of growth hormone and subsequent secretion of insulin-like growth factor 1. Both are produced from a pituitary tumor.

In patients with acromegaly, arthropathy is a common manifestation. It can be an early disease manifestation, affecting peripheral as well as axial joints (cervical and lumbosacral spine). The peripheral joints affected in acromegalic patients are the hips, shoulders, knees, hands, and elbows. Radiographic changes, in the early phase of the disease, show squaring of the enlarged terminal phalanges, widening of the joint space, and periarticular soft tissue hypertrophy. In the later phases, radiographic changes include narrowing of the joint space, osteophyte formation, calcification, and enlargement of the vertebral bodies. Other musculoskeletal manifestations of acromegaly include carpal tunnel syndrome, proximal myopathy, fibromyalgia, and Raynaud's phenomenon.

14. What are the causes and symptoms of osteomalacia?

Osteomalacia is due to impaired bone metabolism and is caused either from insufficient calcium absorption from the intestines or from vitamin D deficiency or resistance to vitamin D action and increased loss of phosphate from the kidneys. In adults, the disorder starts insidiously with pain in the lumbar area as well as in the thighs, and later the aches and pains spread to arms and ribs. Proximal muscle pain and weakness is another manifestation. Characteristics are the "waddling" gait of these patients and the development of spontaneous bone fractures.

15. Which medical conditions may lead to osteomalacia?

- Malnutrition and malabsorption
- Proximal renal tubular acidosis/chronic renal failure
- Hypophosphatemia
- Medications: Cholestyramine, phenytoin, phenobarbital, rifampicin, isoniazid, aluminum-containing antacids, saccharated ferric oxide, cadmium, and lead

16. Which are the differences between osteomalacia and osteoporosis ?

- Serum calcium is decreased in osteomalacia and normal in osteoporosis
- Serum phosphate is decreased in osteomalacia and normal in osteoporosis
- Serum alkaline phosphatase is elevated in osteomalacia and normal in osteoporosis
- Parathormone levels are elevated in osteomalacia and normal in osteoporosis
- Bone softening in osteomalacia and decreased bone mass in osteoporosis

17. What is hypertrophic osteoarthropathy?

Hypertrophic osteoarthropathy (HOA) is characterized by clubbing of the digits, non-inflammatory arthritis, and periostitis of tubular bones. It is classified into:

- Primary HOA (pachydermoperiostosis): with autosomal dominant inheritance, appears in childhood, affects mostly males, and is characterized by digital

  clubbing, pachyderma, coarse facial features, and hyperhidrosis
- Secondary HOA: is associated with intrathoracic malignant neoplasms in 90% of cases. It can also occur secondary to other malignancies (hepatic, gastrointestinal), chronic infections, Graves' disease, inflammatory bowel disease, and cirrhosis
- Platelet and endothelial cell activation with subsequent release of vascular endothelial growth factor and platelet-derived growth factor seem to play a role in the etiopathogenesis of HOA

18. Which hematologic conditions can present rheumatic manifestations?

- Hemophilia A (factor VIII deficiency) and hemophilia B (factor IX deficiency): X-linked coagulation disorders which in males can manifest with arthropathy due to recurrent hemarthroses that lead to accumulation of hemosiderin in the joints, resulting in synovial proliferative response, chronic joint inflammation, and finally cartilage degradation
- Sickle cell anemia: patients may demonstrate polyarthralgias (caused by juxta-articular/periarticular bone microinfarcts), noninflammatory arthritis of large joints, and osteonecrosis. In children with sickle cell anemia, dactylitis, also known as "hand-foot syndrome," can be the first manifestation of the disease. Dactylitis is often self-limited (mean duration of 2 weeks), yet relapsing episodes of pain and edema on the dorsum of the hand, feet, or both simultaneously, often accompanied by increased local temperature and erythema can occur. They rarely cause permanent joint sequelae. Initially, there is no evidence of joint lesions, but later chronic synovitis can develop
- Patients with thalassemia can manifest osteoporosis, pathological bone fractures, and epiphyseal deformities
- Hemochromatosis
- Paraproteinemias (multiple myeloma, Waldenström's macroglobulinemia, and amyloidosis) can present with either rheumatoid arthritis or asymmetric oligoarthritis

19. Which are the articular manifestations of hemochromatosis?

Hemochromatosis is an iron metabolism disorder characterized by excessive deposition of hemosiderin in different organs which can cause them damage and organ malfunction. It is due to a mutation in the hepcidin gene that controls the amount of iron which the body should absorb from food. Usually it begins in men at the age of 50–60 years and in women after 60 years of age. Arthropathy is not an uncommon manifestation in hemochromatosis patients. It presents with chronic indolent pain, joint stiffness, and bony enlargement but without significant signs of inflammation. Small and large joints can be affected symmetrically. A predilection of the disease is the second and third metacarpophalangeal joints. It becomes obvious when the fingers are extended and form the sign of victory "V." In addition, large (hips, knees, elbows) and sacroiliac joints can be affected. Overhanging osteophytes (hooked or beak-like osteophytes projecting from radial ends of 2nd and 3rd metacarpals), chondrocalcinosis (particularly in the knees) and subchondral sclerosis are the main radiologic findings. Acute arthritis from calcium pyrophosphate crystals can occur in hemochromatosis patients since they deposit in the cartilaginous parts of joints. Other organs that can be damaged in patients with hemochromatosis are the liver (cirrhosis), the pancreas (diabetes mellitus), the heart (congestive heart failure), the reproductive system (erectile dysfunction, menopause), and the skin (bronze or gray appearance).

20. Which are the autoimmune manifestations in patients with myelodysplastic syndromes?

Autoimmune disorders or manifestations occur in 10–15% of patients with myelodysplastic syndromes (MDS) [4]. Those include:

- Leukocytoclastic vasculitis
- Systemic vasculitis
- Relapsing polychondritis
- Non-infectious pulmonary infiltrates (interstitial lung disease and bronchiolitis obliterans with organizing pneumonia)
- Symmetric polyarticular synovitis
- Autoimmune cholangitis
- Hashimoto's thyroiditis
- Erythema nodosum
- Livedo reticularis
- Peripheral neuropathy
- Polymyalgia rheumatica

Common laboratory findings in this patient group include hypergammaglobulinemia, positive anti-nuclear antibodies (ANA), and elevated acute-phase proteins (erythrocyte sedimentation rate, C-reactive protein).

Patients with myelodysplasia expressing interferon regulatory factor-1 (IRF-1, a transcription factor involved in interferon signaling) have an increased incidence of autoimmune manifestations [4].

21. What are the etiology and clinical picture of cold agglutinin disease?

Cold agglutinin disease (CAD) is a type of autoimmune hemolytic anemia defined by the presence of cold agglutinins. Cold agglutinins are antibodies that recognize antigens on red blood cells (RBCs) at temperatures below normal body temperature. They can cause agglutination of the RBCs and extravascular hemolysis, resulting in anemia, typically without hemoglobinuria. The vast majority of cold agglutinins are monoclonal IgM kappa. IgM antibodies are pentameric, which allows binding of multiple RBCs by the same IgM molecule causing their agglutination. Cold agglutinin disease can be primary or most commonly secondary, to an underlying condition, such as infection (*Mycoplasma pneumoniae*), lymphoproliferative disorders (low-grade B-cell lymphoma, or lymphocytic lymphoma), systemic autoimmune disease or neoplasm. CAD manifests as acute or chronic hemolytic anemia. A cold environment or a concurrent infection may trigger or exacerbate the condition. Symptoms during hemolytic crises may include severe back and leg pain, headache, vomiting, diarrhea, dark urine, and hepatosplenomegaly. In patients with idiopathic CAD, few clinical symptoms, and mild anemia only avoidance of cold is required. In secondary cases, the underlying cause should be treated.

References

1. Misiorowski W, Czajka-Oraniec I, Kochman M, et al. Osteitis fibrosa cystica—a forgotten radiological feature of primary hyperparathyroidism. Endocrine. 2017;58:380–5.
2. Tagoe CE, Zezon A, Khattri S. Rheumatic manifestations of autoimmune thyroid disease: the other autoimmune disease. J Rheumatol. 2012;39:1125–9.
3. Nicholls JJ, Brassill MJ, Williams GR, Bassett JH. The skeletal consequences of thyrotoxicosis. J Endocrinol. 2012;213:209–21
4. Giannouli S, Kanellopoulou T, Voulgarelis M. Myelodysplasia and autoimmunity. Curr Opin Rheumatol. 2012;24:97–102.

Bone, Cartilage, and Soft Tissue Disorders

12

Haralampos M. Moutsopoulos
and Evangelia Zampeli

Abstract

In most rheumatic diseases, the homeostasis of bone formation and degradation is disrupted through different mechanisms driven by inflammatory mediators, biomechanical factors, and genetic abnormalities. Osteoarthritis (OA) is one of the leading causes of disability in adults worldwide. It is a degenerative disease of the joints secondary to many predisposing factors, most notably age, joint injury, altered mechanical stress, and obesity. All these processes cause a local chronic inflammatory response resulting in the progressive joint failure characteristic of OA. Osteoporosis is the result of cumulative bone loss during aging. Nevertheless, a wide variety of diseases, medications, and lifestyles can cause or contribute to the development of osteoporosis. In addition, the immune system participates in the regulation of bone homeostasis through production of cytokines and inflammatory mediators with subsequent activation of cartilage-degrading proteinases. Paget's disease is a chronic skeletal disorder, caused by enhanced bone resorption followed by abnormal bone formation, in which a potential crosstalk between the bone and the immune system takes place.

Hereditary connective tissue diseases (e.g., Marfan syndrome, Ehlers-Danlos syndromes, and osteogenesis imperfecta) are a heterogeneous group of disorders that result from genetic defects that alter the quantity or structure of extracellular matrix proteins. These disorders can present with various clinical manifestations involving the musculoskeletal, cardiovascular, respiratory, and ocular systems.

H. M. Moutsopoulos (✉)
Athens Academy, Athens, Greece
e-mail: hmoutsop@med.uoa.gr

E. Zampeli
Bioclinic General Hospital of Athens and Institute for Autoimmune Systemic and Neurological Disorders, Athens, Greece
e-mail: ezampeli@bioclinic.gr

1. **What is known to date for the pathogenesis of osteoarthritis?**

   Osteoarthritis (OA) is a particularly common degenerative joint disease; it is characterized by loss of cartilage, remodeling of subchondral bone, and formation of osteophytes. These changes in the joint structure lead to compromised movement, stiffness, and chronic joint pain. Abnormal mechanical loading on the joint triggers an imbalance between cartilage matrix synthesis and degradation, in favor of degradation. Collagen and aggrecan (matrix

H. M. Moutsopoulos, E. Zampeli (eds.), *Immunology and Rheumatology in Questions*,
https://doi.org/10.1007/978-3-030-56670-8_12

proteoglycan) are the main structural components of the cartilage extracellular matrix (ECM). Increased production of matrix metalloproteinases (MMPs) and aggrecanases by chondrocytes has a well-documented role in the degradation of ECM and progression of OA. Although OA is regarded as a non-inflammatory disease, in contrast to rheumatoid arthritis, recent studies suggest that inflammation triggered by factors like biomechanical stress is involved in the development of OA. Various molecules released by the chondrocytes and synoviocytes and infiltrating immune cells (macrophages, T cells, B cells, plasma cells, mast cells, natural killer cells, dendritic cells, and granulocyte), such as cytokines, (interleukin (IL)-1, IL-6) and chemokines are involved in regulating the joint anabolism and catabolism process. Their expressions are in turn governed by the activation of signaling pathways, such as nuclear factor kappa-light-chain enhancer of activated B cells (NF-κB), phosphoinositide 3-kinase/protein kinase B (PI3K/AKT), and mitogen-activated protein kinase (MAPK). These events, in turn, generate more inflammatory molecules and subsequently, MMPs degrade the extracellular matrix. As a result, anatomical and physiological functions of the joint are altered [1, 2].

2. **Which are the risk factors for the development of osteoarthritis?**

- Age
- Family history
- Obesity
- Gender; females are more prone to develop osteoarthritis
- Trauma and repetitive joint stress
- Anatomic joint abnormalities (hip dysplasia or congenital hip dislocation, malposition-varus/valgus, scoliosis)
- Other medical conditions (e.g., hemophilia, sickle cell anemia, Paget's disease, gout, and pseudogout)

3. **Which joints can be more commonly affected by osteoarthritis?**

Knees, hips, lower back (lumbar spine), cervical spine, proximal (Bouchard's nodes), and distal (Heberden's nodes) interphalangeal joints of the fingers, the first carpometacarpal joint, and the first metatarsophalangeal joint.

4. **Which are the characteristic radiographic findings in an osteoarthritic joint?**

- Asymmetric joint space narrowing
- Sclerotic changes at joint margins
- Osteophyte formation
- Subchondral cysts
- Subluxation

5. **Which individuals are primarily affected by shoulder periarthritis? What are the causes and what is evidence-based therapy?**

Shoulder periarthritis refers to the inflammation of the structures (tendons, bursae, and muscles) around the shoulder. It is observed in middle-aged individuals and can be the result of trauma, strain, or inflammation of other organs. It manifests with shoulder pain and limitation of joint motion. Calcific shoulder periarthritis is more commonly seen in patients with long-standing diabetes mellitus. Other plausible risk factors include thyroid disorders, stroke, Parkinson disease, cancer, and complex regional pain syndrome. The goal of therapy for shoulder periarthritis is to relieve pain and to preserve the shoulder's range of motion. Physical therapy is important for pain control and restoration of normal shoulder mobility. Intra-articular corticosteroid injections, especially in the early disease stages, may help decrease pain and improve shoulder mobility. In chronic untreated cases, adhesive capsulitis (frozen shoulder) develops. In such cases, shoulder manipulation, under general anesthesia, is indicated in order to loosen the tightened periarticular tissues.

6. **What are the causes of Milwaukee shoulder? What is its clinical presentation and radiographic findings and how is it treated?**

Milwaukee shoulder is an unusual crystal (calcium hydroxyapatite) deposition disease, which affects women in the late fifth and sixth decades of life. Unilateral, dominant side shoulder joint involvement is more common. The hydroxyapatite crystals are deposited periarticularly or intra-articularly. The intra-articular crystals initiate an acute inflammatory response leading to release of collagenases, elastases, proteases, and interleukin-1. The joint function is compromised and joint anatomy destruction follows. Rupture of the rotator cuff is not unusual. Plain shoulder X-ray shows joint space narrowing, subchondral sclerosis with cyst formation, destruction of subchondral bone, soft-tissue swelling, capsular calcifications, and intra-articular loose bodies. Ultrasonography of the shoulder usually shows fluid collection and marked synovial proliferation. Magnetic resonance imaging demonstrates a large effusion, rotator cuff tears, narrowing of the glenohumeral joint, thinning of the cartilage, and destruction of subchondral bone. The diagnosis is placed with aspiration of the synovial fluid, where hydroxyapatite crystals can be found. In the initial disease stages, nonsteroidal anti-inflammatory drugs, colchicine, or intra-articular corticosteroid injections with physiotherapy are prescribed, while in severe advanced stages, joint replacement is considered.

7. **What is primary and secondary hyperoxaluria and what are its musculoskeletal symptoms?**

Hyperoxaluria occurs when there is an excessive oxalate excretion in the urine. Hyperoxaluria can be primary, caused by an autosomal recessive inherited disease resulting in endogenous overproduction of oxalate, or secondary, resulting from a gastrointestinal disorder associated with fat malabsorption and increased intake of dietary oxalate (spinach, rhubarb, sweet potatoes, and peanuts). In both primary and secondary hyperoxaluria, oxalate crystals are primarily renally eliminated and if in excess, they can deposit in the kidney leading to kidney stone formation and even renal failure. Oxalate crystals may also deposit in bones, joints, heart, eyes, and skin. Bone involvement in hyperoxaluria can manifest as diffuse bone pain. Oxalate arthritis can be clinically indistinguishable from other crystal-induced arthritis; calcium oxalate crystals, however, are detected in the synovial fluid of these patients.

8. **What are the symptoms of sciatica, how is it diagnosed and what are the options of management?**

Sciatica is caused by compression of the L4 through S2 nerve roots mostly due to a herniated or bulging lumbar intervertebral disc. Patients present with unilateral leg pain radiating posteriorly at the leg and below the knee, with or without associated neurological deficits. Sciatica is a clinical diagnosis, and therefore, a thorough history and physical examination (including straight leg raise test/femoral nerve test/slump test) are necessary for a complete evaluation and diagnosis. Imaging is of little value. It should only be requested if pain persists for more than 12 weeks or the patient develops progressive neurological deficits. In general, sciatica should be managed conservatively with exercise, physiotherapy/manual therapy, and/or analgesics. Only patients with signs of urinary retention or decreased anal sphincter tone, which suggest cauda equina syndrome, should be referred urgently. Otherwise, surgical intervention should only be considered in cases when pain does not subside after 6–8 weeks of conservative treatment. Effects of surgery are controversial. In one recent study, it has been shown that the effect of surgery is similar to conservative treatment after one year of follow-up [3], while in another study involving patients with sciatica caused by lumbar disk herniation, microdiscectomy was shown to be superior to nonsurgical treatment with respect to pain intensity at 6 months of follow-up [4].

9. Which initial tests should be ordered to evaluate back pain in a man over 65 years of age?

- X-ray of the lumbar spine and pelvis
- Hematocrit/hemoglobin, serum alkaline phosphatase
- Serum calcium and phosphorus
- Serum protein electrophoresis

10. What is bursitis?

Inflammation of the bursae (small, fluid-filled sacs that alleviate the friction between bones and tendons in the joints). Clinically presents with pain and tenderness over the inflamed bursa and with limited movement of nearby joints.

11. Which are the causes of olecranon bursitis (Fig. 12.1)?

- Trauma, acute blow to the tip of the elbow
- Chronic traumatic pressure by repeated leaning on the point of the elbow
- Infection (from overlying skin or blood borne)
- Rheumatoid arthritis
- Crystal arthritis
- Chronic renal failure and patients on dialysis

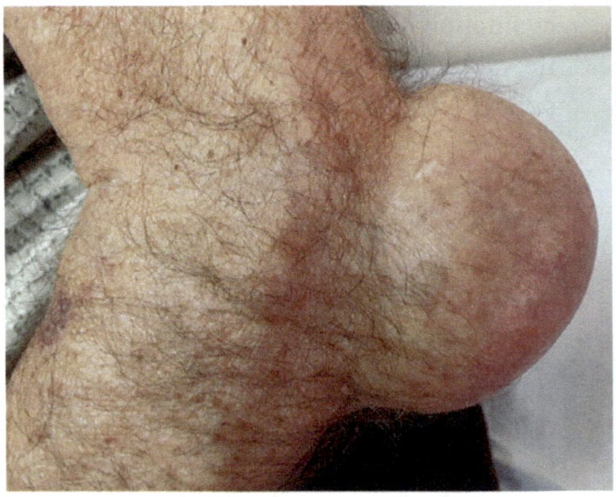

Fig. 12.1 Olecranon bursitis: Painful swelling around the elbow containing inflammatory fluid in a 75-year-old man with long-standing seropositive rheumatoid arthritis (*Figure courtesy of Professor Fotini N.Skopouli, MD*)

12. What is the "Popeye" sign?

It is a painful deformity in the anterior mid-upper arm, due to bulging of the biceps muscle, which becomes more evident when the elbow is flexed. It is due to rupture of the long head of the biceps tendon. It occurs usually in elderly with degenerative lesions in the shoulders, tendons, and ligaments after strenuous effort, e.g., lifting heavy objects or overuse. Infrequently it can occur in athletes. While in elderly, rupture of biceps tendon is treated conservatively (analgesics and anti-inflammatory agents), in athletes it requires surgical correction.

13. Which are the causes of popliteal (Baker's) cyst?

- Trauma
- Rheumatoid arthritis
- Reactive arthritis
- Systemic lupus erythematosus
- Knee osteoarthritis
- Crystal arthritis
- Infectious arthritis
- Hemophilia

14. What is the clinical picture of ruptured Baker's cyst and which easy and cheap method is used to diagnose it?

Ruptured Baker's cyst presents often with acute pain behind the knee and calf as well as swelling of the calf. The method to diagnose ruptured Baker's cyst and differentiate it from other conditions, which produce similar symptoms (deep vein thrombosis, cellulitis, lymphedema, muscle, or tendon tear) is ultrasonography (Fig. 12.2).

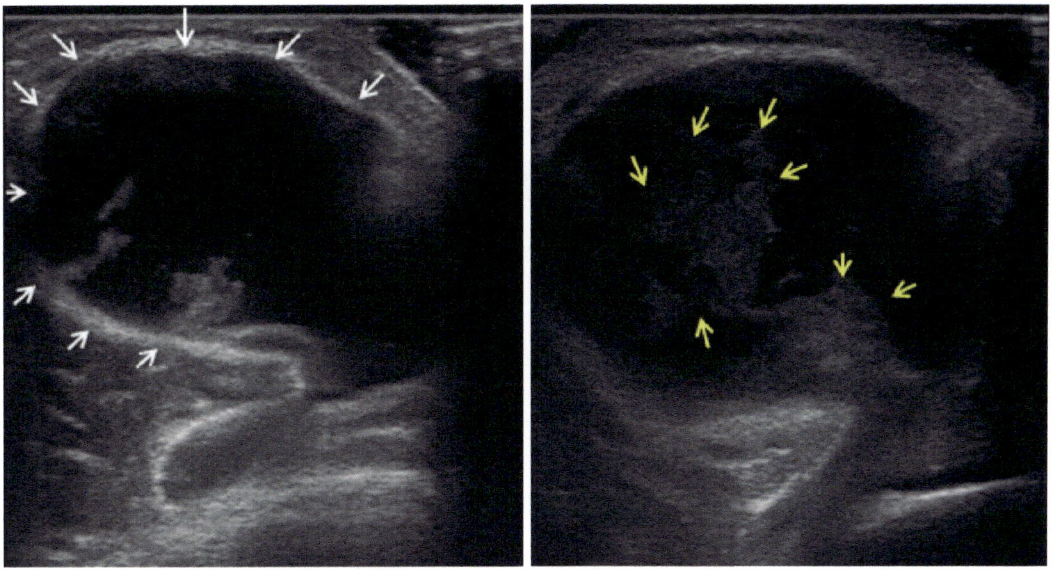

Fig. 12.2 Baker's cyst: Knee ultrasound examination of a 62-year-old male. A well-defined fluid-filled cyst (white arrows), extending into the joint space between the semimembranosus tendon and the medial head of gastrocnemius, and synovial hypertrophy (yellow arrows) are apparent (*Figure courtesy of Professor Paraskevi V. Voulgari, MD*)

15. What is synovial chondromatosis?

Synovial chondromatosis is a rare benign neoplastic condition of unknown etiology, which results in severe disability of the involved synovial joint. Synovial chondromatosis may occur as a primary disease or secondary to active rheumatoid arthritis, osteoarthritis, or osteonecrosis. It occurs more often in men, it is usually mono-articular and the knees are the most commonly affected joints. These joints present as having a large effusion and sometimes appear deformed due to swelling or synovial hypertrophy. They are painful both at rest and in motion, while range of motion is significantly decreased. Joint X-ray reveals multiple loose radio-opaque chondroid bodies of varied sizes in the joint. In primary cases, arthroscopic surgical removal of loose bodies with partial synovectomy of the involved joints is the treatment. In secondary cases, a combination of disease-modifying antirheumatic drugs and arthroscopy should be considered to restore joint function.

16. Which are the causes of carpal tunnel syndrome (median nerve entrapment neuropathy)?

- Repetitive motions, like typing, or any wrist movements that are done over and over
- Trauma
- Conditions like hypothyroidism, obesity, rheumatoid arthritis, and diabetes mellitus
- Pregnancy
- Amyloidosis

17. In which individuals carpal tunnel syndrome is more common?

In women three times more often than in men, in obese individuals, and in the ages between 30 and 60 years.

18. Which are the carpal tunnel syndrome symptoms?

Pain, paresthesia, and sensory loss in the radial side of the palm, the thumb, and the index, middle, as well as ring fingers (distribution of the median nerve). The pain can radiate up to the elbow, the shoulder, and even the neck. Pain is alleviated relatively when the patient walks.

19. Describe a condition in which carpal tunnel syndrome is self-limited.

Carpal tunnel syndrome occurring in the third trimester of pregnancy goes away after delivery. Wrist splints can relieve the symptoms, while local steroid injections are not indicated. Nerve conduction studies should be performed only if symptoms persist after delivery.

20. What is the clinical picture of osteoporosis?

Osteoporosis can progress silently over the years to a low bone mineral density (BMD) level, thereby reducing bone strength in a way that fragility fractures can occur with minimal impact. Fractures of the spine cause pain that is generally self-limited. Multiple vertebral fractures can lead to loss of height, reduced thoracic expansion capacity, progressive thoracic kyphosis, poor functional status, and ultimately frailty. Frailty itself is a risk factor for fractures, thereby creating a vicious cycle. Hip fractures have a much worse impact and prognosis. They require hospitalization and surgery. Usually the elderly suffering from a hip fracture have comorbid conditions which together with prolonged immobilization and rehabilitation required after a hip fracture, decrease their life expectancy.

21. Which are the predisposing factors for the development of osteoporosis in men and women?

In males, besides age, nearly 2/3 of osteoporotic men have an identifiable secondary cause of bone loss, most often alcohol abuse, smoking, low body weight, history of chronic lung disease, history of peptic ulcer disease, endocrine disorders (primary hyperparathyroidism, hyperthyroidism, insulin-dependent diabetes mellitus, hypogonadism) and hematologic disorders (multiple myeloma, lymphoma, leukemia), gastrointestinal tract disorders (celiac disease, malabsorption, Crohn's disease, chronic liver disease, especially cirrhosis). Prolonged exposure to some drugs, mainly glucocorticoids, but also aluminum-containing antacids, proton pump inhibitors, calcineurin inhibitors, antiepileptics, medroxyprogesterone acetate, aromatase inhibitors, GnRH agonists, androgen deprivation therapy use for prostate cancer, selective serotonin reuptake inhibitors and anticoagulants are also among the main identifiable causes of secondary osteoporosis.

Women with early menopause, low body weight/lean built, low dietary calcium intake, estrogen deficiency, and low levels of vitamin D, have the highest risk of developing osteoporosis. Secondary causes of osteoporosis in women are the same as in men.

22. What is the fracture risk assessment tool (FRAX)?

FRAX integrates clinical risk factors (country of origin, age, sex, weight, height, history of previous fracture, hip fracture in the person's mother or father, smoking, glucocorticoid treatment, rheumatoid arthritis, and other diseases associated with osteoporosis, alcohol intake of three or more standard drinks/day) and bone mineral density at the femoral neck in order to calculate the 10-year probability of hip fracture and the 10-year probability of a major osteoporotic fracture (spine, forearm, hip, or shoulder).

23. What are bone marrow edema syndromes?

Bone marrow edema syndromes (BMES) are different clinical conditions characterized by a bone marrow edema pattern with a self-limiting course. Most of them develop in the lower limbs, such as transient osteoporosis of the hip, regional migratory osteoporosis, and transient posttraumatic bone marrow edema syndrome. Transient osteoporosis of the hip is the most frequent one. It generally affects middle-aged men or women in the third trimester of pregnancy. In most cases no triggering events can be found, but an abnormal mechanical stress (such as a long walk) has been described in some cases. The main symptom is acute hip pain, exacerbated by loading, and is often associated with severe functional disability.

The clinical course is often self-limiting, with a resolution in 4–24 months, but a possible evolution toward an osteonecrosis has been proposed. Treatment with bisphosphonates seems to shorten disease duration [5].

24. Which are the clinical/radiological similarities and differences of osteopetrosis and osteoporosis?

Osteopetrosis is a very rare inherited bone disease also called "marble or stone" disease, while osteoporosis is the result of interplay between genetic (family history) and environmental factors (smoking, alcohol abuse, lack of exercise, dietary restriction, etc.). In individuals with mild forms of osteopetrosis as well as in osteoporotic individuals, there are no symptoms. Osteopetrosis can be detected in routine X-rays, where the bones appear denser and harder in contrast to osteoporosis where bones appear brittle and less dense. In osteopetrosis elevated serum alkaline phosphatase levels can be found, while in osteoporosis alkaline phosphatase is within normal limits. In severe cases in both disorders, bone fractures can occur. In osteopetrosis narrowing of bone marrow space occurs, leading to anemia and hepatosplenomegaly. Infections can occur due to bone expansion and extramedullary hematopoiesis. Expanded bones can also put pressure on nerves leading to facial paralysis, blindness, and deafness.

25. How does acute osteonecrosis present? Which are commonly affected areas?

In some patients with bone necrosis, symptoms do not appear until the late stages of the disease process, when collapse of the articular surface occurs. In others, pain is an early symptom, which usually occurs upon weight-bearing but can be present at rest and at night due to increased intraosseous pressure. Range of motion is not affected until degenerative changes occur. Commonly affected areas are those with limited blood supply and restricted collateral circulation and include the femoral head, the carpal bones (scaphoid and lunate), the humeral head, the talus, the femoral condyles, the tarsal navicular bone, the proximal tibia, and the metatarsals [6].

26. Which are the causes of aseptic osteonecrosis (avascular necrosis)?

Corticosteroid administration, alcohol abuse, sickle cell anemia, hemoglobinopathies, hyperlipidemia, hypercoagulable states (thrombophilia, disseminated intravascular coagulopathy), pregnancy, fat emboli, antiphospholipid syndrome, oral contraceptive use, arteriosclerosis/vaso-occlusive disorders, acquired human immunodeficiency syndrome, trauma (fracture of femoral neck), and pancreatitis.

27. Which are the clinical and radiologic findings of an infected intervertebral disc?

Infected intervertebral disc (discitis) is the result of a hematogenous spread of a systemic infection, which can originate from the skin, the lungs, or the urinary tract. It often accompanies vertebral osteomyelitis. Risk factors for discitis include poor nutrition, immune suppression, human immunodeficiency virus (HIV) infection, cancer, diabetes, and obesity. *Staphylococcus aureus* is the most commonly found microorganism, while Gram-negative bacteria (*Escherichia coli* and *Proteus* species) are common in patients with urinary tract infections. *Pseudomonas aeruginosa* or *Klebsiella* species can be the offending microorganisms in intravenous drug abusers. Infrequently discitis can develop post-operatively. Clinically, discitis is presenting with fever (however, not unusually the patient can be afebrile), severe back pain, and inability to move. The diagnosis can be easily placed with an MRI scan that reveals hyperintensity of the affected disc on T2-weighted imaging, presence of paraspinous or epidural inflammation/abscess, and contrast enhancement of the disc and adjacent bone marrow (sensitivity 95%). Biopsy can help the diagnosis but the responsible organism is difficult to be isolated.

28. In which medical conditions shoulder-hand syndrome develops?

The shoulder-hand syndrome (also known as complex regional pain syndrome, Sudeck's atrophy, or reflex sympathetic dystrophy) is characterized by pain and swelling in an extremity, trophic skin changes in the same extremity (skin atrophy/hyperpigmentation, hypertrichosis, hyperhidrosis, nail changes), signs and symptoms of vasomotor changes, altered heat and tactile sensations, limited motion in the proximal joints of the affected limb, and neglect-like symptoms of the affected extremity. It occurs most commonly after stroke, glenohumeral subluxation, and myocardial infarction (especially if associated with prolonged immobilization).

29. What is the Hill-Sachs lesion?

Recurrent anterior shoulder dislocations may lead to posterolateral humeral head compression fractures. This lesion is called Hill-Sachs lesion. It is often associated with a Bankart lesion which is an injury of the anteroinferior aspect of the glenoid labrum. Hill-Sachs lesion itself can predispose to recurrent dislocation/subluxation of the shoulder, by exerting a lever effect during external joint rotation.

30. What is Kienböck's disease?

Kienböck's disease (avascular necrosis of the lunate) is the fracture of the lunate bone in the wrist caused by disruption of its blood supply. It is of unknown etiology and presents with painful and swollen wrist with limited range of motion and decreased grip strength. Tenderness directly above the affected bone is a characteristic finding.

31. What are the Schmorl's nodes?

It is a common finding of an aging spine. The nodes do not cause any symptoms, and plain profile spinal X-ray reveals a defect at the anterior vertebral body which reflects a protrusion of the intervertebral disc, beneath the ring apophysis of the vertebral body.

32. What is the clinical picture of Tietze syndrome?

Tietze syndrome is a benign inflammatory process of the costal cartilages, which is more common in women. It presents with pain, tenderness, as well as swelling of the affected cartilages (the second or third ribs are more frequently affected), at the sternocostal junction. It involves a single joint and is rarely bilateral. The pain increases with pressure application as well as with respiratory movements. Generally, it resolves spontaneously in weeks.

33. Which are the joint/bone findings of Langerhans cell histiocytosis?

A well-circumscribed punched-out lesion of the skull is characteristic of Langerhans cell histiocytosis (LCH). In the mandible, the loss of supporting bone results in the appearance of "floating teeth." When the metaphysis or diaphysis of long bones is affected, the lesion is associated with endosteal scalloping, giving a budding appearance and extensive thick laminated periosteal reaction. LCH is also one of the causes of complete collapse of a vertebral body, known as vertebra plana. In children with LCH, osseous lesions are similar to those seen in multiple myeloma.

34. Which are the clinical features, usual locations and radiologic characteristics of osteoid osteomas?

Osteoid osteomas are benign, small (diameter <1.5 cm) tumors which arise from the osteoblasts. They can be found in any body bone but more frequently are located in the long bones, e.g., the femur or the tibia. Continuous, deep pain, especially at night at the site of the lesion, is the principal symptom of osteoid osteomas. The pain characteristically responds to salicylates. Usually the diagnosis is delayed. Radiographs show a radiolucent area of around 1 cm in diameter, called nidus, with sometimes a calcified center. The nidus is surrounded by radiodense cortical hypertrophy.

35. What is Charcot arthropathy and which disorders can lead to its development?

Charcot arthropathy (neuropathic arthropathy) is a progressive destructive process of the weight-bearing joints which leads to joint dislocations, pathologic fractures, and debilitating deformities. Loss of sensation caused by neuropathies in patients with diabetes mellitus, syphilis, leprosy, alcoholism, spinal cord injuries, and renal dialysis can be responsible for the development of the disorder.

36. Patient with knee monoarthritis with no history of trauma. The aspiration of the synovial fluid of the knee joint yields bloody-appearing synovial fluid. What is your diagnosis?

The most probable diagnosis in a patient with knee monoarthritis in whom arthrocentesis yields a brown-red synovial fluid is pigmented villonodular synovitis. If the synovial fluid is hemorrhagic besides trauma, bleeding disorders (hemophilia, coumarin-induced prolonged bleeding time), Charcot joint, sickle cell anemia, scurvy, and tumors should be considered.

37. What is the clinical picture of pigmented villonodular synovitis and how is it diagnosed?

Pigmented villonodular synovitis (PVNS) is a subtype of slow-growing giant cell tumor that affects the soft tissue lining of joints and tendons. Joints most commonly affected by PVNS are the knees, hips, and ankles, in a monoarticular pattern. Its onset is insidious, with symptoms often being present for years before diagnosis. Patients initially present with painless swelling in the affected joint and as the tumor expands pain and swelling cause a limited range of motion of the affected joint. As PVNS progresses it causes a locally destructive process. Rheumatoid arthritis, septic joints, hemarthrosis, and other neoplasias can mimic the clinical picture of PVNS upon clinical examination. MRI is the most sensitive imaging study to diagnose pigmented villonodular synovitis (PVNS). In the majority of patients inflammatory markers in the serum are not elevated.

38. Which are the genetics and the clinical picture of achondroplasia?

Achondroplasia is a common cause of asymmetric dwarfism. The affected individuals present with a short stature (male adults average height 131 cm, females 123 cm), short proximal limbs, short fingers and toes, large head with prominent forehead and small midface with flattened nasal bridge, spinal kyphosis, and knees with "varus" or "valgus" deformities. It is caused by a sporadic or inherited mutation of the receptor 3 of fibroblast growth factor. This receptor when mutated is constantly active and leads to extremely shortened bones. Achondroplasia can be detected prenatally with ultrasound or

DNA test. If the embryo carries two copies of the mutant gene, this leads to stillbirth.

39. Which are the bone and cartilage findings of alkaptonuria (ochronosis)?

Alkaptonuria is a rare inherited disorder caused by a mutation of the gene responsible for the production of the enzyme homogentisate 1,2-dioxygenase. Individuals who inherit two abnormal gene copies accumulate homogentisic acid in their blood and tissues. Children and young adults are usually asymptomatic, but when their urine is left exposed to open air, it turns to black or inky black color. Accumulation of homogentisic acid in the ears, cartilage, and eyes sclera produces pigmentation, in the bone cartilages leads to osteoarthritis, and in the heart valves of the affected individuals causes regurgitation primarily of mitral and aortic valves. Stones consisting of homogentisic acid can be found in the gallbladder, the kidneys, the prostate, and the major salivary glands. Almost half of the affected individuals suffer from hearing loss. The weight-bearing joints (spine, hips, and knees) are commonly affected, and severe articular pain starts after the age of 30 years. The pain is severe and interferes with the individuals' daily activities. Involvement of the spinal joints limits the ability of rib cage movements and thus affects lung gas exchange. Bone mineral density is affected leading to osteoporotic bone fractures.

40. Which are the prominent manifestations of pseudoxanthoma elasticum?

Skin: Small, yellowish papules are evident on the neck, axillae, and groin and inside the surface of elbows and knees. The skin may become lax and redundant.

Retina: On fundoscopic examination, angioid streaks are present. These develop because Bruch's membrane, which separates the blood vessel-rich layer from the pigmented retina layer, is mineralized creating cracks (angioid streaks) that radiate out from the optic disc. The retinal blood vessels sometimes leak, and the hemorrhages may lead to the loss of central vision.

The gastrointestinal (GI) and cardiovascular systems can also be involved in pseudoxanthoma elasticum (PXE); the principal GI symptom is GI bleeding, usually from the stomach. This occurs in a very small number of patients. Peripheral arteries can be affected and the patient presents with intermittent claudication. In later disease stages coronary artery disease may develop. Joint hypermobility and chronic synovitis can be seen in patients with PXE.

41. Which proteins are affected by gene mutations and for which hereditary connective tissue disorders are they responsible?

Hereditary connective tissue diseases (HCTD) are a heterogeneous group of disorders that result from genetic defects that alter the quantity or structure of extracellular matrix (ECM) proteins including collagens, fibrillins, elastin, and non-collagenous matrix proteins. Depending on the ECM protein involved, the tissues most likely to be affected can be predicted, e.g., osteogenesis imperfecta, collagen type I defect; Ehlers-Danlos, collagen type I, III, or V defects/fibronectin defects; and Marfan syndrome, fibrillin-1 defect.

42. Which are the major clinical findings of Marfan syndrome?

Patients with Marfan syndrome have a characteristic phenotype: Tall stature, long-thin extremities, abnormally low upper/lower body segment ratio, diminished subcutaneous fat, arachnodactyly, pectus excavatum or carinatum, loss of thoracic kyphosis, scoliosis, reduced elbow extension (<170°), and pes planus. Scoliosis is a major problem in Marfan patients which might be rapidly progressive during adolescence requiring surgery. Joint hypermobility leading to arthralgias, spinal pain, and ligament injuries are common manifestations in adult patients with the syndrome. Facial characteristics include a high arched palate, long-narrow face, retrognathia, and enophthalmos. Ectopia lentis occurs in 50–80% of patients. Cardiovascular complications include aneurysmal dilatation of the ascending aorta with dissection, which is the most common cause of death in these patients. Mitral valve prolapse with regurgitation or aortic insufficiency are common. Pulmonary manifestations can be cystic disease or spontaneous pneumothorax.

43. Which are the major clinical findings of Ehlers-Danlos syndrome?

Ehlers-Danlos syndrome (EDS) is a group of 13 subtypes of hereditary connective tissue disorders. Patient presentations vary widely based on the respective underlying subtype; however, the major clinical manifestations of the syndrome include:

- Skin hyperextensibility, smooth and velvet-like texture, fragility, delayed wound healing leaving thin atrophic scars after healing
- Joint hypermobility leading to repeated subluxation and dislocation
- Mitral valve prolapse and aortic root dilation
- Classic facies include down slanting palpebral fissures, epicanthal folds, blue sclera, the appearance of premature aging, and micrognathia
- Spontaneous and traumatic rupture or perforation of hollow and solid internal organs. Hernias are common

44. What is the benign joint hypermobility syndrome?

Benign joint hypermobility syndrome is a connective tissue disorder characterized by chronic musculoskeletal pain due to joint hyperextensibility. Its prevalence is estimated to be around 3% of the general population. Its etiopathogenesis is not clear. Genetic and biomechanical defects (decreased proprioceptive acuity and muscle mass/strength) seem to play a role. Patients with benign hypermobility syndrome present with generalized and symmetric polyarthralgias exacerbated by repetitive use or physical activity. Weight-bearing joints like the knees and ankles are more commonly involved. Accompanying symptoms or findings in these patients are fatigue, in the majority of patients, recurrent headaches, abdominal and pelvic pain, mitral valve prolapse, pes planus, genu valgum, patellar subluxation, and marfanoid habitus. Differential diagnosis should include Marfan syndrome, Ehlers-Danlos syndrome, and fibromyalgia [7].

45. What is osteogenesis imperfecta? Which are the major clinical findings of osteogenesis imperfecta?

Osteogenesis imperfecta is a group of genetic disorders that mainly affect the bones. Individuals with this condition have bones that break easily, often from mild trauma or with no apparent cause. There are at least 19 recognized forms of osteogenesis imperfecta, designated type I through type XIX. Type I (also known as classic nondeforming osteogenesis imperfecta with blue sclerae) is the mildest form. Type II is the most severe. Other types of this condition, including types III (progressively deforming osteogenesis imperfecta) and IV (common variable osteogenesis imperfecta with normal sclerae), have signs and symptoms that fall somewhere between the two extremes. The most common clinical findings of all types include:

- Fragile bones (Fig.12.3a)
- Blue sclerae (Fig. 12.3b)
- Short stature
- Scoliosis
- Loose joints, joint contractures
- Decreased hearing
- Disorders of tooth development

Osteogenesis imperfecta has most of the time an autosomal dominant pattern of

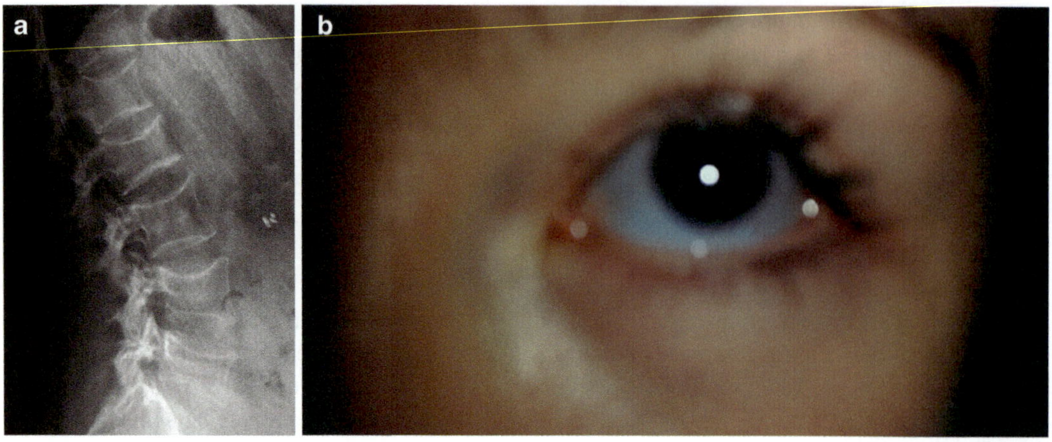

Fig. 12.3 Osteogenesis imperfecta: (**a**) Multiple vertebral fractures (L1-L5) on a lumbar spine X-ray of a 34-year-old lady two months after delivery. The patient had a positive family history from her father suffering from severe osteoporosis with spontaneous fractures since his youth. In order to confirm the diagnosis of osteogenesis imperfecta a whole genome sequencing analysis on chromosome 12 was performed. Whole exome sequencing analysis with Illumina NextSeq-500 system showed that on chromosome 12 (12q13.1), a heterozygous mutation, in COL2A1 (collagen type II α1 chain) gene and exon 45 were detected. A nucleotide replacement of c.3136C>T, which causes an amino acid replacement p. Pro1046Ser was noted (*Reproduced from Boutzios G et al. 2020*) [8]. (**b**) Osteogenesis imperfecta: blue sclera is evident in a 16-year-old young lady with a long history of multiple bone fractures after minimal trauma (*Figure courtesy of Professor Fotini. N. Skopouli, MD*)

inheritance, caused by mutations in the COL1A1 or COL1A2 (collagen type I) genes. Less commonly, osteogenesis imperfecta has an autosomal recessive pattern of inheritance and only type XIX has an X-linked recessive pattern [9, 10].

46. What is the clinical picture of Paget's bone disease?

Paget's disease of bone is the result of an excessive bone breakdown and formation which is followed by disorganized bone remodeling. The affected bones become fragile. The most commonly affected bones are the pelvis, the skull, the spine, and the legs. The diagnosis of the disease is based on the patient's clinical picture, the elevated serum alkaline phosphatase levels, and the characteristic bone appearance on X-rays. Bone reabsorption, enlargement of the affected bone, and bowing of the long bones are evident. Complications of Paget's disease of the bone include bone fractures, hearing loss, and pinched nerves of the spine. There is no curative therapy for the disease, but bisphosphonates can relieve bone pain and disease progression. In severe cases, surgery may be necessary.

References

1. de Lange-Brokaar BJ, Ioan-Facsinay A, van Osch GJ, Zuurmond AM, Schoones J, Toes RE, et al. Synovial inflammation, immune cells and their cytokines in osteoarthritis: a review. Osteoarthr Cartil. 2012;20:1484–99.
2. Chow YY, Chin KY. The role of Inflammation in the pathogenesis of osteoarthritis. Mediators Inflamm. 2020;2020:8293921.
3. Jensen RK, Kongsted A, Kjaer P, et al. Diagnosis and treatment of sciatica. BMJ. 2019;367:l6273.
4. Bailey CS, Rasoulinejad P, et al. Surgery versus conservative care for persistent sciatica lasting 4 to 12 months. N Engl J Med. 2020;382:1093–102.
5. Manara M, Varenna M. A clinical overview of bone marrow edema. Reumatismo. 2014;66:184–96 .
6. Mont MA, Cherian JJ, Sierra RJ, Jones LC, Lieberman JR. Nontraumatic osteonecrosis of the femoral head: where do we stand today? A ten-year update. J Bone Joint Surg Am. 2015;97:1604–27.
7. Kumar B, Lenert P. Joint hypermobility syndrome: recognizing a commonly overlooked cause of chronic pain. Am J Med. 2017;130:640–7.

8. Boutzios G, Moutsopoulos HM. Severe osteoporosis in a premenopausal woman. Scand J Rheum. 2019;48:424–5.
9. Fratzl-Zelman N, Misof BM, Roschger P, et al. Classification of osteogenesis imperfecta. Wien Med Wochenschr. 2015;165:264–70.
10. Augusciak-Duma A, Witecka J, Sieron AL, et al. Mutations in the COL1A1 and COL1A2 genes associated with osteogenesis imperfecta (OI) types I or III. Acta Biochim Pol. 2018;65:79–86.

Rheumatic Manifestations: A Compilation

13

Haralampos M. Moutsopoulos
and Evangelia Zampeli

Abstract

Autoimmune diseases present with a wide range of symptoms able to affect nearly all body organs. Differential diagnosis of these symptoms can be difficult, as a particular presenting symptom may be encountered in distinct autoimmune diseases, and at the same time many non-rheumatic diseases may share similar clinical manifestations. In the large overlapping field of infections and rheumatology, many autoimmune diseases may present as fever of unknown origin, and on the other hand, many different infectious agents cause signs and symptoms mimicking a systemic autoimmune disease. Clinical manifestations affecting the skin and its annexes, oral cavity, joints, and periarticular structures but also major organs such as the heart and vascular system, lung, liver, spleen, and gastrointestinal tract can be initial symptoms of a systemic autoimmune disease. The use of immune checkpoint inhibitors for the treatment of different types of cancers has radically changed the scenery in cancer therapy. Nevertheless, their use is often limited by the development of immune-related adverse events (iRAEs). Among these rheumatologic iRAEs are relatively common. It is important for rheumatologists to recognize and manage them early. The good knowledge of underlying pathogenetic mechanisms of particular clinical manifestations, the thorough physical examination, and the accurate use and interpretation of laboratory, serological, and imaging findings are necessary skills in overcoming the challenging differential diagnosis.

1. **Which autoimmune disease patients have the highest incidence to drug allergies?**

Patients with systemic and organ-specific autoimmune disorders have higher incidence of allergies compared to age-, sex-, and race-matched healthy individuals. It appears that a common variation of the BACH2 gene (the BACH2 protein plays a crucial role in T-lymphocyte maturation) accounts for the coexistence of allergies and autoimmune diseases.

H. M. Moutsopoulos (✉)
Athens Academy, Athens, Greece
e-mail: hmoutsop@med.uoa.gr

E. Zampeli
Bioclinic General Hospital of Athens and Institute for Autoimmune Systemic and Neurological Disorders, Athens, Greece
e-mail: ezampeli@bioclinic.gr

H. M. Moutsopoulos, E. Zampeli (eds.), *Immunology and Rheumatology in Questions*,
https://doi.org/10.1007/978-3-030-56670-8_13

2. **What is the association of systemic autoimmune disorders with autoimmune thyroid diseases?**

Rheumatoid arthritis, polymyalgia rheumatica, Sjögren's syndrome, psoriatic arthritis, systemic lupus erythematosus, scleroderma, celiac disease, diabetes mellitus, and HCV-related cryoglobulinemia are encountered with increased prevalence in patients with thyroid autoimmune diseases [1].

3. **With which connective tissue diseases can celiac disease be associated?**

Celiac disease (CD) has been described in patients with Sjögren's syndrome (SS), Systemic Lupus Erythematosus (SLE), and Juvenile Idiopathic Arthritis (JIA). Several studies have shown an increased prevalence of CD, confirmed by small bowel biopsy, in patients with SS which ranges between 4.5 and 15%. Treatment of CD did not relieve, however, the sicca complains or manifestations of SS patients. In SLE patients CD has been described in some case reports, while prevalence of CD in JIA ranges from 2.5 to 7%.

4. **In which conditions can Raynaud's phenomenon manifest?**

- Autoimmune disorders: Scleroderma, mixed connective tissue disease, Sjögren's syndrome, rheumatoid arthritis, systemic lupus erythematosus, and anti-aminoacyl-tRNA synthetase inflammatory myopathies
- Interstitial pneumonia with autoimmune features
- Hyperviscosity syndromes
- Use of certain medications (ergotamine/β-blockers)
- Buerger's disease
- Smoking
- Mechanical reasons (repeated action/vibration)
- Anatomic reasons, such as excessive seventh cervical rib [2]

5. **In which diseases can subcutaneous nodules be observed?**

- Rheumatoid arthritis
- Rheumatic fever
- Systemic lupus erythematosus
- Adult-onset Still's disease
- Erythema nodosum
- Tophaceous gout
- Multicentric reticulohistiocytosis
- Granulomatosis with polyangiitis (Wegener's granulomatosis)
- Eosinophilic granulomatosis with polyangiitis (Churg-Strauss syndrome)
- Polyarteritis nodosa
- Sarcoidosis
- Type II hyperlipoproteinemia
- Limited scleroderma (calcinosis cutis)
- Weber Christian panniculitis (Fig. 10.5)

6. **In which autoimmune conditions can localized lipodystrophy (lipoatrophy) be seen?**

Lipodystrophy (lipoatrophy) is the local lack of adipose tissue production, as a result of panniculitis. It has been described in patients with autoimmune thyroiditis, autoimmune hepatitis, systemic lupus erythematosus, Sjögren's syndrome, juvenile dermatomyositis, Celiac disease, and morphea.

7. **Which are the oral manifestations of connective tissue diseases?**

- **Rheumatoid arthritis:**
  - Increased prevalence of periodontitis
  - Temporomandibular joint (TMJ) involvement
  - Aphthous stomatitis related to methotrexate use
  - Gingival overgrowth due to prolonged use of cyclosporine-A
  - Sicca manifestations
- **Sjögren's syndrome (SS):** Patients with severe xerostomia present
  - Dry and friable oral mucosa with superficial ulcerations

- Erythematous, fissured (scrotal) tongue with atrophic papillae
- Oral Candidiasis
- Angular cheilitis
- Halitosis

• **Systemic lupus erythematosus (SLE):** In patients with active and severe disease oral mucosa lesions include hard palate erythematous macules or plaques, blisters, and asymmetric erosions anywhere in the oral mucosa and less frequently erythematous-purpuric macules appearing on the lips. Infrequently lupus erythematosus patients present sicca manifestations, recurrent aphthous stomatitis, lichen planus- or leukoplakia-like lesions and discoid lesions

• **Systemic sclerosis (SSc):**
  - Microstomia/Microcheilia
  - Fixation of the TMJ joint (pseudoankylosis) owing to fibrosis of periarticular soft tissues resulting in difficulty in opening the mouth
  - Telangiectasias can be seen, particularly in the mucosal site of the lips
  - Loose periodontal ligaments lead to early teeth loosening
  - Rarely, appearance of asymptomatic pigmented fungiform papillae on the dorsal and lateral aspects of the tongue as scattered hyper-pigmented spots
  - Tongue cancer has a significantly increased frequency in patients with SSc that present a mouth opening <30 mm

• **Vasculitides:**
  - *Granulomatosis with polyangiitis (GPA, Wegener's granulomatosis):* deep painful ulcers can appear anywhere in the oral mucosa including the lateral aspects of the tongue. A typical form of gingival overgrowth is "strawberry-like gingivitis", which is characterized by reddened, swollen and somewhat granular tissue that is often covered with petechiae and small punctate lesions. It is an almost pathognomonic oral manifestation of GPA
  - *Giant cell arteritis:* may present with jaw claudication and rarely with tongue ulceration and necrosis

8. In which autoimmune conditions can painless mouth ulcers be observed?

Painless mouth ulcers can be seen in patients with systemic lupus erythematosus, Sjögren's syndrome, and post-infectious arthritis (Reiters'syndrome).

9. Which are the subjective and objective findings of mouth ulcers in patients with systemic lupus erythematosus, granulomatosis with polyangiitis (Wegener's granulomatosis), and post-infectious arthritis?

• Systemic lupus erythematosus: Irregularly shaped, raised white plaques, silvery-white scarred lesions, and ulcers with surrounding erythema on the soft and hard palate (Fig. 4.7) or buccal mucosa and lips. Oral ulcers are usually painless, and there is not always temporal association with disease activity. Typical discoid lupus lesions with erythema, atrophy, and depigmentation can also occur
• Granulomatosis with polyangiitis: Two classic mouth lesions can be seen; gum inflammation (strawberry gums) and tongue ulcers, which typically occur on the lateral sides of the tongue (Fig. 8.4). Gum inflammation and tongue ulcers are both painful
• Sjögren's syndrome: Xerostomia and altered saliva properties promote oral mucosa lesions. Frequent aphthae and non-specific, shallow, painless ulcers are common
• Post-infectious arthritis: oral ulcers are usually shallow and painless

10. Which are the causes of saddle nose deformity?

Saddle nose is characterized by a loss of nose height. The depressed nasal dorsum may be due to destruction of bony, cartilaginous, or both components of the nasal dorsum. It is observed after nasal trauma (most common cause) or in patients with:

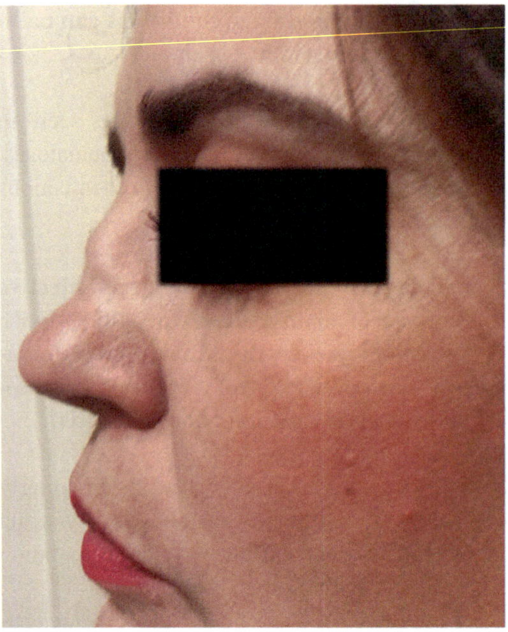

Fig. 13.1 Saddle nose deformity: in a 35-year-old female patient with granulomatosis with polyangiitis (Wegener's granulomatosis)

- Congenital syphilis/leprosy
- Relapsing polychondritis
- Granulomatosis with polyangiitis (Fig. 13.1)
- Cocaine abuse

11. Which conditions are associated with perforation of the nasal diaphragm?

Conditions associated with perforation of the nasal diaphragm include systemic lupus erythematosus, granulomatosis with polyangiitis (Wegener's granulomatosis), syphilis, leprosy, sarcoidosis, tuberculosis, neoplastic causes (nasopharyngeal carcinoma, middle line lethal granuloma), and cocaine sniffing.

12. Which patients with rheumatic disease develop oral candidiasis?

- Immunosuppressed patients with systemic connective tissue diseases
- Sjögren's syndrome patients with severe xerostomia

13. What are the telangiectasias and under which conditions can they develop?

Telangiectasias form gradually and often in clusters. They are widened venules which cause threadlike red lines or patterns on the skin and mucosae. They are also called "spider veins" because of their fine and weblike appearance. Conditions in which telangiectasias are observed include alcoholism, pregnancy, aging, rosacea, habitual corticosteroid use, limited scleroderma (Fig. 7.2), dermatomyositis, and, in some patients, systemic lupus erythematosus.

14. Which autoimmune disorders can present with Bell's palsy and uveitis?

These are sarcoidosis and Sjögren's syndrome.

15. Which inflammatory arthritis can affect distal interphalangeal joints?

Psoriatic arthritis and gout can affect distal interphalangeal joints.

16. What is the clinical picture and etiopathogenesis of fibromyalgia?

Fibromyalgia (FM) is a non-autoimmune, non-inflammatory disorder characterized by generalized pain (comprising 19 different areas of the body where the patient might feel the pain), fatigue, unrefreshing sleep, cognitive disturbances, and somatic symptoms. FM presents with a wide range of manifestations, yet physical examination reveals no signs of articular or muscular disease. FM may accompany rheumatic diseases and various disorders, such as hypothyroidism, can mimic FM. Many other painful diseases (e.g., osteoarthritis, spinal stenosis, and mood and anxiety disorders) may co-occur in patients with FM. Furthermore, different medications may contribute to the development of generalized pain, such as statins, aromatase inhibitors, and opioids (i.e., opioid-induced hyperalgesia).

The multifaceted symptoms and comorbidities associated with FM make the diagnosis sometimes difficult, and FM can be underdiagnosed and undertreated [3]. The etiopathogenesis of FM is controversial. Genetic predisposition, environmental factors (diet, social distress, and poor social relationships), and neuromodulation are considered as possible triggering and perpetuating factors. Reduction of intraepidermal nerve fiber density in the skin biopsies of patients with fibromyalgia has been recently detected, but the association of this finding with the disease-related symptoms remains to be elucidated.

17. Which arthritides can affect the temporomandibular joint?

Degenerative arthritis, rheumatoid arthritis, juvenile idiopathic arthritis, and psoriatic arthritis can affect the temporomandibular joint.

18. Which nerve root is affected if a patient presents with back pain and numbness around the left knee, medial shin, and calf and absence of the left knee reflex?

The L3/L4 root since the knee reflex is mediated by the L3/L4 nerve root. L3 nerve root supplies the dermatome of the anterior aspect of the knee, and the L4 nerve root supplies the medial aspect of calf muscles and skin.

19. Which are the symptoms and causes of plantar fasciitis?

The principal symptom of plantar fasciitis is pain in the heel and bottom of the foot. The pain is usually most severe in the morning when the individual gets up from the bed or after a rest period. The symptoms typically come on slowly. The causes of plantar fasciitis are unclear. Risk factors include long periods of standing, strenuous exercise, and obesity. Other conditions in which plantar fasciitis symptoms can manifest include flat feet, osteoarthritis, ankylosing spondylitis, and reactive arthritis. In only one-third of patients, both feet are affected.

20. Which are the therapeutic measures for the management of plantar fasciitis?

The symptoms of plantar fasciitis resolve with time. Rest, changing the individual's activities, and pain medications can be sufficient to alleviate the symptoms. If, however, these are not effective, physiotherapy, orthotics, or splinting, can be applied. Corticosteroid injection has been frequently used for plantar fasciitis pain, although there is limited high-quality evidence to support this treatment. [4].

21. Which systemic rheumatic diseases can affect the aortic valve?

- Ankylosing spondylitis
- Cogan syndrome
- Relapsing polychondritis
- Marfan syndrome
- Giant cell arteritis
- Granulomatosis with polyangiitis (Wegener's granulomatosis)
- Reactive arthritis
- Rheumatoid arthritis
- Rheumatic fever
- Antiphospholipid syndrome

22. Which clinical picture of autoimmune diseases resembles that of the subacute endocarditis?

Libman-Sacks endocarditis that manifests in systemic lupus erythematosus and antiphospholipid syndrome patients can resemble the clinical picture of subacute endocarditis.

23. Which cardiac tumor can present as an inflammatory disorder?

Atrial myxomas, primary non-cancerous tumors of the heart, can cause symptoms associated with obstruction due to size and location of the tumor, symptoms associated with pulmonary and systemic embolization, or constitutional symptoms. Constitutional symptoms occur in around 50% of patients and include malaise, anorexia, fever, arthralgia, weight loss, and Raynaud's phenomenon often mimicking connective tissue diseases. Laboratory abnormalities such as raised acute phase proteins (C-reactive protein, erythrocyte sedimentation rate), anemia, leukocytosis, thrombocytopenia, elevated gamma globulins, and ferritin levels are usually found in these patients. These clinical and laboratory inflammatory features are attributed to overproduction and secretion of interleukin (IL)-6 by cardiac myxoma cells. Serum IL-6 levels are predictors of cardiac myxoma recurrence in these patients. Two-dimensional echocardiography is the diagnostic procedure of choice. Surgical removal is the therapy of choice.

24. **In which diseases are arterial microaneurysms found?**

- Polyarteritis nodosa
- Ehlers-Danlos disease
- Fibromuscular dysplasia (Fig. 8.7a, b)
- Pseudoxanthoma elasticum
- Neurofibromatosis
- Segmental arterial mediolysis

25. **In which systemic autoimmune disorders can pleurisy be the first disease manifestation?**

In men with rheumatoid arthritis, in systemic lupus erythematosus, and rarely in granulomatosis with polyangiitis (Wegener's granulomatosis).

26. **Which findings characterize a body fluid as exudate?**

Appearance: Cloudy
- Specific gravity >1020
- Fluid/serum protein ratio >0.5
- Fluid/serum LDH ratio >0.6

27. **Which autoimmune patients are at the highest risk to develop Pneumocystis jiroveci pneumonia?**

Pneumocystis jiroveci (formerly known as *Pneumocystis carinii*) pneumonia occurs frequently in patients with autoimmune inflammatory diseases older than 60 years of age and on steroid treatment.

28. **Which autoimmune diseases may present with alveolar hemorrhage?**

Alveolar hemorrhage should be suspected in patients with progressive dyspnea accompanied by alveolar opacities on chest imaging that cannot be otherwise explained. Hemoptysis is a typical sign but is often absent. A drop of blood hemoglobin over a few days without hemolysis or any overt blood loss should raise the suspicion of diffuse alveolar hemorrhage. Bright red fluid obtained from bronchoalveolar lavage is diagnostic. It can occur in the following autoimmune diseases:
- Systemic lupus erythematosus
- Different types of vasculitis (mainly microscopic polyangiitis or granulomatosis with polyangiitis and, exceptionally, eosinophilic granulomatosis with polyangiitis)
- Antiphospholipid syndrome
- Goodpasture syndrome
- Isolated pauci-immune capillaritis
- Idiopathic pulmonary hemosiderosis

29. **When should a physician think that a patient has pulmonary arterial hypertension?**

Pulmonary arterial hypertension (PAH) should be ruled out in a patient presenting with dyspnea and fatigue, which cannot be attributed to heart, lung, or blood disorders. There are few signs of early PAH, but there are several important physical examination findings that suggest the presence of advanced PAH, such as features of right heart dysfunction, including lower extremity edema, murmur of tricuspid regurgitation, jugular vein distension, ascites, and hepatomegaly. Right heart catheterization is the gold standard for the diagnosis of PAH.

30. **In which autoimmune rheumatic disorders can pulmonary arterial hypertension develop?**

It can develop in scleroderma patients and less frequently in patients with systemic lupus erythematosus, mixed connective tissue disease, and Sjögren's syndrome.

31. **What is macrophage activation syndrome?**

It is a secondary (reactive) syndrome which can occur in patients with adult-onset Still's disease and systemic juvenile idiopathic arthritis and in patients with active Epstein-Barr, cytomegalovirus, and recently with SARS-COV-2 infection. It is a life-threatening condition with poor prognosis and presents with:

- High fever
- Hepatosplenomegaly
- Very high serum ferritin levels
- Sudden drop of the high fibrinogen levels
- Elevated liver function tests
- Pancytopenia
- Hypertriglyceridemia
- Oliguric renal dysfunction
- Acute respiratory distress
- Altered mental status
- Consumptive coagulopathy
- Hypotension and biventricular systolic dysfunction
- Central nervous system involvement

Diagnosis is confirmed by a bone marrow aspiration which shows phagocytosis of hemopoietic cells by macrophages.

32. **Which conditions (autoimmune and others) may present with macrophage activation syndrome (reactive hemophagocytic lymphohistiocytosis)?**

- Adult-onset Still's disease
- Systemic-onset juvenile rheumatoid arthritis
- Systemic lupus erythematosus
- EBV/CMV/SARS Cov-2 infection
- Brucellosis
- Tuberculosis
- Leishmaniasis

33. **In which autoimmune patient group is the incidence of splenomegaly higher?**

Incidence of splenomegaly is higher in patients with adult-onset Still's disease, autoimmune hemolytic anemia, and Felty's syndrome.

34. **Which autoimmune disorders can manifest clinical, laboratory, and histopathologic features of autoimmune hepatitis? What autoantibodies can these individuals have in their serum?**

Autoimmune hepatitis (AIH) is classified as type 1 and type 2 based on the expression of different autoantibodies. Patients with type 1 AIH are mainly females and can have other associated autoimmune disorders like rheumatoid arthritis, Sjögren's syndrome, systemic lupus erythematosus, inflammatory bowel disease, and autoimmune thyroid diseases. In their serum autoantibodies against nuclear antigens, cellular antigens (particularly against anti-Ro/SSA), and smooth muscle antigens (ASMA) are present. Type 2 AIH is mainly a pediatric disease. It is characterized by the presence of anti-liver kidney microsomal antibody type 1 (LKM-1) and/or anti-liver cytosol type 1 (LC-1) autoantibodies. Recent clinicopathological studies have identified an immunoglobulin (Ig) G4-associated AIH as a subtype of AIH. Confirmation of hepatic accumulation of IgG4-expressing plasma cells is absolutely required for the diagnosis of IgG4-AIH on the condition that the patient meets the diagnostic criteria for AIH [5].

35. Which drugs can be responsible for the development of autoimmune liver disease?

Well-established associations are minocycline, nitrofurantoin, oxyphenisatin, alpha-methyl-dopa, clometacin, statins, alpha and beta interferons, infliximab and etanercept. Less compelling associations (infrequent reports) include diclofenac, fenofibrate, dihydralazine, and benzarone.

36. In which rheumatic diseases can esophageal motility disorders be seen?

They can be seen in the majority of systemic sclerosis patients, but they can also be seen in patients with polymyositis/dermatomyositis, undifferentiated connective tissue diseases/mixed connective tissue disease, and Sjögren's syndrome.

37. In which rheumatic disorders can microscopic colitis develop?

Microscopic colitis is a clinicopathologic entity of middle-aged, predominantly female, patients who present with chronic, intermittent, or recurrent episodes of watery diarrhea and abdominal cramps. The colonic mucosa of patients with microscopic colitis appears normal in colonoscopy, while the tissue taken during colonoscopy reveals two distinct histopathologic forms: the collagenous and the lymphocytic. Patients with celiac disease, autoimmune thyroid disease, rheumatoid arthritis, systemic lupus erythematosus, scleroderma, and spondyloarthropathies can manifest symptoms and signs of microscopic colitis. In these rheumatic disorders, collagenous microscopic colitis is the most frequent histopathologic form.

38. What is the clinical picture of ischemic colitis and which are possible underlying causes?

Ischemic colitis is the result of reduced blood flow in the colon. The colon tissue damage can range from inflammation and superficial injury to necrosis of the full wall thickness. Classically ischemic colitis affects individuals in their sixties to seventies. Clinically it presents acutely with colicky abdominal pains accompanied with bloody bowel movements.

Underlying causes of ischemic colitis can be:

- Atherosclerosis/diabetes mellitus leading to: thrombosis/emboli
- Arterial hypoperfusion/hypovolemia (septic shock, hemorrhagic shock, cardiopulmonary bypass, hemodialysis, hemorrhagic pancreatitis)
- Hypercoagulable state (severe dehydration, thrombophilia, sickle cell disease)
- Drugs (antihypertensives, digitalis, estrogens, pseudoephedrine, simvastatin, interferon-ribavirin)
- Cocaine abuse
- Cardiac myxoma
- Polyarteritis nodosa and systemic lupus erythematosus
- Amyloidosis
- Postradiation

39. In which systemic autoimmune diseases can mesenteric vasculitis occur?

Mesenteric vasculitis is defined by inflammation of medium- and small-size mesenteric arteries. Most often it affects branches of the celiac, superior, and inferior mesenteric arteries. Vasculitis of medium-size arteries occurs in patients with polyarteritis nodosa (PAN), while in patients with systemic lupus erythematosus, Sjögren's syndrome, and rheumatoid arthritis small-size vessels are inflamed. The diagnosis of PAN mesenteric arteritis is placed with selective mesenteric artery angiography, while for the small vessel vasculitis contrast-enhanced abdominal computed tomography is the diagnostic test of choice.

40. Which are the characteristic contrast-enhanced CT findings in systemic lupus

erythematosus patients with mesenteric vasculitis?

In systemic lupus erythematosus (SLE) mesenteric vasculitis the small bowel wall vessels are involved, which cannot be visualized by mesenteric angiography. Because of these limitations, contrast-enhanced computed tomography of the abdomen is the most useful modality for diagnosis. The characteristic features of mesenteric SLE vasculitis are best seen on cross-sectional images: the "target" sign which is produced by the bowel wall edema and the "thumb-like" sign produced by the projections of the intestinal mucosa into the lumen. On longitudinal sections "thumb-printing" is evident which indicates bowel wall ischemia, while prominence of mesenteric vessels resembles the teeth of a comb, producing the so-called "comb" sign.

41. Which autoimmune conditions are responsible for nephrocalcinosis?

Sjögren's syndrome with chronic untreated interstitial kidney disease and sarcoidosis are the autoimmune conditions responsible for nephrocalcinosis.

42. What can be the causes of interstitial nephritis?

- Drugs: Nonsteroidal anti-inflammatory drugs, antibiotics (penicillin, fluoroquinolones), proton-pump inhibitors, rifampicin, sulfa drugs, diuretics, allopurinol, and phenytoin
- Metabolic (hyperuricemia, hypercalcemia, and hyperoxaluria)
- Heavy metals (lead, cadmium, arsenic, mercury)
- Autoimmune diseases: Sjögren's syndrome (early in the disease), sarcoidosis (granulomatous interstitial nephritis), granulomatosis with polyangiitis and IgG4-related diseases
- Acute transplant rejection
- Infections: Bacterial (obstructive uropathy), viral (CMV, HIV, HBV), parasitic (leishmaniasis), mycobacterial, and fungal (histoplasmosis)
- Hematologic disorders (multiple myeloma, sickle-cell anemia, paroxysmal nocturnal hemoglobinuria)
- Genetic: Alport syndrome
- Endemic: Balkan nephropathy

43. In which autoimmune conditions is interstitial cystitis observed? What are the main clinical manifestations?

Interstitial cystitis can be associated with Sjögren's syndrome, inflammatory bowel disease, and systemic lupus erythematosus. Common symptoms include urgency/frequency to urinate, bladder pressure and pain that gets worse when the bladder is full, as well as pain in the lower abdomen and lower back, pelvis, or urethra. In women pain in the vulva/vagina occurs during intercourse.

44. What is fibrillary glomerulonephritis?

Fibrillary glomerulonephritis (FGN) is a rare glomerular disease, more common in adults aged 45–65 years. Although it has long been considered an idiopathic glomerular disease, it can be associated with underlying malignancy (most commonly lymphoproliferative disorders and carcinoma), hepatitis C infection, or autoimmune diseases (15%), such as systemic lupus erythematosus, Sjögren's syndrome, rheumatoid arthritis, Graves' disease, Crohn's disease, and idiopathic thrombocytopenic purpura. Presenting manifestations include nephrotic-range proteinuria, hematuria, hypertension, and renal insufficiency. The most common histologic pattern is mesangial proliferative/sclerosing glomerulonephritis followed by membranoproliferative glomerulonephritis. Because of the universal presence of IgG and complement components in the glomerular deposits, the pathogenesis of FGN is thought to result from glomerular localization of immune complexes that have the ability to undergo fibrillogenesis. Disease remission occurs spontaneously in a minority of patients while nearly one-half of patients progress, within four years, to end-stage renal disease. Older age, elevated serum creatinine, and higher degree of glomerulosclerosis at diagnosis are bad prognostic factors for renal survival [6, 7].

45. In which systemic autoimmune diseases can autoimmune orchitis develop?

Autoimmune orchitis can develop in patients with polyarteritis nodosa, IgA vasculitis (Henoch-Schönlein purpura), and can be a manifestation of IgG4-related diseases. Infrequently autoimmune orchitis can be seen in patients with systemic lupus erythematosus, rheumatoid arthritis, scleroderma, inflammatory muscle diseases, relapsing polychondritis, and inflammatory bowel disease. In contrast to patients with primary autoimmune orchitis, patients with the secondary form do not have in their sera autoantibodies against sperm autoantigens. In order to place the diagnosis testicular ultrasound and biopsy is of paramount importance [8].

46. What is the etiology and clinical picture of Alport syndrome?

Alport syndrome is a hereditary disease caused by mutations that affect the production and/or function of type IV collagen, the major constituent of mature basement membranes in the glomerulus, cochlea, cornea, lens, and retina. It is a rare syndrome, yet it accounts for about 1% of patients on hemodialysis. The earliest clinical manifestation of Alport syndrome is hematuria. Anterior lenticonus, discolored retina, and hearing loss are extrarenal manifestations.

47. What is Balkan nephropathy?

Balkan nephropathy is a familial chronic tubulointerstitial disease. It presents insidiously and slowly progresses to end-stage renal disease. It is frequently related to upper urothelial cancer. Its cause remains largely unknown. Polygenic susceptibility to the disease in interaction with multiple environmental factors is assumed. Chronic intoxication with Aristolochia (family of plants) or long-term exposure to organic toxins (lignite) is considered a major environmental risk factor [9].

48. Which are the rheumatic manifestations of amyloidosis and in which type of amyloidosis can they occur more often?

Rheumatic manifestations occur more frequently in AA amyloidosis (previously known as secondary amyloidosis), and they include muscle weakness (myopathy); arthropathy of shoulders, knees, wrists, as well as of the small hand joints; bone lesions (osteopathy); and carpal tunnel syndrome. In contrast to light-chain (AL, primary) amyloidosis, transthyretin (ATTR), and beta-2 microglobulin (A beta-2M) types of amyloidosis, musculoskeletal manifestations due to amyloid A deposition are subtle, subclinical, and only apparent in tissue biopsy. Rarely, sicca syndrome can develop.

49. In which chronic medical conditions can AA amyloidosis develop?

- Chronic infections: Tuberculosis
- Autoimmune-inflammatory diseases: Rheumatoid arthritis, inflammatory bowel disease, and periodic fever syndromes (Familial Mediterranean fever, Tumor necrosis factor receptor-associated periodic syndrome, Cryopyrin-associated periodic syndromes, Hyper IgD syndrome)

50. Which autoimmune diseases can develop in individuals with IgA deficiency?

- Rheumatoid arthritis
- Systemic lupus erythematosus
- Immune thrombocytopenic purpura
- Thyroid autoimmune disorders
- Inflammatory bowel disease

51. In which other autoimmune diseases, in addition to Sjögren's syndrome, can trigeminal neuralgia manifest?

Trigeminal neuralgia can manifest in scleroderma, sarcoidosis, systemic lupus erythematosus, and multiple sclerosis.

52. In which autoimmune conditions is leukopenia prevalent?

Leukopenia is prevalent in systemic lupus erythematosus, Sjögren's syndrome, autoimmune thyroiditis, and Felty's syndrome.

53. In which systemic autoimmune diseases can migraine headache manifest?

- Systemic lupus erythematosus
- Antiphospholipid syndrome
- Sjögren's syndrome
- Limited scleroderma

54. In which autoimmune diseases can Devic's syndrome (neuromyelitis optica) manifest?

Devic's syndrome can manifest in systemic lupus erythematosus, Sjögren's syndrome, sarcoidosis, rheumatoid arthritis, myositis, antiphospholipid syndrome, autoimmune hypothyroidism, immune thrombocytopenic purpura, inflammatory bowel disease, myasthenia gravis, and pemphigus.

55. In which disorders can cerebrospinal fluid monoclonal bands be found? Are they disease specific?

They can be found in the cerebrospinal fluid (CSF) of patients with multiple sclerosis but also of patients with systemic lupus erythematosus and acquired immunodeficiency syndromes, particularly when the patients from the two later groups have central nervous system involvement.

56. In which autoimmune patients can pseudo-pseudo Meigs syndrome develop?

Pseudo-pseudo Meigs Syndrome (PPMS) is a very rare and of uncertain etiology phenomenon seen in patients with active systemic lupus erythematosus. It manifests with ascites, pleural effusions, and elevated serum CA-125 levels. PPMS is not associated with benign or malignant pelvic tumors. Due to the rarity of the condition, the underlying pathophysiology of ascites in PPMS is still uncertain. It is suggested that severe, uncontrolled inflammation related to the underlying systemic lupus erythematosus could be the cause. Therefore immunosuppressives to treat lupus flare are used for treating PPMS [10].

57. In which autoimmune patients are contraceptives contraindicated?

Contraceptives containing estrogens can exacerbate systemic lupus erythematosus and can increase the risk of thrombosis in patients with antiphospholipid syndrome.

58. Which autoimmune conditions can develop in individuals with silicone breast implants?

Sjögren's syndrome, rheumatoid arthritis, systemic sclerosis, undifferentiated connective tissue disease, sarcoidosis, and Raynaud's phenomenon can develop in these individuals [11].

59. What is the impact of bariatric surgery on patients with rheumatoid arthritis?

Obesity is one of the described risk factors for rheumatoid arthritis (RA) onset; it negatively affects disease activity and treatment outcome. The benefit of bariatric surgery on disease risk, outcome, and prognosis is still controversial. In one study [12], RA patients who underwent bariatric surgery lost substantial weight twelve months following surgery, RA disease activity and inflammatory indexes significantly improved, and the patients were on less rheumatoid arthritis-related medications. In another prospective study [13] obese RA patients who underwent bariatric surgery had significant weight loss and a better response to treatment after 12 months of follow up, yet RA-related medication usage, had no difference between the obese RA patients who underwent bariatric surgery and those who did not. Interestingly, in a Swedish study with a follow-up of 29 years, there was no association between bariatric surgery and the incidence of RA in obese patients [14], which might demonstrate that bariatric surgery has no preventive effect on the occurrence of RA.

60. Which are the rheumatic manifestations in HIV-infected individuals?

The most common rheumatic manifestations among HIV-infected patients prior to the introduction of the highly active antiretroviral therapy were rheumatoid arthritis, sicca syndrome, reactive arthritis, and psoriatic arthritis.

In the era after the advent of the highly active antiretroviral therapy, although the incidence and prevalence of rheumatic manifestations associated to HIV infection have significantly declined, other rheumatic disorders have emerged in HIV infected patients, namely systemic and discoid lupus erythematosus, polymyositis, Behçet's disease, autoimmune hemolytic anemia, adult-onset Still's disease, osteoporosis, and avascular bone necrosis [15].

61. What adverse musculoskeletal effects are caused by the use of performance-enhancing drugs?

Performance-enhancing drugs (PEDs) are pharmacologic agents that athletes and non-athlete weight lifters use to enhance performance. There are several categories of PEDs that are currently popular. The most frequently used anabolic drugs causing musculoskeletal disorders are:

- Androgenic-anabolic steroids (AAs): Can cause rhabdomyolysis and tendon ruptures (attributable both to the disproportionate strength of hypertrophied muscles and to possible deleterious effects of AAs on the architecture of the tendons themselves)
- Growth hormone: Can cause acral enlargement, arthropathy, and carpal tunnel syndrome

62. Which are the clinical manifestations and histopathologic findings of Kikuchi-Fujimoto disease (histiocytic necrotizing lymphadenitis)?

Kikuchi-Fujimoto disease (KFD) is a rare benign and self-limiting cause of lymphadenopathy, mainly cervical. It classically affects young women during the third decade of life. Although an infectious etiology has been suggested, a definitive causative agent has not been recognized. Typical symptoms include localized lymphadenopathy, fever, and odynophagia. Laboratory findings are usually normal except for mild increase of inflammatory markers and/or mild cytopenias. Biopsy of affected lymph nodes is useful to rule out malignant lymphoma [16].

63. With which autoimmune systemic disease is Kikuchi-Fujimoto disease associated?

Kikuchi-Fujimoto disease is associated with the development of systemic lupus erythematosus (SLE). Indeed, these two entities can manifest in the same patient, perhaps reflecting shared pathophysiology. Presence of weight loss, arthralgias, skin manifestations, and high titers of antinuclear antibodies in patients with Kikuchi-Fujimoto disease have been shown to be associated with the development of SLE.

64. What immunophenotyping features distinguish lymphadenopathy of systemic

lupus erythematosus (SLE) and Kikuchi-Fujimoto disease (KFD) from malignant or infectious processes?

In a recent study, investigators analyzed routine diagnostic flow cytometry of 975 benign and malignant lymph nodes to evaluate whether KFD/SLE has an immunophenotype distinct from other lymphadenopathies. This signature was then evaluated in 1198 fine-needle aspiration specimens. A flow cytometry signature was identified that can distinguish KFD/SLE from a wide variety of benign and malignant entities. The most discriminatory feature of this signature consists of CD38 expression by the majority of $CD19^+$ small B cells. Another discriminatory feature is the decreased T-cell expression of CD57 in the KFD/SLE setting. $CD4^+CD57^+$ T cells are germinal center T cells that play a significant role in promoting B-cell immunoglobulin production and this is in line with the observed lack of germinal centers in lymph nodes involved by KFD/SLE. Finally, IgD positivity on small B cells also supports a diagnosis of KFD/SLE when a B-cell–predominant area is sampled by FNA [17].

65. What rheumatic and/or autoimmune manifestations can develop in cancer patients receiving immunotherapy with checkpoint inhibitors?

Cancer immunotherapy with checkpoint inhibitors is the latest therapeutic modality used for cancer treatment. Cancer patients treated with checkpoint inhibitors (CPIs) can exhibit the following rheumatic and autoimmune adverse events:

- Arthralgias, tenosynovitis, myalgias
- Polymyalgia rheumatica-like syndrome
- Rheumatoid and psoriatic-like arthritis
- Myositis
- Sicca syndrome
- Vitiligo, psoriasiform or lichenoid reactions, bullous pemphigoid
- Autoimmune hypothyroidism more common than hyperthyroidism
- Hypophysitis
- Type 1 diabetes mellitus
- Inflammatory bowel disease, enteritis/colitis
- Pneumonitis
- Multiple sclerosis
- Myasthenia gravis

The use of CPIs may result in disease exacerbation in approximately one-quarter of patients with pre-existing autoimmune disease [18, 19].

66. Does immune checkpoint inhibitor-induced inflammatory arthritis persist after cessation of immunotherapy for cancer?

Inflammatory arthritis develops as a side-effect of checkpoint inhibitor (CPI) immunotherapy. It has been shown that after 9 months of CPI discontinuation inflammatory arthritis in the majority of patients can still be active, particularly in cancer patients who received for a prolonged period of time CPI. The patients in whom arthritis persists were treated with immunomodulatory agents who did not appear to affect tumor outcome [20].

67. What are the clinical characteristics of immune checkpoint inhibitor-associated myositis and how is it different from idiopathic inflammatory myopathies (IIM)?

Checkpoint inhibitor (CPI)-related myositis represents a rare (<1%) yet potentially life-threatening side effect of CPI therapy. Most CPI-related myositis cases occur with anti-Programmed Death Ligand (PDL)-1 or anti-Cytotoxic-T-Lymphocyte-Associated Protein (CTLA)-4 monotherapies. CPI-related myositis differs greatly from IIM in that it may frequently occur with bulbar symptoms, ptosis, and oculomotor impairment—manifestations seen in myasthenia gravis—and with myocarditis (in 15-30% of CPI-related myositis patients) which is lethal in up to 50% of cases. The majority of patients do not carry in their sera myositis-specific autoantibodies (MSAs). In some reported CPI-related myositis cases MSAs strongly associated with cancer (such as anti-TIF1-γ, anti-NXP2, and anti-SAE1 antibodies) can be found [21].

References

1. Fallahi P, Ferrari SM, Ruffilli I, Elia G, Biricotti M, Vita R, et al. The association of other autoimmune diseases in patients with autoimmune thyroiditis: review of the literature and report of a large series of patients. Autoimmun Rev. 2016;15:1125–8.
2. Wigley FM, Flavahan NA. Raynaud's phenomenon. N Engl J Med. 2016;375:556–65.
3. Salaffi F, Di Carlo M, Farah S, et al. Diagnosis of fibromyalgia: comparison of the 2011/2016 ACR and AAPT criteria and validation of the modified fibromyalgia assessment status. Rheumatology (Oxford). 2020;pii:keaa061. [Epub ahead of print]
4. Whittaker GA, Munteanu SE, Menz HB, et al. Corticosteroid injection for plantar heel pain: a systematic review and meta-analysis. BMC Musculoskelet Disord. 2019;20:378.
5. Minaga K, Watanabe T, Chung H, Kudo M. Autoimmune hepatitis and IgG4-related disease. World J Gastroenterol. 2019;25:2308–14.
6. Touzot M, Terrier CS. Groupe Coopératif sur le Lupus Rénal (GCLR). Proliferative lupus nephritis in the absence of overt systemic lupus erythematosus: a historical study of 12 adult patients. Medicine (Baltimore). 2017;96:e9017.
7. Nasr SH, Valeri AM, Cornell LD, et al. Fibrillary glomerulonephritis: a report of 66 cases from a single institution. Clin J Am Soc Nephrol. 2011;6: 775–84.
8. Silva CA, Cocuzza M, Carvalho JF, Bonfá E. Diagnosis and classification of autoimmune orchitis. Autoimmunity Reviews. 2014;13:431–4.
9. Stefanovic V, Toncheva D, Polenakovic M. Balkan nephropathy. Clin Nephrol. 2015;83(7 Suppl 1):64–9.
10. Zampeli E, Skopouli FN, Moutsopoulos HM. Polyserositis in a Patient with Active Systemic Lupus Erythematosus: A Case of Pseudo-pseudo Meigs Syndrome. J Rheumatol. 2018;45(6):877–78.
11. Watad A, Rosenberg V, Tiosano S, et al. Silicone breast implants and the risk of autoimmune/rheumatic disorders: a real-world analysis. Int. J. Epidemiol. 2018;47:1846–54.
12. Sparks JA, Halperin F, Karlson JC, Karlson EW, Bermas BL. Impact of bariatric surgery on patients with rheumatoid arthritis. Arthritis Care Res (Hoboken). 2015;67:1619–26.
13. Xu F, Yu C, Li D-G, et al. The outcomes of bariatric surgery on rheumatoid arthritis disease activity: a prospective cohort study. Sci Rep. 2020;10:3167.
14. Maglio C, Zhang Y, Peltonen M, et al. Bariatric surgery and the incidence of rheumatoid arthritis – a Swedish obese subjects study. Rheumatology (Oxford). 2020;59:303–9.
15. Vega LE, Espinoza LR. Human immunodeficiency virus infection (HIV)–associated rheumatic manifestations in thepre- and post-HAART eras. Clin Rheumatol. 2020 Apr 15:1–8. [Epub ahead of print].
16. Dumas G, Prendki V, Haroche J, Amoura Z, Cacoub P, Galicier L, et al. Kikuchi-Fujimoto disease: retrospective study of 91 cases and review of the literature. Medicine (Baltimore). 2014;93:372–82.
17. Scott GD, Kumar J, Oak JS, et al. Histology-independent signature distinguishes kikuchi-fujimoto disease/systemic lupus erythematosus-associated lymphadenitis from benign and malignant lymphadenopathies. Am J Clin Pathol. 2020 pii: aqaa036. [Epub ahead of print].
18. Abdel-Wahab N, Shah M, Lopez-Olivo MA, Suarez-Almazor ME. Use of immune checkpoint inhibitors in the treatment of patients with cancer and preexisting autoimmune disease: a systematic review. Ann Intern Med. 2018;168:121–30.
19. Tocut M, Brenner R, Zandman-Goddard G. Autoimmune phenomena and disease in cancer patients treated with immune checkpoint inhibitors. Autoimmun Rev. 2018;17:610–6.
20. Braaten TJ, Brahmer JR, Forde PM, et al. Immune checkpoint inhibitor-induced inflammatory arthritis persists after immunotherapy cessation. Ann Rheum Dis. 2020;79:332.
21. Nguyên T, Maria ATJ, Ladhari C, et al. Rheumatic disorders associated with immune checkpoint inhibitors: what about myositis? An analysis of the WHO's adverse drug reactions database. Ann Rheum Dis. 2020; pii: annrheumdis-2020-217018. [Epub ahead of print].

Part IV

Treatment and Management of Rheumatic Diseases

14 Medications, Therapeutic Modalities, and Regimens Used in the Management of Rheumatic Diseases

Haralampos M. Moutsopoulos
and Evangelia Zampeli

Abstract

Therapy of systemic autoimmune rheumatic diseases can still be a challenge for clinicians despite enormous progress made in the last decades on the understanding of the pathophysiological mechanisms involved in these diseases. The use of biologic targeted therapies as an adjunct to disease-modifying antirheumatic drugs (DMARDs) for the treatment of autoimmune rheumatic diseases has completely changed the standard of care and is still expanding.

Indications, therapeutic schemes, and specific side effects are presented for the classical disease-modifying anti-rheumatic drugs (DMARDs). In addition, contemporary therapeutic modalities and biologic therapies targeting key effector cells and cytokines implicated in different autoimmune diseases are thoroughly addressed. The major targets of most biologic therapies that we now possess to treat systemic autoimmune diseases are cytokines, B cells, and co-stimulation molecules. Tumor necrosis factor (TNF)-α, interleukin (IL)-1, IL-6, and IL-17 belong to the cytokines targeted. B-cell depletion includes the use of anti-CD20 antibodies and B-cell receptor modulation by the B-lymphocyte stimulator (BLyS). Although some of the biologic therapies have been found to be useful in more than one disease, others are specific for a single disease. Latest indications and therapeutic schemes involving biologic therapies in autoimmune rheumatic as well as in autoinflammatory diseases are given in this chapter. Up-to-date treatment guidelines for osteoporosis in men and women are presented. Finally, questions and answers addressing matters of special interest, such as the use of anti-inflammatory and immunosuppressive agents during pregnancy and lactation as well as vaccination recommendations in immunocompromised patients, are an interesting part of this chapter.

H. M. Moutsopoulos (✉)
Athens Academy, Athens, Greece
e-mail: hmoutsop@med.uoa.gr

E. Zampeli
Bioclinic General Hospital of Athens and Institute for Autoimmune Systemic and Neurological Disorders, Athens, Greece
e-mail: ezampeli@bioclinic.gr

H. M. Moutsopoulos, E. Zampeli (eds.), *Immunology and Rheumatology in Questions*,
https://doi.org/10.1007/978-3-030-56670-8_14

Main Therapeutic Agents Used in Rheumatic Diseases: Mode of Action, Specific Side-Effects, and Considerations

1. How do glucocorticoids exert their anti-inflammatory/immunosuppressive action?

Glucocorticoids (GCs) are small lipophilic hormones that can diffuse into cells and exert their main actions by binding to their intracellular receptor. GCs act upon almost every immune cell type:

- Prevent monocytes from entering apoptosis and inhibit the liberation of pro-inflammatory mediators
- In macrophages, promote phagocytosis and motility, while they inhibit adhesion, apoptosis, and oxidative burst
- Inhibit the rolling, adhesion, and activation of neutrophils
- Promote maturation, survival, migration, and motility of dendritic cells
- Inhibit the ability of dendritic cells to activate T cells by suppressing the production of pro-inflammatory molecules
- Act on Th1 cells by suppressing the production of pro-inflammatory molecules such as interleukin (IL)-2 and interferon (IFN)-γ
- Suppress globin transcription factor (GATA) 3 activity in Th2 cells by inhibiting the expression of IL-4 and IL-5
- Upregulate enzymes that degrade bradykinin resulting in vasoconstriction, suppress the production of prostaglandins and inhibit nuclear factor (NF)κB which suppresses cyclooxygenase (COX)-2 synthesis

2. How does methotrexate exert its anti-inflammatory/immunosuppressive action?

Methotrexate (MTX) is an antimetabolite which exerts its anti-inflammatory action through:

- Inhibition of purine and pyrimidine synthesis
- Suppression of transmethylation reactions with accumulation of polyamines
- Inhibition of T-cell activation
- Suppression of intercellular adhesion molecule expression by T cells
- Selective downregulation of B cells
- Increase of the CD95 sensitivity of activated T cells [CD95 (Fas/Apo1) and CD95 ligand (CD95L) have been known as the death receptor/death system which induces apoptosis (programmed cell death), maintains immune homeostasis, and eliminates virally infected and neoplastic cells]
- Inhibition of methyltransferase activity

All these actions lead to deactivation of enzyme activity relevant to immune system function, which stimulates adenosine release. Adenosine is a potent neutrophil function inhibitor and has strong anti-inflammatory properties. Another mechanism of methotrexate action is the inhibition of interleukin-1 beta binding to its cell surface receptor. Possibly, the combination of these mechanisms is responsible for the anti-inflammatory effects of methotrexate. The adenosine-mediated methotrexate's anti-inflammatory effect is supported by in vitro, in vivo, and clinical data

3. How does leflunomide exert its anti-inflammatory/immunosuppressive action?

Leflunomide exerts its immunomodulatory action by inhibiting the mitochondrial enzyme dihydroorotate dehydrogenase, which plays a key role in the *de novo* synthesis of uridine monophosphate. Uridine monophosphate is required for the synthesis of DNA and RNA. Through this mechanism leflunomide inhibits the reproduction of rapidly dividing cells, especially lymphocytes.

4. How does cyclosporine-A exert its anti-inflammatory/immunosuppressive action?

Cyclosporine-A exerts its immunosuppressive action by binding to the cytosolic protein cyclophilin (immunophilin) of lymphocytes, especially T cells. This cyclosporine/cyclophilin complex binds to calcineurin and inhibits calcineurin–calmodulin interaction, which, under normal circumstances, is responsible for activating the transcription of interleukin (IL)-2. In T cells, T-cell receptor activation normally increases intracellular calcium, which via calmodulin activates calcineurin. Calcineurin thereafter dephosphorylates the nuclear transcription factor of activated T cells, which translocates to the T-cell nucleus and increases the activity of gene coding for IL-2, leading to a reduced function of effector T cells. Cyclosporine-A does not have cytostatic activity.

5. How does tacrolimus exert its anti-inflammatory/immunosuppressive action?

Tacrolimus is a macrolide calcineurin inhibitor. Its action resembles that of cyclosporine-A, although the cellular receptors differ. Tacrolimus binds to an intracellular receptor and subsequently binds to calcineurin and inhibits the calcineurin pathway that stimulates the nuclear factor of activated T-cells (NFAT). By inhibiting the action of NFAT, tacrolimus inhibits synthesis of inflammatory cytokines, in particular of interleukin-2 (IL-2), which results in decreased activation of T-lymphocytes. Furthermore, tacrolimus inhibits release of mast cell and basophil mediators and decreases inflammatory mediator expression. It is 10–100 times more potent than cyclosporine-A.

6. How does hydroxychloroquine its anti-inflammatory/immunosuppressive action?

- Hydroxychloroquine (HCQ) accumulates in lysosomes where it increases the lysosomal pH resulting in inhibition of lysosomal enzymes. This counteracts MHC class II-mediated autoantigen presentation
- It also accumulates in endosomes where it binds to double-stranded DNA. It inhibits Toll-like receptor (TLR) signaling by altering the pH of endosomes and thus preventing TLR7 and TLR9 from binding their ligands (RNA and DNA, respectively). HCQ can also inhibit the activity of the nucleic acid sensor cyclic GMP-AMP (cGAMP) synthase (cGAS) by interfering with its binding to cytosolic DNA. By preventing TLR signaling and cGAS—stimulator of interferon genes (STING) signaling, HCQ can reduce the production of pro-inflammatory cytokines, including type I interferons
- In antigen-presenting cells, such as plasmacytoid dendritic cells and B cells, HCQ inhibits antigen processing and MHC class II presentation to T cells, thereby preventing T cell activation, differentiation, and expression of co-stimulatory molecules and also reducing the production of cytokines (such as IL-1, IL-6, and TNF) by both T cells and B cells

7. How does D-penicillamine exert its anti-inflammatory action?

- Decreases the serum levels of circulating rheumatoid factors and immune complexes
- Affects macrophage functions, and decreases the ability of lymphocytes to proliferate
- Increases the rates of apoptosis through a p53 oncogene-mediated mechanism and arrests angiogenesis by chelating with copper which is a cofactor for this process
- Interferes with fibroblast proliferation and inhibits the cross-linking of collagen and elastin fibers

8. How does thalidomide exert its anti-inflammatory action?

- Inhibits leukocyte chemotaxis to the site of inflammation
- Decreases phagocytosis by polymorphonuclear leukocytes
- Increases production of interleukin (IL)-4 and IL-5 by mononuclear cells
- Inhibits interferon-γ production
- Selectively inhibits tumor necrosis factor (TNF)-α production by monocytes and macrophages

9. **How does dapsone exert its anti-inflammatory action?**

Dapsone belongs to the group of synthetic sulfones. Its effects on inflammatory effector cells, cytokines, and/or mediators have been investigated mainly *in vitro*:

- Inhibition of the enzyme myeloperoxidase accounts for dapsone's anti-inflammatory action
- It inhibits chemotaxis, but only when certain stimuli are applied
- It has an inhibitory effect on prostaglandin synthesis and release
- It inhibits leukotriene C4 production, which could explain its corticosteroid-sparing effect in asthma patients

10. **How does danazol exert its anti-inflammatory action?**

Danazol is a synthetic anabolic steroid with androgenic properties. It can be beneficial in the treatment of hereditary angioedema, refractory autoimmune hemolytic anemia and thrombocytopenia complicating systemic lupus erythematosus, or when there are contraindications to splenectomy and/or corticosteroids. It is relatively well tolerated and may decrease the duration of glucocorticoid therapy. The effects of danazol are based on several immunomodulatory properties:

- Downregulates the expression of Fcγ receptor on monocytes, which in turn decreases platelet phagocytosis
- Reduces the proliferation of lymphocytes
- Alters lymphocyte differentiation by increasing the percentage of helper T lymphocytes
- In mice, danazol decreases the production of pro-inflammatory cytokines (IL-2, IFN-γ) and increases anti-inflammatory cytokines (IL-10)

11. **How does azathioprine exert its immunosuppressive action?**

Azathioprine is a purine analog, and the accepted mechanism of its action is at the level of DNA. Both *in vitro* and *in vivo*, azathioprine is metabolized to 6-mercaptopurine. Ultimately, azathioprine can be incorporated into replicating DNA, blocking the *de novo* pathway of purine synthesis and thus leading to both cytotoxicity and reduced cellular proliferation. This action is thought to contribute to the relative specificity of azathioprine for lymphocytes due to their lack of a salvage pathway.

12. **How does mycophenolate mofetil exert its immunosuppressive action?**

Mycophenolate mofetil (MMF) is a prodrug of mycophenolic acid. Mycophenolic acid:

- Decreases the synthesis of guanine nucleotides, hinders DNA synthesis and consequently reduces lymphocyte proliferation, antibody production, and even microRNA expression
- Reduces CD40L-mediated co-stimulation of antigen-presenting cells, thereby diminishing cell-mediated immune responses
- Inhibits the recruitment of lymphocytes and monocytes into sites of inflammation
- Has antiproliferative effects on fibroblasts probably through inhibition of guanine nucleosides' formation

13. **How does cyclophosphamide exert its immunosuppressive action?**

Cyclophosphamide is a nitrogen mustard, one of the most potent immunosuppressive drugs available. It is an inactive prodrug that is metabolized via the cytochrome-P450 enzymatic system. Phosphoramide mustard and acrolein are its main active and inactive metabolites, respectively. The former is spontaneously degraded, whereas the latter is excreted into the urine. Acrolein, the main inactive metabolite of cyclophosphamide, is responsible for the unwanted drug effects such as hemorrhagic cystitis and bladder neoplasia.

Cyclophosphamide exerts its immunosuppressive action through:

- Attachment of alkylated bases to DNA, resulting in DNA fragmentation by repair

enzymes and ultimately stopping DNA synthesis and RNA transcription from the affected DNA
- Formation of cross-links in the DNA, which prevents DNA from being separated for synthesis or transcription
- Induction of mispairing of the nucleotides leading to mutations

14. Which are the specific side-effects of the commonly used antirheumatic drugs?

The majority of antirheumatic, immunomodulatory, and immunosuppressive medications can cause gastrointestinal discomfort, allergic reactions, bone marrow suppression and increased susceptibility to infections. The specific side effects of the commonly used antirheumatic drugs are:

(a) *Glucocorticoids*: Glucose intolerance, osteoporosis, osteonecrosis, skin manifestations (striae, hirsutism, bruising, delayed wound healing), peptic ulcer disease, higher risk of infections (pneumocystis jiroveci, tuberculosis, fungal-candida, viral-especially herpes zoster) with increasing doses, hypertension, mental disturbances at higher doses, muscle weakness (worse with fluorinated glucocorticoids), posterior subcapsular cataract formation, glaucoma

(b) *Methotrexate*: Oral ulcers, hepatotoxicity, acute pneumonitis, flu-like symptoms, worsening nodulosis and leukocytoclastic vasculitis in seropositive rheumatoid arthritis patients, and teratogenicity

(c) *Leflunomide*: Hypertension, hepatotoxicity, skin rash, neutropenia/thrombocytopenia, alopecia, and teratogenicity

(d) *Cyclosporine-A*: Hypertension, decreased renal function, hirsutism, gum hypertrophy, hyperuricemia, anemia, lymphoma (EBV-related), and bone pain

(e) *Tacrolimus*: Hyperglycemia, diabetes mellitus, hyperkalemia headaches, tremors, hypertension, renal impairment, diarrhea, and nausea

(f) *Hydroxychloroquine*: Retinal toxicity, hyperpigmentation of skin, myopathy, and cardiac toxicity, which although rare can be severe. The most common cardiac complications are conduction disorders (bundle or atrioventricular block), but other non-specific cardiac events can include ventricular hypertrophy, hypokinesia, heart failure, pulmonary arterial hypertension, or valvular dysfunction. The risk for cardiac toxicity increases with a higher cumulative dose of hydroxychloroquine

(g) *D-penicillamine*: Dysgeusia, drug-induced lupus, membranous glomerulonephritis, antibody-mediated myasthenia gravis and Lambert-Eaton myasthenic syndrome, which can persist even after its withdrawal

(h) *Thalidomide*: Sensory polyneuropathy, blood clot formation, teratogenic (phocomelia), sedation, and constipation

(i) *Dapsone*: Hemolysis, leucopenia, liver toxicity, and peripheral neuropathy

(j) *Danazol*: Androgenic side effects: hirsutism, acne, irreversible deepening of the voice, adverse blood lipid profiles, breast atrophy and decreased breast size, hot flashes, elevation of liver enzymes, and mood changes

(k) *Azathioprine*: Hepatotoxicity, pancreatitis, hypersensitivity syndrome (rash, fever, hepatitis, renal failure within the first 2 weeks of use), and warfarin resistance. Azathioprine is converted to its active metabolite 6-mercaptopurine by xanthine oxidase and thiopurine methyltransferase (TPMT). In patients concomitantly treated with allopurinol (inhibits xanthine oxidase), it should be used with caution or not at all due to increased toxicity of azathioprine. The activity of TPMT is affected by genetic polymorphisms. Individuals with low enzymatic activity are at risk for severe myelosuppression, in particular, 4–10 weeks after onset of treatment with azathioprine, and in these patients TPMT phenotype activity should be measured

(l) *Mycophenolate mofetil (MMF)*: Gastrointestinal side effects (mainly diarrhea), leukopenia, anemia, hepatotoxicity, infections, and lymphoproliferative diseases (EBV-associated)
(m) *Cyclophosphamide*: Bladder toxicity (hemorrhagic cystitis, carcinoma), premature menopause, and amenorrhea

15. Pneumocystis jiroveci prophylaxis in patients with rheumatic diseases exposed to prolonged high-dose glucocorticoids. When to start, when to stop, and what are the benefits of prophylaxis?

Pneumocystis jiroveci pneumonia (PJP) can be lethal in severely immunosuppressed patients. It is suggested that in patients with rheumatic diseases on high-dose glucocorticoids (prednisone ≥30 mg/day) for 4 or more weeks and particularly in those starting at higher doses (60 mg/day) where the short-term risk of PJP is much greater, prophylaxis with trimethoprim/sulfamethoxazole (TMP/SMX) should be initiated. In these patients stopping prophylaxis with TMP/SMX should be considered once doses have been tapered to 15 mg/day. In cases where other PJP risk factors (e.g., cyclophosphamide use, lymphopenia, or underlying vasculitis) are present, prophylaxis should continue until lower doses are achieved. Incidence of PJP among the non-prophylaxed immunosuppressed patients is significantly higher regardless of the underlying disease, although patients with vasculitis are at even greater risk. The use of TMP/SMX has been shown to associate with a 93% decrease in the incidence of PJP in patients on high-dose glucocorticoids [1].

16. Which anti-rheumatic drugs are implicated in the development of DRESS syndrome?

Drug reaction with eosinophilia and systemic symptoms (DRESS) syndrome is a rare hypersensitivity reaction to many drugs which manifests 2–6 weeks after drug exposure. It presents with fever, rash, lymphadenopathy and involvement of the liver, kidney, heart and lung which can lead to affected organ failure. The commonly responsible anti-rheumatic drugs for its development are allopurinol, sulfasalazine and dapsone. Rarely, leflunomide, hydroxychloroquine, nonsteroidal anti-inflammatory drugs, febuxostat, bosentan and solcitinib have been reported as the offending drugs for the development of the syndrome [2].

17. Hydroxychloroquine retinopathy: What are the risks of toxicity and how often is screening recommended?

The risk of hydroxychloroquine (HCQ) toxicity is dependent on the daily dose and duration of treatment. At recommended doses (≤5.0 mg/kg/day), the risk of toxicity at 10 years is less than 2%, but it rises to 20% after 20 years of use. Patients should have baseline ophthalmic examination to rule out preexisting maculopathy. For most patients annual screening should begin after they have been on therapy for 5 years. Patients at increased risk of toxicity (i.e., HCQ dose >5 mg/kg/day, concomitant tamoxifen use, impaired renal function) should commence annual screening from the outset [3].

18. Based on which scientific grounds was anti-tumor necrosis factor-α (TNF-α) therapy established for the treatment of inflammatory arthritis?

The rationale for the development of anti-TNF-α therapy was based on the following laboratory, experimental animal, and clinical studies.

Initially, abundance of TNF-α was found in inflamed synovial tissues from rheumatoid arthritis patients. Subsequently, it was observed that synovial membrane cell cultures from rheumatoid arthritis patients produce, over several days, in the absence of extrinsic stimulation, pro-inflammatory cytokines. The addition of anti-TNF-α antibodies to the cultures markedly reduced the production of other pro-inflammatory cytokines, including interleukin (IL)-1, IL-6, IL-8, and granulocyte-macrophage colony-stimulating factor (GM-CSF). These observations led to the concept that TNF-α holds a dominant position in a pro-inflammatory cytokine within the rheumatoid arthritis joint.

Another group of investigators constructed TNF-α transgenic mice which develop arthritis resembling human rheumatoid arthritis. Treatment of these animals with anti-TNF-α antibodies resulted in amelioration of arthritis. An independent group of investigators treated mice with collagen-induced arthritis using anti-TNF-α antibodies, resulting in amelioration of disease activity. All the above studies indicated that TNF-α drives a multi-cytokine, multicellular chronic disease and can be an ideal therapeutic target. Initially, anti-TNF-α antibodies were administered, in an open-label study, in rheumatoid arthritis patients, and the encouraging results led to the development of controlled multicenter studies that documented the therapeutic efficacy of anti-TNF-α antibodies for rheumatoid arthritis. The success of anti-TNF-α treatment efficacy in rheumatoid arthritis prompted its study in other related diseases such as juvenile rheumatoid arthritis, ankylosing spondylitis, psoriatic arthritis, Crohn's disease, ulcerative colitis, and psoriasis. In all of these, the effect on patients has been very satisfactory and has greatly improved their quality of life. The limitations for the use of this biologic agent are the high cost and the unwanted side-effects.

19. What is the rationale for the use of CTLA4-Ig as a therapeutic agent in patients with rheumatoid arthritis?

Following antigen recognition via the major histocompatibility complex on antigen-presenting cells by the T-cell receptor, T cells require a second, co-stimulatory signal to become activated. CTLA4-immunoglobulin-Fc (CTLA4-Ig) fusion protein selectively modulates T-cell co-stimulation. It binds to both CD80 and CD86 (B7 molecules) and prevents interaction with their counter-receptors, expressed on T cells, CD28, and CTLA4, respectively. This interferes with T-cell-antigen-presenting cell interaction and limits T-cell activation, a process that plays a central role in the immunopathogenesis of rheumatoid arthritis. In addition, CTLA4-Ig can bind to B7 molecules expressed on dendritic cells and activate a pathway of tryptophan catabolism that indirectly leads to inhibition of lymphocyte activation and T-cell death. Recently, it has been shown that the effects of CTLA4-Ig are mediated by regulatory T cells (Tregs) and transforming growth factor β and require macrophage-derived nitric oxide.

20. What is the rationale of interleukin-6 signaling pathway blockade for the treatment of patients with inflammatory arthritis?

Interleukin (IL)-6 has many physiologic functions and plays an active role in inflammatory responses, bone metabolism, arthritis, and neoplasia. In several inflammatory disorders such as rheumatoid arthritis and systemic-onset juvenile idiopathic arthritis, overproduction of IL-6 has been documented. Interruption of the IL-6 signaling pathway was evaluated as a treatment option for these diseases. Furthermore, mice lacking the IL-6 gene were protected from collagen-induced arthritis and in susceptible mice strains antibodies with specificity for IL-6 receptor ameliorated collagen-induced arthritis. On the basis of these studies and observations, clinical trials were initiated with humanized monoclonal anti-IL-6 receptor antibody and indicated that this biologic therapy dramatically improves disease activity and is rather well tolerated.

21. Are JAK inhibitors effective therapeutic agents for rheumatoid arthritis?

Janus kinases (JAKs) are intracellular enzymes transmitting signals from cytokines binding to their receptors on the cell surface, in order to recruit signal transducers and activators of transcription (STATs), which will, in turn, initiate pro-inflammatory cellular responses. Four members of the JAK family have been identified: JAK1, JAK2, JAK3, and tyrosine kinase 2. JAK–STAT pathway plays a significant role in the pathogenesis of rheumatoid arthritis (RA). Two JAK inhibitors are approved by FDA/EMA for the treatment of active RA: tofacitinib (selective JAK1/JAK3 inhibitor) was the first JAK inhibitor approved as a therapeutic agent for active RA and the approval of baricitinib (selective JAK1/JAK2 inhibitor) followed. Both of these JAK inhibitors were shown, in combination with methotrexate or as monotherapy, to improve symptoms and signs of active RA. Furthermore, both JAK inhibitors seem to affect structural joint damage progression [4, 5]. Recently, tofacitinib has also been approved for the treatment of psoriatic arthritis. Nonetheless, given the lack of direct head-to-head comparisons of JAK inhibitors with biologics, the recently published 2019 update of EULAR recommendations for the management of RA [6] has itemized different JAK inhibitors among drugs suitable to be started in patients failing conventional synthetic DMARD therapy, but no priority was highlighted, even with respect to biologic DMARDs.

22. On what basis inhibition of IL-17A or IL-17 led to its use as a therapeutic agent for rheumatoid arthritis?

Two experimental observations suggested that IL-17A may play an important role in mediating joint degradation in rheumatoid arthritis. Firstly, in collagen-induced arthritis, a widely accepted experimental arthritis mouse model, IL-17A overexpression accelerated development, enhanced severity of synovial inflammation and bone erosions. Blocking IL-17A with a soluble IL-17 receptor fusion protein suppressed arthritis development and joint damage. Secondly, in human rheumatoid synovial and bone explants, IL-17A enhanced collagen degradation, bone resorption, blocked collagen synthesis and bone formation. Blocking IL-17A protected against all these effects. In human studies, however, IL-17 inhibition either with anti-IL-17 monoclonal antibodies or with a monoclonal antibody against IL-17 receptor failed to show a significant therapeutic effect. The therapeutic failure of IL-17 inhibition in rheumatoid arthritis contrasts the significant therapeutic effect of IL-17 inhibition in psoriasis, psoriatic arthritis, and ankylosing spondylitis.

23. What is the rationale of IL12/23 signaling pathway inhibition for the treatment of patients with psoriatic arthritis?

The rationale for developing IL-12 antagonists was driven by observations that IL-12p40-deficient mice are resistant to experimentally induced inflammatory arthritis, ocular inflammation, and gut inflammation [7]. In mice and humans, IL-12 is composed of the p40 subunit and the p35 subunit. This heterodimer signals through the IL-12 receptor (IL-12R), which is composed of the β1 and β2 subunits. IL-23 is composed of the p19 and the p40 subunits, which signals through IL-23R and IL-12Rβ1. Following the recognition, that IL-12 and IL-23 share the p40 subunit but only IL-23 uses the p19 subunit [8], it was determined that mice deficient in IL-23 but not IL-12 are resistant to experimental immune-mediated diseases [7]. In addition to the data from preclinical disease models, family genetic studies, large-scale genome-wide association studies (GWAS) and next-generation sequencing approaches have underlined that IL-23 may contribute to the risk of inflammatory disease. GWAS for psoriasis, psoriatic arthritis, and ankylosing spondylitis reported a protective association for a particular single-nucleotide polymorphism (SNP, rs11209026 (c.1142G>A; p.

Arg381Gln)) residing in the IL-23R protein-coding sequence [9–11]. All this provided the rationale to develop the human IL-12–neutralizing antibodies. Ustekinumab is a fully human IgG1 monoclonal antibody that binds with high affinity to the shared p40 subunit of human IL-12 and IL-23, inhibiting their binding to the IL-12Rβ1 receptor on the surfaces of T cells, NK cells, and antigen-presenting cells. Therapeutic use of ustekinumab for moderate to severe psoriasis, and psoriatic arthritis was associated with improvements on, related enthesitis, dactylitis, pain, quality of life, physical function, and inhibition of radiological damage [12, 13].

24. What is the rationale of cAMP phosphodiesterase-4 inhibition for the treatment of psoriasis and psoriatic arthritis?

Phosphodiesterase-4 (PDE-4) is an intracellular enzyme that catalyzes the hydrolysis of cyclic adenosine 3', 5'-monophosphate (cAMP) into the intracellular second messenger, AMP. Increased levels of intracellular cAMP lead to inhibition of NFκB, which is involved in pro-inflammatory responses. cAMP is degraded by phosphodiesterases (PDEs) and increased expression of PDE4 isoforms is seen in patients with psoriasis [14]. By decreasing levels of intracellular cAMP, PDE4 promotes increased production of pro-inflammatory mediators and decreased production of anti-inflammatory mediators [14]. Apremilast is an orally administered, targeted synthetic agent that inhibits PDE4. *In vitro*, it has been shown to inhibit the expression and/or production of pro-inflammatory cytokines and chemokines from various cell types, such as TNF-a, IL-12, and IL-23 from stimulated peripheral blood mononuclear cells [15, 16], TNF-a by natural killer cells, keratinocytes [17] and human rheumatoid synovial cells [16]. *In vivo*, apremilast demonstrated beneficial activity in murine models of psoriasis [17] and arthritis [16].

25. What is the rationale of interleukin-1 signaling pathway blockade for the treatment of patients with inflammatory arthritis and autoinflammatory syndromes?

Interleukin (IL)-1 (IL-1α and IL-1β) is a master pro-inflammatory cytokine implicated in both local and systemic inflammation. Both IL-1α and IL-1β act on IL-1 receptor and are inhibited by IL-1 receptor antagonist (IL-1Ra). IL-1Ra is a naturally occurring member of the IL-1 family, which blocks the IL-1 receptor type 1. This receptor is expressed on all nucleated cells; therefore, IL-1Ra hinders systemic inflammation induced by IL-1. Infants born with a loss of function mutation in the naturally occurring endogenous IL-1 receptor antagonist (IL-1Ra), a condition called deficiency of interleukin-1 receptor antagonist (DIRA), present overwhelming sterile inflammation of the skin, joints, and bone. This constituted unequivocal evidence of the role of IL-1 in orchestrating inflammation. Mice deficient in IL-1Ra are similarly affected in that they develop spontaneous inflammation resembling rheumatoid arthritis and can succumb to lethal arteritis. The best evidence for the role of IL-1 (either IL-1α or IL-1β) in disease comes from specific blockade, and inhibiting IL-1 by manipulating IL-1Ra became an attractive therapeutic strategy in rheumatoid arthritis (RA) and other chronic inflammatory diseases. The IL-1Ra receptor antagonist (anakinra) blocks the IL-1 receptor and therefore reduces the activity of IL-1α and IL-1β. Canakinumab is a fully human monoclonal antibody targeting IL-1β, while rilonacept is a soluble decoy receptor. IL-1α is expressed as a precursor and is constitutively present in most cells of healthy subjects. In contrast, IL-1β is not detected in health; it is a product of blood monocytes, tissue macrophages, and dendritic cells; and is first synthesized as an inactive precursor. The precursor requires cleavage by caspase-1, which is activated following the oligomerization of the intracellular protein complex termed inflammasome. Autoinflammatory diseases are due to mutations in the intracellular proteins that control caspase-1, and they constitute a group of rare genetic disorders, which are effectively treated with IL-1 blocking therapies. Amyloidosis is a destructive process affecting several organs due to the deposition of amyloid fibrils. IL-1, which is commonly elevated in several chronic inflammatory diseases, is an inducer of serum amyloid A (SAA). Left untreated, IL-1-mediated diseases result in organ failure due to amyloid deposits.

A growing number of chronic inflammatory disorders without a known genetic basis, where IL-1 contributes significantly to the inflammation, respond to reducing IL-1 activity. In adult-onset Still's disease, monotherapy with anakinra is highly effective. Systemic-onset juvenile idiopathic arthritis and macrophage activation syndrome are affectively treated with anakinra. Crystal arthritides (gout and calcium pyrophosphate crystal arthritis) with recurrent attacks and unresponsive to other standards of therapy are highly responsive to anakinra or canakinumab.

26. On the basis of which facts were anti-CD20 antibodies developed as therapeutic agents for rheumatoid arthritis patients?

Rituximab, a monoclonal chimeric anti-CD20 antibody originally used in non-Hodgkin's lymphoma, recognizes a determinant expressed on intramedullary pre-B- to B-memory stage lymphocytes. It induces antibody-dependent cell-mediated cytotoxicity, complement-dependent cytotoxicity, and apoptosis of B cells in various developmental stages leading to their transient but almost complete depletion in peripheral blood, although only partially in the bone marrow and synovial tissue niches. Eliminating B cells by targeting the CD20 cell surface differentiation antigen may remove a large population of cells loaded with pathophysiologically important cytokines, such as TNF-α and IL-6. Concurrent depletion of CD20+ non-B cells and prevention of antigen presentation by eliminating B cells may offer additional effect by leading to a reduction in T-cell activation without primarily affecting co-stimulation. In many rheumatoid arthritis patients, synovial extra-follicular germinal centers develop, where B cells play an important role in local inflammation and the generation of memory B cells and plasma cells. These local processes lead to activation of the immune system and ultimately to joint destruction in rheumatoid arthritis. Administration of anti-CD20 monoclonal antibodies in rheumatoid arthritis patients appears to influence many B-cell functions, such as depletion of memory B cells, interruption of immune activation, antigen-presentation, and production of inflammatory cytokines. The beneficial effect of B-cell depletion therapy of rheumatoid arthritis patients substantiates the notion that B cells are important players in the pathogenesis of the disease.

27. What evaluations are mandatory prior to anti-CD20 (Rituximab) monoclonal antibody administration?

Exclude hepatitis B and C as well as latent tuberculosis infections, and make sure that the patient has been immunized with influenza and pneumococcal vaccines.

28. On what basis was inhibition of B-lymphocyte-activating factor developed as a therapeutic agent for systemic lupus erythematosus?

B-lymphocyte-activating factor (BAFF), also known as B-lymphocyte stimulator (BLyS), belongs to the family of tumor necrosis factor ligands. It is expressed by many cell types including hematopoietic and stromal cells. Increased circulating levels of BAFF were found in the sera of patients with systemic autoimmune disorders. Furthermore, inhibition of BAFF in murine experimental systemic lupus erythematosus models resulted in delayed disease onset. These observations led to the development of a human monoclonal antibody (belimumab) which inhibits soluble but not transmembrane BAFF.

29. Which are the specific side-effects of the commonly used biologic and targeted synthetic antirheumatic drugs?

(a) *Anti-TNF drugs* (infliximab, adalimumab, etanercept, golimumab, and certolizumab pegol): Injection site reactions (for subcutaneous administration of TNF inhibitors), infusion reactions for infliximab (hypotension, headache, nausea, and vomiting), infections (reactivation of latent tuberculosis, hepatitis B/C, varicella zoster virus, and *Pneumocystis jiroveci*), demyelinating syndromes (multiple sclerosis-like, Guillain-Barré polyradiculopathy), autoimmune phenomena (some patients will develop positive ANA, anti-dsDNA, and a small number of drug-induced lupus), anti-drug antibodies in patients treated with infliximab (patients may lose response to infliximab and may experience more severe infusion reactions), and psoriasiform rashes
(b) *CTLA4-Ig* (abatacept) upper and lower respiratory tract infections, local and systemic injection site reactions, elevated liver enzymes
(c) *Anti-IL6 receptor antibody* (tocilizumab): Infusion reactions (intravenous administration), infections (rheumatoid arthritis patients with increased baseline DAS28 and peripheral blood absolute neutrophil counts, negative anti-citrullinated peptides, and concomitant leflunomide treatment are at higher risk to develop serious infections after initiation of treatment with anti-IL-6 antibody [18]), elevated hepatic enzymes, neutropenia, lipid elevations (LDL), gastrointestinal tract perforation (rare), and macrophage activation syndrome (in 3% of treated systemic juvenile idiopathic arthritis patients)
(d) *JAK inhibitors* (tofacitinib and baricitinib): Neutropenia, lymphocytosis, anemia, liver enzyme elevation, increases in lipid parameters, increased risk of herpes zoster infection, and increased risk of thromboembolism
(e) *Anti-IL17A, anti-IL17RA antibodies* (secukinumab, ixekizumab, brodalumab): Nasopharyngitis, upper respiratory tract infections, injection site reactions, headache, arthralgia, depression, suicidal ideation (brodalumab)
(f) *Anti-IL12/23* (ustekinumab): Injection site reactions, flu-like symptoms, headache, fatigue
(g) *Anti-PDE4* (apremilast): Mostly gastrointestinal side-effects with nausea and emesis
(h) *IL-1 receptor antagonist* (anakinra): Injection site reactions, neutropenia, and infections
(i) *Anti-CD20* (rituximab): Infusion reactions, serum sickness, infections, viral infections (reactivation of hepatitis B, JC virus, VZV), hypogammaglobulinemia (after repeated infusions), and late-onset neutropenia (3–4 month post-therapy)
(j) *Anti-BlyS* (belimumab): Fever, anaphylactic reaction, infusion site reaction, nausea, diarrhea

30. Are low doses of glucocorticoids associated with increased infection risk in patients with rheumatoid arthritis (RA)?

A very recent retrospective study used Medicare and commercial claims data from 2005–2016, to compare patients with RA who had been receiving stable doses of disease-modifying anti-rheumatic drugs (DMARDs), including biologics, for six months according to whether they were receiving glucocorticoids. Associations between glucocorticoid dose (prednisone: none, ≤5 mg/d, 5 to 10 mg/d, and >10 mg/d) and hospitalizations for infections were recorded. According to the results of this study the one-year cumulative incidence of hospitalizations due to infection was significantly increased with increasing daily doses of glucocorticoids. RA patients receiving higher-dose glucocorticoids (>10 mg/d) had more than twice the risk of serious infection compared to patients not receiving glucocorticoids. The risk of infections in patients receiving prednisone 5 mg/daily or less was smaller but still significant [19].

31. Which biologic agent(s) produce the most serious infections in patients with rheumatoid arthritis (RA)?

In RA patients who switch from one biological disease-modifying anti-rheumatic drug (bDMARD) to another the risk of serious infections is higher compared to patients who have not been exposed to biological agents before. Infliximab seems to carry a higher risk for serious infections including reactivation of latent tuberculosis, pneumonia, soft and skin tissue infections, septicemia, and genitourinary tract infections. Other biological agents, including abatacept, adalimumab, etanercept, and rituximab carry lower risk, varying between patients with baseline low or high risk of infections [20]. In a Japanese study, there were no statistically significant differences of risk for serious infections among patients treated with different biological agents [21]. These data do not clearly point which biologic agent used for RA treatment carries the highest risk of infections.

32. How should the therapeutic regimen of adult patients on traditional disease-modifying antirheumatic drugs, biologic agents, and glucocorticoids be modified if they undergo elective total hip or total knee arthroplasty?

- For patients with rheumatoid arthritis (RA), spondyloarthropathies (SpA, including ankylosing spondylitis and psoriatic arthritis), juvenile idiopathic arthritis (JIA), or systemic lupus erythematosus (SLE) undergoing elective total hip arthroplasty (THA) or total knee arthroplasty (TKA):
  - The current dose of methotrexate, leflunomide, hydroxychloroquine, and/or sulfasalazine should be continued
- For SLE patients not treated (induction or maintenance) for severe organ manifestations:
  - The current dose of mycophenolate mofetil, azathioprine, cyclosporine-A, or tacrolimus should not be given 1 week prior to elective THA or TKA surgery
- For RA, SpA, JIA, or SLE patients on biologic agents:
  - All biologic agents should be discontinued prior to surgery in patients undergoing elective THA or TKA, and the surgery should be planned at the end of the dosing cycle for each specific biologic
  - Biologics in these patients can be restarted once wound healing is established (approximately after 14 days), all sutures/staples are out, and there is no clinical evidence of surgical and non-surgical site infections
- For RA, SpA, or SLE patients on glucocorticoids:
  - The current daily dose should be continued in these patients undergoing THA or TKA, rather than administering perioperative supraphysiologic glucocorticoid doses (the so-called stress dosing)
  - An increased arthroplasty-related infection risk exists with long-term use of prednisone (or equivalent) dose >15 mg/day. Therefore careful tapering of prednisone dose prior to surgery to <20 mg/day, when possible, is advisable [22]

33. Do biologics and/or corticosteroids increase the risk of infection in rheumatoid arthritis (RA) patients with hip or knee arthroplasty?

It is known that RA patients have an increased risk for infection after arthroplasty. It is not known though if this risk increases in patients who underwent arthroplasty while on therapy with biologic agents. In a retrospective cohort study data between January 2006 through September 2015, on adult RA patients who had elective knee or hip arthroplasty (primary or revision) with recent therapy including one of the following biologic agents: abatacept, adalimumab, etanercept, infliximab, rituximab, or tocilizumab before surgery, were included. In this study, 9911 RA patients were treated with biologics and had undergone 10923 surgical procedures. No statistically significant differences were observed on the incidents of infections between patients who received different biologic agents. In contrast, the risk of infection almost doubled (13%) in RA patients who received in addition to biologics corticosteroids (>10 mg prednisolone a day) and had arthroplasty [23]. The results of this study should be reexamined in a multination, multicenter study since in the present one the number of patients on rituximab and tocilizumab treatment was rather small.

34. What is the impact of immunosuppression with biologic or targeted synthetic disease-modifying anti-rheumatic drug (bDMARDS or tsDMaRDs) on postoperative mortality and readmission in patients with rheumatoid arthritis?

This question was addressed by a recent retrospective study that included adult rheumatoid arthritis (RA) patients who underwent hip fracture, abdominopelvic surgery (cholecystectomy, hysterectomy, hernia, appendectomy, colectomy) or cardiac surgery (coronary artery bypass graft, mitral/aortic valve) through 2006–2015. RA patients on conventional synthetic DMARDs (methotrexate) and RA patients on bDMARDs or tsDMARDs had the same risk of 90-day mortality or 30-day readmission after any kind of surgery. Risk of mortality and readmission was higher with 5–10 mg/day of glucocorticoids, when compared to RA patients who did not receive any glucocorticoids, especially for cardiac surgery. Based on these results, the common practice to hold biologics before surgery could be reconsidered. Furthermore, necessary non-elective surgeries do not need to be delayed in RA patients receiving bDMARs, since delaying these surgeries has its own consequences [24].

35. How do high doses of intravenous immunoglobulins exert their immunomodulatory action?

Intravenous immunoglobulins (IVIg) therapy is widely used and is an effective treatment for many autoimmune disorders (idiopathic thrombocytopenia, Kawasaki disease, and inflammatory myopathies). The exact immunomodulatory mechanism(s) of IVIg high doses remains speculative. The proposed immunomodulatory mechanisms include modulation of complement activation, suppression of idiotypic antibodies, saturation of Fc receptors on macrophages, blockade of IgG receptors on phagocytic cells, and blockade of FcRn receptors on endothelial cells, which prevent internalization and catabolism of immunoglobulins in the endosome; thus IVIg by saturating FcRn receptors enables rapid catabolism of endogenous and possibly pathogenic immunoglobulins in the endosome; in addition IVIg decreases MHC I molecule expression and cytokines, downregulates transforming growth factor β1, and suppresses various inflammatory mediators, including cytokines, chemokines, as well as metalloproteinases. These mechanisms are not mutually exclusive and may act simultaneously in order to modulate the immune system response.

36 In which diseases can intravenous immunoglobulin therapy be considered?

- Kawasaki disease
- Guillain–Barré syndrome
- Idiopathic thrombocytopenic purpura

- Chronic inflammatory demyelinating polyneuropathy
- Idiopathic inflammatory myopathies (steroid-resistant or aggressive)
- ANCA-positive vasculitis (in patients with refractory disease)
- Motor neuron peripheral neuropathy in patients with Sjögren's syndrome

37. Which are the specific side effects of intravenous immunoglobulins?

Specific side-effects of intravenous immunoglobulins (IVIg) include: headache, hypotension, flushing, aseptic meningitis, serum sickness, severe anaphylactic reaction in patients with IgA deficiency, acute renal failure especially when sucrose is used as an excipient to stabilize the protein in the solution (sucrose-containing IVIgs) and when the patient is concurrently treated with angiotensin-converting enzyme inhibitors or angiotensin receptor antagonists, and pseudohyponatremia (due to hyperproteinemia and increased serum viscosity following IVIg infusion).

38. Which drugs used for the therapy of rheumatic diseases can cause gynecomastia?

- Methotrexate
- Cyclophosphamide
- Prednisone
- H2 histamine receptor blockers (cimetidine)

39. To which patients should acetylsalicylic acid not be given?

Patients most at risk to develop hypersensitivity reactions to acetylsalicylic acid (ASA) are severe asthmatics with nasal polyps (Samter's triad = asthma, nasal polyps, and aspirin sensitivity). Up to 78% of these patients may have a reaction to aspirin. This is considered sensitivity and not allergy because it is not IgE mediated. Inhibition of COX-1 by aspirin diverts the arachidonic precursors down the leukotriene (LT) pathway resulting in excessive production of LTC4, LTD4, and LTE4, which are effective chemoattractants and activators of inflammatory cells. This induces topically chronic sinonasal inflammation resulting in mucosal overgrowth characterizing nasal polyps.

40. What are the risks of long-term use of proton pump inhibitors?

Proton pump inhibitors (PPIs) are medications very frequently prescribed in patients with rheumatic diseases to prevent possible side effects of drugs and are often used for a long time. Absolute indications for PPI use include infection with helicobacter pylori, erosive esophagitis, gastric ulcers, and stress ulcer prevention in high-risk critically ill patients. Several studies have suggested a possible association between long-term use of PPI and progression of chronic kidney disease, deficiencies of various micronutrients, such as hypomagnesemia, low serum vitamin B12 and osteoporosis with increased fracture risk, especially hip fractures [25, 26].

Therapeutic Agents in Pregnancy and Lactation

41. Which nonsteroidal anti-inflammatory and immunosuppressive agents are permitted in pregnant patients?

Based on current evidence, nonsteroidal anti-inflammatory drugs (NSAIDs) and disease-modifying anti-rheumatic drugs (DMARDs) are recommended to be used during pregnancy as follows:

- Nonselective cyclooxygenase (COX) inhibitors can be continued during the first and second trimesters
- Glucocorticoids can be continued at the lowest effective dose (preferably less than 10 mg daily) throughout pregnancy. Fluorinated glucocorticoids are less metabolized by the placenta and should

be used with caution only to treat fetal problems. Intravenous glucocorticoids can be given, when required

- Conventional synthetic DMARDs compatible with pregnancy are hydroxychloroquine, chloroquine, sulfasalazine, azathioprine, and cyclosporine–A
- Colchicine can be used throughout pregnancy
- Intravenous immunoglobulin (IVIg) can be used throughout pregnancy
- Tacrolimus can be continued throughout pregnancy at the lowest effective dose

42. Which nonsteroidal anti-inflammatory and immunosuppressive agents should be avoided in pregnant patients?

- Selective COX II inhibitors should be avoided in pregnancy
- Targeted synthetic DMARDs (apremilast, tofacitinib, baricitinib) should be avoided during pregnancy until data are gathered on the risks associated with their use. Given their short half-lives (3–12 h), discontinuation 1 month before conception should be sufficient
- Leflunomide has been recently shown not to be associated with significantly increased risk of major congenital malformations, prematurity, low birth weight, or spontaneous abortions when used during pregnancy [27]. Nevertheless, given that relatively few women were exposed to leflunomide during pregnancy in this particular cohort, leflunomide should be avoided
- Methotrexate should be withdrawn 1–3 months before a planned pregnancy
- Cyclophosphamide must be withdrawn before a planned pregnancy
- Mycophenolate mofetil (MMF) should be withdrawn 1.5 months before a planned pregnancy
- Tofacitinib should be stopped 2 months before conception

43. Has azathioprine long-term side effects in embryos exposed to this drug during pregnancy?

A recent PubMed search showed that the risk of newborns, delivered from mothers on azathioprine (AZA) therapy, for congenital anomalies, was similar to those found in the general population. Nevertheless, a higher incidence of prematurity, lower birth weight, and intrauterine developmental delay, as well as increased maternal-embryo cytomegalovirus infections, were noted in these newborns in comparison with the general population. It has been questioned, however, if these newborns present neurocognitive impairments. A long follow-up of these offsprings is of paramount importance in order to answer the question on the long-term outcomes of children born by mothers treated with AZA during pregnancy [28].

44. How does hydroxychloroquine affect disease flares in patients with systemic lupus erythematosus during pregnancy and postpartum?

A recent study of a large cohort of systemic lupus erythematosus (SLE) patients including 398 pregnancies, in whom the definition of flares was carefully defined, showed an increased SLE flare rate during pregnancy which was modified by hydroxychloroquine (HCQ) therapy. The risk of flare in pregnancy compared to non-pregnant/non-postpartum periods was higher for patients not taking HCQ than for patients under HCQ therapy. The risk of flare in the 3-months postpartum was lower in women taking HCQ after delivery. This work suggests that HCQ if continued during pregnancy and postpartum diminishes the risk of flare in SEL patients [29].

45. Which biologic agents are permitted in pregnant patients?

Biologics differ significantly in structure, half-life, and placental passage. Their placental transfer is low during organogenesis but increases steadily after the 13th week of gestation. Those biologic agents that extensively transfer through the placenta reach high serum levels in the fetus when administered after the 30th week of gestation, thus increasing the risk of postnatal infection.

- Infliximab and adalimumab can be continued up to the 20th week of gestation. If absolutely indicated, they can be used throughout pregnancy
- Etanercept can be used up to 30–32 weeks of gestation, and if strongly indicated, it may be considered for use throughout pregnancy due to its low rate of transplacental passage
- Certolizumab may be considered for use throughout pregnancy due to its low rate of transplacental passage

It should be noted that neonates exposed to biologics before gestational week 22 can receive vaccinations according to standard protocols including live vaccines. Whereas, children exposed to biologics at the late second and during the third trimester can follow vaccination programs but should not receive live vaccines in the first 6 months of their life.

46. Which biologic agents should be avoided in pregnant patients?

- Golimumab should not be considered for treatment during pregnancy because of limited evidence
- Rituximab can be used early in gestation only in exceptional cases. Its use at later stages of pregnancy bares the risk of B-cell depletion and other cytopenias in the neonate
- Anakinra and canakinumab can be used before and during pregnancy only when there are no other options available for treatment
- Tocilizumab, abatacept, ustekinumab, and belimumab should be avoided during pregnancy

47. Are vitamin K antagonists indicated during pregnancy?

Vitamin K antagonists (VKAs), such as warfarin, cross the placenta. During the first trimester of pregnancy, especially beyond the eighth week after last menstrual period, VKAs at doses >5 mg daily may account for adverse outcomes, such as miscarriage, stillbirth, and embryopathy. Although warfarin has much lower fetal toxicity at doses ≤5 mg/day than at higher doses, when the dose to achieve the target INR exceeds 5 mg/day, substitution with low molecular weight heparin (LMWH) during the first trimester, the critical phase of organogenesis, is recommended [30].

LMWH does not cross the placenta and is cleared entirely by the kidneys. In that sense fixed, weight-based dosing tends to underperform as the pregnancy advances, due to the increase in glomerular filtration rate (and clearance of LMWH) throughout pregnancy. Therefore, when LMWH is used during pregnancy, peak anti-Xa level should be checked 4–6 h post-dose, and LMWH carries a low risk of thromboembolic complications when the levels are kept between 1.0 and 1.2 U/ml [31]. Evidence is lacking regarding the safety of the direct oral anticoagulants apixaban, rivaroxaban, dabigatran, and fondaparinux in pregnancy and use of these drugs is therefore not recommended.

48. Which nonsteroidal anti-inflammatory drugs and immunosuppressive agents are permitted and which should be avoided in lactating patients?

- Nonselective COX inhibitors are compatible with breastfeeding, while from the selective COX II inhibitors, only celecoxib should be used during lactation
- Glucocorticoids are compatible with lactation, yet they should be taken 2–4 h before breastfeeding
- Hydroxychloroquine, cyclosporine-A, sulfasalazine (caution in cases of premature children, G6PD deficiency, and hyperbilirubinemia), tacrolimus, colchicine, and intravenous immunoglobulin are compatible with breastfeeding
- Methotrexate, leflunomide, cyclophosphamide, MMF, and tofacitinib should be avoided during breastfeeding

49. Which biologic agents are permitted and which should be avoided in lactating patients?

- Infliximab, adalimumab, golimumab, etanercept, and certolizumab are compatible with breastfeeding
- Rituximab, belimumab, anakinra, canakinumab, tocilizumab, abatacept, and ustekinumab should be avoided during breastfeeding

Vaccination Recommendations for Patients with Autoimmune Rheumatic Diseases

50. Which precautions and measures should be taken before vaccination is administered in adult patients with autoimmune rheumatic diseases?

- The vaccination status of the patients should be assessed and documented at the earliest after diagnosis, and recommended vaccinations should be administered as soon as possible, preferably before initiation of immunosuppressive therapy
- It is generally safe to administer inactivated vaccines to patients with autoimmune rheumatic diseases under immunosuppressive treatment; the immunogenicity may be reduced
- Live attenuated vaccines (MMR, measles, mumps, rubella, varicella zoster) should only be given before initiation of immunosuppressive treatment (at least 4 weeks)
- BCG vaccination should not be administered to patients with autoimmune rheumatic diseases under immunosuppressive treatment
- In already treated autoimmune patients, vaccines should ideally be administered when immunosuppressive therapy is at the lowest levels and during stable disease

51. Which vaccines are recommended for adult patients with autoimmune rheumatic diseases?

For adult patients with autoimmune diseases the following inactivated (non-live) vaccines are recommended [32]:

- Seasonal influenza vaccine: For all autoimmune patients annually
- Pneumococcal vaccination: Ideally, both PCV13 and PPSV23 should be given ≥2 weeks before the beginning of any immunosuppressive treatment and in particular anti-CD20 (rituximab), abatacept, tofacitinib, and methotrexate
  - Patients who have not received either vaccine previously should receive the 13-valent pneumococcal vaccine (PCV13) first followed by the 23-valent pneumococcal polysaccharide vaccine (PPSV23)
  - Patients who have received either vaccine previously:

    If one dose of PCV13 has been received and no/unknown PPSV23 status: give first dose PPSV23 ≥8 weeks after PCV13 and second PPSV23 at least 5 years after first PPSV23

    If one dose of PPSV23 has been received and no/unknown PCV13 status: give PCV13 ≥1 year after first PPSV23. The second dose of PPSV23should be given 5 years later
- Vaccination against hepatitis B is encouraged in all patients
- Vaccination against human papillomavirus in female patients aged 11–26 years should be considered
- Other inactivated vaccines (e.g., tetanus, diphtheria, pertussis, and meningococcal vaccines) should be given per the same indications and schedules as the general adult population
- In hyposplenic/asplenic patients, influenza, pneumococcal, hemophilus influenza B, and meningococcal C vaccinations are recommended

52. For how long methotrexate administration should be discontinued prior to influenza vaccination?

Discontinuing methotrexate (MTX) for 2 weeks after seasonal influenza vaccination, regardless of the time the RA patient has received the last MTX dose, improved vaccine responses to a similar extent to those who discontinued MTX for 4 weeks, without increasing RA disease activity [33, 34].

53. Can immunization provoke a gouty attack?

It is known that trauma, dehydration, heavy alcohol consumption, and diuretics are precipitating factors of gouty attacks. Interestingly, the aluminum adjuvants contained in more than 50% of the routinely administered adult vaccines have been shown to activate the NLRP3 inflammasome. A recent study showed that two days after immunization the risk of a gouty attack doubles [35].

54. What are the vaccination recommendations before elective splenectomy and what antibiotic prophylaxis scheme is recommended post-splenectomy?

In patients with thrombocytopenia (SLE/APS/ITP) not responsive to steroids and newer immunosuppressives (anti-CD20 antibodies and thrombopoietin mimetics), at times elective splenectomy is performed. In these patients it is important to follow a strict pre- and post-splenectomy vaccination schedule in order to minimize the risk of severe infections.

Pre-splenectomy: Initial vaccinations to be given 4–6 weeks before elective splenectomy:

Pneumococcus: If there is no record of previous vaccination in the patient's medical file: Conjugate vaccine (Prevenar 13) 0.5 mL IM and after 8 weeks Polysaccharide (Pneumovax 23) 0.5 mL IM/SC. One more dose of Polysaccharide (Pneumovax 23) 0.5 mL IM/SC 5 years later.
Meningococcus: Conjugate ACWY (Menveo, Menactra, Nimenrix) 0.5 mL IM and Recombinant B + (Bexsero) 0.5 mL IM followed by a second dose of both 8 weeks later.
Hemophilus influenza type b: Conjugate Hib (Liquid PedvaxHIB, Hiberix) 0.5 mL IM single dose.
Influenza: Quadrivalent Influenza vaccine and thereafter yearly every October.

Post-splenectomy:

Antibiotic Prophylaxis: If in the patient's medical history penicillin allergy is mentioned—roxithromycin 150 mg once daily or erythromycin 250 mg once daily or clarithromycin 250 mg twice daily should be given life-long (immunocompromised patient).
Emergency plan: Instruct/educate the patient to immediately increase roxithromycin to 300 mg a day or erythromycin 1g four times a day (and take all capsules at once) if signs of bacterial infection occur, especially if not able to receive prompt medical review [36].

Therapeutic Modalities and Regimens for Inflammatory Arthritides

55. Which is the therapeutic algorithm for the treatment of seropositive and seronegative rheumatoid arthritis?

The cornerstone therapeutic agent used initially for both entities is methotrexate (0.2–0.3 mg/kg/week) alone or in combination with small prednisone doses (<7.5 mg/day). If this therapeutic scheme after 3 months of follow-up does not place arthritis into remission, then another disease-modifying agent should be added to the above therapeutic scheme; either leflunomide (20 mg/day) or sulfasalazine 2 mg/day or cyclosporine-A (1–3 mg/kg/day) can be used. If this combination is not effective, then in the seropositive arthritis group, an anti-CD20 monoclonal antibody or an anti-TNF biologic agent can be prescribed. In the seronegative group, an anti-TNF biologic agent is the preferred therapeutic modality. In a small percentage of either seropositive or seronegative polyarthritis patients that do not respond to the above therapeutic schemes, anti-interleukin-6 receptor monoclonal antibody therapy can be beneficial.

56. What principles should guide the treatment of psoriatic arthritis?

Psoriatic arthritis (PsA) can have a very heterogeneous presentation. Therefore, the type of treatment depends on particular manifestations, including peripheral arthritis, enthesitis, dactylitis, axial disease, and skin/nail disease.

- In patients with mono/oligoarthritis accompanied by structural damage and increased inflammatory markers as well as in patients with polyarthritis (≥4 joints), a conventional synthetic (cs) DMARD (methotrexate, leflunomide, sulfasalazine) should be initiated early, with methotrexate preferred in patients with skin involvement. If remission is not achieved within 6 months, treatment with a biologic (b) DMARD (TNF inhibitor, IL-12/IL-23 inhibitor, or IL-17 inhibitor) should be initiated. TNF inhibitors are recommended over IL-17 inhibitors, IL-12/23 inhibitors, abatacept, or tofacitinib. If this therapeutic approach fails a JAK inhibitor or a PDE4 inhibitor may be considered
- In patients with enthesitis and insufficient response to NSAIDs or local glucocorticoid injections, therapy with a TNF inhibitor should be considered
- In patients with axial disease therapy with a TNF inhibitor should be instituted. If there is extended skin involvement, an IL-17 inhibitor is preferred
- In patients with PsA and inflammatory bowel disease (IBD) TNF inhibitors are preferred over IL-12/23 inhibitors. Of note, with IL-17 inhibitors adverse effects including possible new-onset or exacerbation of IBD have been reported, although causality has not yet been established
- Local injections of glucocorticoids can be considered as adjunctive therapy in PsA. Systemic glucocorticoids in high doses should be used cautiously, as there is a risk of inducing a flare of psoriasis during rapid tapering [37]

57. Which are the predictors of methotrexate inefficacy in patients with inflammatory polyarthritis?

Although Methotrexate (MTX) therapy is the cornerstone therapeutic intervention for inflammatory polyarthritis, its effectiveness in this patient population, is not universal. MTX failure has been observed more frequently in female than in male inflammatory polyarthritis patients, in smokers and those with longer disease duration. Recently it was shown that MTX failure is additionally associated with rheumatoid factor positivity, younger age, and higher baseline disease activity score (DAS-28) at the onset of symptoms. Patients with these characteristics may benefit from an early combination therapy as a first-line therapeutic option [38].

58. What is the cause of secondary treatment failure of anti-TNF biologic agents in patients with inflammatory arthritis?

Factors which have been proposed to lead to secondary treatment failure of anti-TNF agents in patients with inflammatory arthritis include patient compliance, obesity, monotherapy with biologic agents, and development of antibodies against anti-TNF agents. The rate of antibody development against anti-TNF agents is similar in rheumatoid arthritis (RA) and seronegative spondyloarthritis (SpA) patients treated with either infliximab or adalimumab [39]. In contrast, antibodies do not develop in patients treated with etanercept. In the majority of patients with antibodies against anti-TNF agents, the anti-TNF agent itself is not detected in the patients' sera. Thus, the development of antibodies against anti-TNF agents, is the main factor involved in reducing the serum concentration of the biologic agent and subsequently leading to secondary treatment failure in patients with inflammatory arthritis [40].

59. Which laboratory indices could predict if a patient with rheumatoid arthritis will respond better to IL-6R targeted therapy or to anti-TNF therapy?

Nowadays clinicians have a great number of biologic agents in their armamentarium for therapeutic intervention in rheumatoid arthritis (RA) patients. Precise clinical, biochemical, or molecular parameters are not available in order to direct the clinician to select the most appropriate biologic agent for a given individual patient with RA. A recent study aimed to develop a scoring system that could discriminate between RA patients more likely to respond to either tocilizumab (TCZ) or an anti-TNF agent. The expression of IL-6 and TNF-α mRNA in peripheral blood from 45 newly diagnosed RA patients was measured by DNA microarrays to evaluate cytokine activation. A significant inverse correlation between the expression of IL-6 and TNF-α mRNA was found. Subsequently, simple clinical and laboratory parameters were evaluated prior to the initiation of anti-IL-6 receptor or anti-TNF therapies. After 6 months of therapy, it was shown that RA patients who prior to therapy initiation had higher platelet numbers, lower hemoglobin and lower aspartate aminotransferase (AST), and alanine aminotransferase (ALT) levels responded better to TCZ treatment than to anti-TNF inhibitors [41].

60. Does anti-TNF therapy increase the risk of lymphoma in rheumatoid arthritis patients?

Patients with rheumatoid arthritis (RA) have a two times higher risk for lymphoma (both Hodgkin's and non-Hodgkin's lymphomas) development compared to the general population. To date, there is no evidence whether treatment with anti-TNF agents influences the risk of lymphoma development over the background risk in subjects with rheumatoid arthritis or whether it affects the risk of specific lymphoma subtypes. In a recent large collaborative prospective analysis of European registries, it was shown that cases of non-Hodgkin's lymphoma (NHL) were more frequent than Hodgkin's lymphoma in RA patients and diffuse large B-cell lymphoma (DLBCL) was the most frequent B-cell NHL subtype. Nevertheless, although the lymphoma subtype distribution was different between RA patients and the general population, there was no evidence of any change in the distribution of lymphoma subtypes among patients with RA treated with anti-TNF agents and those never having received biologics [42].

61. Which are the recent recommendations for the treatment of ankylosing spondylitis (AS) and non-radiographic axial spondyloarthropathies (SpA)?

A panel of experts developed recommendations by voting (70% agreement) for the therapy of AS and non-radiographic axial SpA. For both entities recommendations were the same. Anti-TNF agents were recommended over secukinumab or ixekizumab as the first biologic to be used. Secukinumab or ixekizumab was recommended over the use of a second anti-TNF in patients with primary unresponsiveness to the first anti-TNF. Anti-TNF, secukinumab, and ixekizumab are favored over tofacitinib. Methotrexate co-administration with anti-TNF was not recommended. In contrast, sulfasalazine was recommended only for persistent peripheral arthritis when anti-TNF was contraindicated. Patients in whom the disease responded to biologic therapies are advised to continue their therapy without tapering the dose of the biologic agent. Evaluation of the disease progress with serial pelvis or spine X-rays or magnetic resonance images is not advised [43].

62. Which form of exercise the physician should recommend to a patient with rheumatoid arthritis (RA), and why?

In RA aerobic conditioning exercise can reduce articular pain and stiffness, increase range of joint motion and muscle strength. In addition, exercise programs can increase cardiovascular fitness and probably improve physical function. It can also lead to weight loss, which will reduce stress on painful joints. The best exercises for people with arthritis are those that place the least stress on the joints, such as exercising in water, swimming, walking, stretching, and using weight machines as well as stationary cycling. Before beginning any new exercise program, the patient should consult the treating physician.

63. Which form of exercise the physician should recommend to a patient with ankylosing spondylitis (AS), and why?

Physiotherapy in patients with AS brings short-term improvements in spinal and hip range of motion. Spinal mobility exercises slow down the loss of mobility over the long-term, but controlled studies are needed to confirm this. Exercise for improvement of respiratory function relates more to cardiopulmonary fitness. It possibly also improves the diaphragmatic respiration, rather than changes the thoracic cage mobility. Furthermore, in a recent randomized controlled study it was shown that exercise in conjunction with pharmacological therapy three times weekly for three months, significantly improved mood, vitality and general health of patients with axial spondyloarthritis in comparison to the control group but didn't affect the poor quality of sleep [44].

64. An adult patient with rheumatic fever: For how long should the patient be on prophylactic antibiotic therapy?

All individuals who have had an initial attack of rheumatic fever, whether or not they have rheumatic heart disease, should receive chronic administration of an antibiotic to prevent infection of the upper respiratory tract by group A streptococci. Secondary prophylaxis has been documented to reduce significantly the risk of recurrent attacks and associated morbidity and mortality. Regular intramuscular injection of repository penicillin (benzathine benzylpenicillin) is the most effective available treatment. Although classically given every 4 weeks, recent data indicate that 1,200,000 units of benzathine benzylpenicillin given every 3 weeks is more effective in preventing recurrences of rheumatic fever, especially in high-risk patients.

65. Which are the therapeutic steps to treat adult-onset Still's disease?

In mild to moderate disease, prednisolone 0.5–1 mg/kg/day in combination with methotrexate (0.2–0.3 mg/kg/week) is initiated. Methotrexate is added as an anti-inflammatory and steroid-sparing agent. In severe disease with poor prognostic factors, high doses of steroids (prednisolone 1 mg/kg/day) in combination with methotrexate (0.2–0.3 mg/kg/week) and biologic agents, either anti-IL-1 receptor antagonist (anakinra) or anti-IL-6 receptor antibody (tocilizumab), should be given [45, 46].

Therapeutic Modalities and Regimens for Systemic Lupus Erythematosus and Antiphospholipid Syndrome

66. In which systemic lupus erythematosus manifestations is methotrexate indicated?

It is predominantly indicated in patients with arthritis. The administration of methotrexate significantly reduces systemic lupus erythematosus disease activity index (SLEDAI) and the average daily dose of corticosteroids in adult patients with systemic lupus erythematosus [47].

67. In which systemic lupus erythematosus patients is anti-BLyS (belimumab) monoclonal antibody administration indicated?

Belimumab administration is indicated in systemic lupus erythematosus (SLE) patients that display a mild-to-moderate active disease with acute mucocutaneous and musculoskeletal manifestations, active serology, and disproportionate corticosteroid intake, having overall a relapsing-remitting course despite receiving standard therapy. It is not indicated for SLE patients with active neuropsychiatric lupus, severe lupus nephritis, or life-threatening-related manifestations. It has not been studied in combination with other biologics or cyclophosphamide [48].

68. In which systemic lupus erythematosus patients are monthly intravenous cyclophosphamide pulses indicated alone or in combination with methylprednisolone?

Monthly intravenous cyclophosphamide pulses are indicated in systemic lupus erythematosus patients with life- or major organ-threatening disease, like proliferative glomerulonephritis, central nervous system involvement, mesenteric vasculitis, and diffuse pulmonary hemorrhage. It is more effective when given in combination with methylprednisolone intravenous pulses.

69. Which are the predictors of sustained amenorrhea from intravenous cyclophosphamide pulses in premenopausal women with systemic lupus erythematosus?

Sustained amenorrhea is difficult to be avoided in women 32 years or older, even with very short intravenous cyclophosphamide courses. In these patients alternative regimens should be considered. In younger women treated with a monthly intravenous cyclophosphamide regimen, sustained amenorrhea may occur predominantly in those with the recognized adverse predictors like longer systemic lupus erythematosus disease duration and autoantibodies to Ro/SSA and U1RNP autoantigens [49].

70. What is the evidence-based therapeutic intervention for the induction therapy of lupus nephritis classes III, IV, and V?

In general, for the treatment of lupus nephritis, immunosuppressive agents are recommended in class III_A or $III_{A/C}$ and IV_A or $IV_{A/C}$ nephritis and also in pure class V nephritis if proteinuria exceeds 1 g/24 h despite the optimal use of renin–angiotensin–aldosterone axis blockers. Treatment should aim for a complete renal response with proteinuria <0.5 g/24 h and normal or stable glomerular filtration rate (GFR). Response to treatment defined as ≥50% reduction in proteinuria and stability or improvement in GFR should be achieved by 6–12 months after initiation of treatment.

Induction therapy

- *Class III/class IV lupus nephritis:*
  - IV pulse methylprednisolone (0.5–1 g) daily for 3 days followed by oral prednisolone
  - 1 mg/kg/day (if crescents are present in the biopsy) or 0.5 mg/kg/day (if no crescents present in the biopsy) tapered after a few weeks to lowest effective dose

    plus
  - Mycophenolate mofetil (MMF) 2–3 g/day for 6 months (preferred to cyclophosphamide in African-American and Hispanic patients)

    or
  - Cyclophosphamide (CYC): High dose IV (0.5–1 g/m² body surface area monthly × 6 doses) or low-dose IV (500 mg every 2 weeks × 6 months)
  - Patients who fail to improve on MMF should be switched to CYC. Patients who fail to improve on CYC are switched to MMF. Patients who fail to respond to both are candidates for rituximab (RTX) or calcineurin inhibitors (cyclosporine-A and tacrolimus)
  - Combination of MMF (1–2 g/day) with a calcineurin inhibitor (especially tacro-

limus) is an alternative, particularly in patients with nephrotic-range proteinuria

- *Class V lupus nephritis*:
  - Oral prednisolone 0.5 mg/kg/day for 6 months plus MMF 2–3 g/day for 6 months
  - Alternative options include high dose CYC IV for 6 months, or calcineurin inhibitor (especially tacrolimus) either as monotherapy or in combination with MMF, particularly in patients with nephrotic-range proteinuria

71. **What is the evidence-based therapeutic intervention for maintenance therapy of lupus nephritis classes III, IV, and V?**

Maintenance therapy

Azathioprine (2 mg/kg/day) or MMF (2 g/day). Each of these drugs is given in association with a dose of prednisolone to control extra-renal manifestations, and prednisolone is tapered over time. Although there are no strict guidelines on the duration of maintenance treatment, it is recommended for at least 3 years. RTX has also been used as maintenance therapy when patients fail or cannot tolerate azathioprine or MMF.

Adjunctive therapy

In cases of active lupus nephritis, the following should be added to treatment:

- Hydroxychloroquine
- Angiotensin-converting enzyme inhibitor or angiotensin-receptor blocker if proteinuria ≥0.5 g/24 h
- Control blood pressure (≤130/80)
- Statin therapy if LDL >100 mg/dL
- Counsel against pregnancy while nephritis is active [50, 51]

72. **What is the therapy for subacute cutaneous lupus erythematosus?**

If the cutaneous lesions are limited on extend or severity local application of tacrolimus can be recommended. Oral antimalarials—hydroxychloroquine, chloroquine, and quinacrine—are the first-line agents used for systemic therapy of all subacute cutaneous lupus erythematosus (SCLE) subtypes. Half of the patients respond to this regimen. In non-responders thalidomide or dapsone can be used providing that the physician attends their side effects and follows-up the patient carefully. Alternatively, immunosuppressive agents like methotrexate, mycophenolate mofetil, or even anti-CD20 therapy can be used [52].

73. **What is the oral anticoagulation treatment used in a patient with primary antiphospholipid syndrome?**

Treatment for antiphospholipid syndrome (APS) patients is based on the patient's clinical status, levels of antiphospholipid (aPL) antibodies, and history of thrombotic events.

- In case of an asymptomatic patient with aPL positivity without previous thrombotic events, the treatment is mainly focused on the reduction of modifiable vascular risk factors (smoking, lipid profile, hypertension, diabetes mellitus, birth control pills). In these patients the use of acetylsalicylic acid (ASA) is controversial
- APS patients who have had a venous thrombosis, after initial low molecular weight heparin (LMWH) therapy, should be placed on life-long anticoagulation with warfarin at a target INR of 2.5 (range 2.0–3.0)
- In APS patients with a history of cerebral arterial thrombosis, combination of antiplatelet agents (ASA plus clopidogrel) or warfarin plus ASA is used based on the risk assessment for recurrence
- In APS patients with a previous non-cerebral arterial thrombotic event, ASA plus clopidogrel or ASA plus warfarin is used in cases of noncardiac arterial thrombus, while in cases of cardiac arterial thrombus and high risk of recurrence

warfarin, ASA and clopidogrel are the combination treatment preferred

74. **Are direct oral anticoagulants an alternative to vitamin K antagonists for the treatment of thrombotic antiphospholipid syndrome?**

Anticoagulation is the cornerstone therapeutic intervention for thrombotic antiphospholipid syndrome (APS). During the past decade, direct oral anticoagulants (DOACs) provided a novel approach to oral anticoagulation more than 50 years after the introduction of warfarin. Rivaroxaban, an oral direct factor Xa inhibitor is approved for the treatment of venous thromboembolism and for stroke prevention in patients with atrial fibrillation, without the need for laboratory monitoring. Two randomized trials [53, 54], including high-risk APS patients (i.e., with previous arterial events and/or triple APS antibody positivity), compared the efficacy and safety between rivaroxaban and vitamin K antagonists (VKAs) for secondary prophylaxis in the setting of thrombotic APS. Both studies failed to demonstrate non-inferiority of rivaroxaban to VKAs and showed a greater proportion of arterial events in the rivaroxaban patient groups. In line with these randomized trials, a systematic review indicated a higher thrombosis recurrence rate among APS patients with previous arterial thrombosis and those with triple antibody positivity who were receiving any DOAC [55]. As such, the data available up to date suggest that DOACs should not be prescribed for patients with high-risk APS. Whether there is a lower-risk subset of patients with APS who might be eligible for DOAC therapy is still questionable.

75. **What is the evidence-based therapeutic intervention in order to prevent maternal morbidity in a female antiphospholipid syndrome patient?**

As soon as pregnancy is achieved in an antiphospholipid syndrome patient, in order to prevent abortion, fetal intrauterine growth retardation, or stillbirth, acetylsalicylic acid (aspirin) 80 mg/day should be started in combination with heparin (unfractionated or low molecular weight heparin, LMWH) and hydroxychloroquine 200–400 mg/day. According to a recent systematic Cochrane review the combination of heparin (unfractionated or LMWH) plus aspirin during the course of pregnancy may reduce the risk of pregnancy loss and increase the live birth rate in women with persistent antiphospholipid antibodies when compared with aspirin treatment alone [56].

76. **What are the benefits of hydroxychloroquine administration in patients with primary antiphospholipid syndrome?**

Hydroxychloroquine (HCQ) is an effective adjuvant treatment for thrombosis and pregnancy morbidity prevention, possibly via an antiphospholipid antibody titer reduction [57, 58].

Therapeutic Modalities and Regimens for Inflammatory Muscle Disease

77. **Which therapeutic agents can be used for the treatment of idiopathic inflammatory myopathies?**

Standard therapeutic approach for most types of idiopathic inflammatory myopathies (IIM) consists of high prednisolone dose (1 mg/kg) either orally or intravenously in combination with immunosuppressive agents (methotrexate or azathioprine or cyclosporine-A) which will reduce inflammation and will permit to taper the prednisolone dose.

- Methotrexate 1.5–3 mg/kg/week and cyclosporine-A 3 mg/kg/day have similar therapeutic effects. Azathioprine 2 mg/kg/day is equally effective to methotrexate, but its therapeutic effects are delayed by 2–3 months
- In IIM resistant to other immunosuppressants (methotrexate or azathioprine), or in IIM associated with refractory interstitial

lung disease (ILD) tacrolimus, at a dose of 0.1 mg/kg/day can be used

- Mycophenolate mofetil (MMF) at a dosage of 30 mg/kg/day has been demonstrated to be effective in improving muscle and skin disease in dermatomyositis and polymyositis. Furthermore, MMF in IIM patients with ILD has been shown to ameliorate lung function tests' parameters, while permitting prednisolone tapering
- Cyclophosphamide at a dose of 1–2 mg/kg/day orally or as intravenous pulse therapy (up to 1 g/m^2 body surface area per pulse) is particularly effective in IIM-related ILD
- In serious cases, monthly administration of intravenous immunoglobulin (IVIg) pulses (2 g/kg) in 2 consecutive days for 6 months should be added to the above regimen and can speed recovery. Dysphagia appears to respond particularly well to IVIg
- Rituximab has been tested in a randomized controlled trial and its efficacy has also been documented in several case series and reports as well as systematic reviews. In case series of patients with refractory ILD secondary to the anti-synthetase syndrome, rituximab has shown promising results
- Exercise, especially endurance exercise, should be an integral part of the treatment of IIM [59]

Therapeutic Modalities and Regimens for Sjögren's Syndrome and IgG_4-Related Disorders

78. Which are the therapeutic interventions for keratoconjunctivitis sicca of Sjögren's syndrome?

Medications which exacerbate eye dryness such as anticholinergics, antihistamines, and diuretics, as well as dust and cigarette smoke, should be discouraged. Additionally, the maintenance of a humid environment, the use of spectacle side shields, and taking regular breaks while reading or working on a computer should be recommended. Artificial tears (preservative-free) and ophthalmic lubricant ointments, stimulation of tear secretion (e.g., pilocarpine hydrochloride 5 mg t.i.d.), tear retention treatment (punctual occlusion), and local application of immunomodulatory agents with anti-inflammatory activity, like cyclosporine-A, may be used for keratoconjunctivitis sicca in Sjögren's syndrome according to disease severity.

79. How can pilocarpine hydrochloride be effective in Sjögren's syndrome patients and which are its commonest side effects?

Oral pilocarpine, a cholinergic parasympatheticomimetic agonist, at a dose of 5 mg three times daily can be beneficial for the treatment of sicca symptoms (xerostomia and xerophthalmia) in Sjögren's syndrome patients. Specific side effects include flushing, increased sweating, dizziness, diarrhea, headaches, increased or frequent urge to urinate, and exacerbation of peptic ulcer.

80. Which are the therapeutic interventions for xerostomia of Sjögren's syndrome?

Routine dental care and preventive dental treatment are of major importance. Meticulous oral hygiene and frequent dental visits should be encouraged. The use of fluoride is essential to enhance mineralization of the hydroxyapatite structure of the enamel, rendering it less susceptible to decay. Common fluoride-containing dentifrices, preferably with mild taste should be used. Upon progressive hyposalivation, fluoride gels, prescription-strength fluoride toothpaste, and/or oral rinses containing 0.4–1.25% fluoride are highly recommended. For the treatment of oral candidiasis, topical antifungal treatment is the first line of treatment followed by systemic antifungals for persisting or recurrent episodes.

81. In which Sjögren's syndrome patients can hydroxychloroquine be beneficial?

It is usually prescribed for fatigability and arthralgias/arthritis in Sjögren's syndrome patients, despite the fact that double-blinded, placebo-controlled studies have shown that hydroxychloroquine is not superior to placebo. The only definite hydroxychloroquine effect is the decrease of serum immunoglobulin levels in Sjögren's syndrome patients with hypergammaglobulinemia [60].

82. Can immunosuppressive agents alleviate symptoms or disease manifestations of Sjögren's syndrome?

A number of immunosuppressive agents (azathioprine, cyclosporine-A, and methotrexate) have been evaluated in various trials of Sjögren's syndrome patients in order to alleviate the symptoms or to alter the natural disease process, but the results were mostly unsatisfactory and questionable. Thus, their use for the main manifestations of Sjögren's syndrome, i.e., keratoconjunctivitis sicca or xerostomia is not recommended. However, despite the fact that there are no double-blind controlled studies, corticosteroids along with conventional immunosuppressive agents or anti-CD-20 are used to combat extraglandular Sjögren's syndrome manifestations like interstitial lung disease, glomerulonephritis, and vasculitis.

83. What is the therapy for IgG4-related diseases?

IgG4-related diseases respond well to systemic corticosteroids as a first-line treatment at initial prednisolone doses of 0.6–1.0 mg/kg per day. Relapses occur in two-third of patients during steroid tapering or withdrawal, within a mean of 3.5 months. About 72% of patients may require long-term steroids and/or immunosuppressive agents such as azathioprine, methotrexate, and mycophenolate mofetil. Therapy with rituximab has been particularly effective as a second or third-line treatment, with possible high rates of remission in IgG4-related disease [61].

Therapeutic Modalities and Regimens for Systemic Sclerosis

84. Which therapeutic agents are used in the treatment of rapidly progressive systemic sclerosis?

- Cyclophosphamide (CYC) treatment has been shown to stabilize or mildly improve—in terms of lung volume measurements in pulmonary function tests—systemic sclerosis (SSc) patients with rapidly progressive interstitial lung disease (ILD). However, the beneficial effects of CYC do not persist more than 12 months following its cessation
- D-Penicillamine is known to exert a strong anti-fibrotic effect by interfering with collagen cross-linking and by accelerating collagen turnover even at low doses and is used for rapidly progressive cutaneous involvement in SSc
- Mycophenolate mofetil (MMF) has been effectively used for rapidly progressive cutaneous involvement in SSc. Of note, SSc patients with shorter disease duration seem to obtain greater benefit from MMF therapy, showing more pronounced improvement in skin fibrosis
- Methotrexate can be used for less severe skin progression and for patients unable to tolerate MMF
- Rituximab (RTX) has been shown to induce improvement in SSc-cutaneous and lung involvement. A recent head-to-head randomized trial between RTX and CYC showed similar efficacy of the two treatments in skin fibrosis and SSc-ILD with RTX having a better safety profile [62]
- Tocilizumab (TCZ) treatment for diffuse systemic sclerosis in the phase II and III tri-

als showed a substantial stabilization of skin involvement and ILD, especially in patients with early disease and lung involvement [63]

85. What are possible therapeutic options for calcinosis cutis?

Calcinosis cutis is extremely difficult to be treated. Therapies that have been used include low-dose (1 mg/day) warfarin (inhibits the vitamin K-dependent γ-carboxyglutamic acid matrix protein, found to be high in areas of calcinosis), colchicine (suppresses local inflammation in calcinosis lesions), topical sodium thiosulfate, and aluminum hydroxide, administration of diltiazem (doses up 360 mg/day) and probenecid (500 mg b.i.d), and high doses of bisphosphonates (e.g., alendronate 10 mg/day). All, however, have limited success. Preliminary studies have shown that intravenous immunoglobulins (2 g/kg) in a 4-day protocol once a month seem to have a beneficial effect after the third monthly dose.

86. What is the potential pharmacological treatment of Raynaud's phenomenon associated with systemic sclerosis?

Besides general measures, such as avoidance of cold exposure, maintaining high core body temperature, use of gloves and socks, and cessation of smoking, systemic sclerosis (SSc) patients with Raynaud's phenomenon could benefit from some pharmacological intervention:

- Calcium channel blockers (e.g., nifedipine) demonstrate a moderate reduction in frequency and severity of attacks of Raynaud's phenomenon in patients with SSc and do not seem to reduce digital ulceration. Common side effects include hypotension, headache, and peripheral edema
- Intravenous iloprost (prostacyclin), is a potent vasodilator that is effective in the treatment of Raynaud's phenomenon, reduces the frequency and severity of attacks and the development of digital ulcers. The most common side effects are headache, flushing, hypotension, and nausea, which can be controlled by reducing the rate of infusion
- Phosphodiesterase type 5 inhibitors (sildenafil, vardenafil, and tadalafil) increase cyclic guanosine monophosphate-dependent microvascular and macrovascular vasodilation. They have shown only a moderate reduction in attacks in patients with secondary Raynaud's phenomenon to SSc and are given to patients not responding to calcium channel blockers. Adverse side effects include headache, flushing, and dizziness, but they are generally well tolerated
- The endothelin receptor antagonist bosentan is used for the treatment of pulmonary arterial hypertension. It has an emerging role in the treatment of Raynaud's phenomenon and digital ulcers in SSc patients. A multicenter, randomized, placebo-controlled, double-blind study showed that bosentan may be effective in preventing new digital ulcers; however, no benefit was demonstrated for healing of existing ulcers [64–66]

87. Is a single dose on demand of phosphodiesterase-5 (PDE5) inhibitor effective therapy for Raynaud's phenomenon?

A recent study examined in a randomized double-blind controlled manner if a single PDE5 inhibitor dose (40 or 80 mg) before or during exposure to cold may be an alternative to chronic therapy. The results of the study showed a high probability that sildenafil is superior to placebo. However, a significant therapeutic response heterogeneity was observed in patients with Raynaud's phenomenon raising doubts if a single PDE5 inhibitor dose has clinically relevant efficacy [67].

Therapeutic Modalities and Regimens for Vasculitides and Related Diseases

88. What is the treatment of polymyalgia rheumatica?

The cornerstone for polymyalgia rheumatica (PMR) treatment are glucocorticoids (GC). In line with consensus-based recommendations, initial therapy for PMR is 12.5–25 mg/day prednisone or equivalent followed by individualized tapering regimens. Intramuscular methylprednisolone can be considered as an alternative to oral GCs in some cases of PMR [68]. There are some studies supporting the use of methotrexate in addition to GCs, particularly in patients with severe disease, peripheral arthritis, at risk for relapse and/or prolonged therapy as well as in cases with risk factors, comorbidities, and/or concomitant medications where GC-related adverse events are more likely to occur. There is no evidence yet for TNF-blocking agents in the treatment of PMR.

89. What is the management of large vessel vasculitis?

Giant cell arteritis (GCA) and Takayasu's arteritis (TKA) affect both large vessels.
Glucocorticoids (GC) are still the cornerstone of treatment for large vessel vasculitis (LVV). They should be initiated immediately at a dose 40–60 mg/day of prednisone-equivalent and if clinical improvement is seen after 2–4 weeks glucocorticoid dose should be tapered by 10 mg every 2 weeks to <5 mg/day by 12 months from diagnosis [69]. If a flare occurs, glucocorticoids should be increased to pre-relapse dose and tapered within 4–8 weeks to pre-relapse dose. Subcutaneous tocilizumab 162 mg/week or methotrexate 7.5–15 mg/week can be considered in GCA patients with relapsing disease [69].

Adjunctive therapy with tocilizumab (TCZ) was approved for GCA treatment by the US and European regulatory authorities in 2017 on the basis of two randomized clinical trials [70, 71]. However, a recent systematic review on the efficacy and safety profile of TCZ in TKA showed that existing evidence from randomized control trials is promising but limited [72]. Tumor necrosis factor (TNF)-α blockers are ineffective in GCA, yet they can be considered in TKA patients with relapsing disease [73]. Recent real-world data on the use of MTX in GCA show its effectiveness in reducing the relapse rate compared to patients taking GC alone [73]. Preliminary results from the use of leflunomide as a corticosteroid-sparing agent are promising both in CGA [74] and in TKA [75] in the induction of remission and decrease of relapse rates, yet they need to be confirmed in larger cohorts or clinical trials.
Also, recently it was shown that JAK/STAT signaling pathway plays an important role in the pathogenesis of TKA and as such JAK inhibitors could be a promising therapeutic modality [76, 77].

90. Can Interleukin (IL)-6 receptor antagonist therapy be discontinued in giant cell arteritis patients who went into remission and in which ones?

The duration of therapy with tocilizumab (TCZ) in giant cell arteritis (GCA) and the long-term unwanted effects are not known. A small prospective observational study attempted to answer this question. Seventeen GCA patients, who were in remission after 52 weeks of treatment from the tocilizumab arm of a randomized clinical trial were followed up. After 6 months of TCZ discontinuation almost half of these patients relapsed. The rest of the patients stayed in remission for the 28 months observational period. Aorta magnetic resonance imaging angiography was performed in all patients and revealed that the enhancement of the vessel wall remained regardless of the patients being in remission or relapse. The results of this study did not indicate neither which GCA patient should discontinue TCZ therapy nor which is the optimal time for continuation of TZC therapy [78].

91. **How is granulomatosis with polyangiitis treated?**

The induction therapy for granulomatosis with polyangiitis (GPA) with major organ involvement consists of: IV methylprednisolone pulses (1 g) for 3 consecutive days plus monthly IV pulses of cyclophosphamide (0.5–1 mg/m^2 body surface area) for 6 months. Another equally effective alternative to cyclophosphamide is rituximab (two doses of 1000 mg given 2 weeks apart). After 6 months of induction therapy and if remission has been achieved, less toxic immunosuppressives can be used to maintain remission, such as azathioprine (2 mg/kg/day). In addition to immunosuppressive therapy, oral trimethoprim/sulfamethoxazole should be used prophylactically for recurrent *Staphylococcus aureus* sinus infections that can exacerbate GPA.

92. **Which is the preferred therapeutic agent for induction therapy in eosinophilic granulomatosis with polyangiitis (EGPA, Churg-Strauss vasculitis) and which agent is prescribed to spare steroid side effects?**

The treatment of choice for induction therapy in Churg-Strauss vasculitis are glucocorticoids. In patients with more than one risk factor (serum creatinine >1.6 mg/dL, proteinuria >1 g/24 h, central nervous system involvement, gastrointestinal tract involvement, and myocardial involvement), cyclophosphamide monthly pulses should be added (0.5–1 mg/m^2 body surface area). Those with severe presentations may benefit from plasmapheresis. Milder cases may be treated with azathioprine (2 mg/kg/day), methotrexate (0.2–0.3 mg/kg/week), or mycophenolate mofetil (2–3 g/day). In refractory cases, rituximab and interferon-a have been used with some success.

93. **Is plasma exchange an effective therapeutic intervention in patients with ANCA-associated vasculitis?**

In severe ANCA-associated vasculitis (AAV) patients, plasma exchange (PE) traditionally is used in order to lower the incidence of organ damage, by removing ANCA autoantibodies. However, the benefit of PE applied along with the classical immunosuppressive medications, versus immunosuppressive therapy alone, in long-term survival or end-stage renal disease (ESRD) is questionable. Recently, it was proven that in patients with severe AAV with findings of kidney injury or diffuse alveolar hemorrhage plasma exchange had no impact either on progression to ESRD or survival [79].

94. **How is panuveitis of Behçet's syndrome treated?**

If the patient has severe eye disease defined as >2 lines of drop in visual acuity on a 10/10 scale and/or retinal disease (retinal vasculitis or macular involvement), it is recommended to receive either cyclosporine-A (2–3 mg/kg body weight/day) or infliximab in combination with azathioprine (1–3 mg/kg body weight/day) and corticosteroids. Alternatively, interferon (IFN)-α with or without corticosteroids can be used.

Therapeutic Modalities and Regimens for Crystal Arthritides, Osteoarthritis, and Fibromyalgia

95. **How are the acute episodes of gout treated?**

- Nonsteroidal anti-inflammatory drugs, e.g., Indomethacin 50 mg, four times daily for 24–48 h, and then 50 mg, three times daily for

48 h; taper and discontinue after the attack subsides

- Oral colchicine: 1 mg followed by 0.5 mg 1 h later. Most effective within the first 36 h of the attack. Contraindicated in elderly with significant renal/hepatic insufficiency, avoid concomitant use with other P450 inhibitors (e.g., cyclosporine-A)
- Systemic corticosteroids: Prednisolone 0.5 mg/kg/day for 5–10 days or for 2–5 days and then taper for 7–10 days or triamcinolone acetate IM 60 mg (can be repeated once)
- Intra-articular steroids: First septic arthritis should be excluded, and then triamcinolone or methylprednisolone (40 mg for large joints, 10–20 mg for small joints/bursae) can be administered. Effective within the first 24 h of the attack
- Canakinumab as an IL-1β blocking agent has been shown to reduce the risk of acute gouty arthritis flares during initiation of allopurinol treatment and has been proven to be a valuable therapeutic agent for patients with limited treatment options

96. How are the acute episodes of pseudogout treated?

Administration of nonsteroidal anti-inflammatory drugs, or colchicine, or intra-articular/intra-muscular triamcinolone. All the above agents are known to interrupt acute pseudogout attacks. In addition, treatment or elimination of offending agents or pathologies (hyperparathyroidism, hypomagnesemia, hemochromatosis, hypophosphatasia, drugs causing hypercalcemia/hypophosphatemia: loop-thiazide diuretics, proton pump inhibitors, cyclosporine-A, tacrolimus, and intravenous bisphosphonates) is mandatory.

97. Is the maintenance therapy for gout and pseudogout similar or different? What are the sequelae if these disorders are left untreated?

Gout: life-long therapy with an anti-hyperuricemic drug is indicated in cases of (a) more than two to three acute gouty attacks occurring in 1–2 years, (b) renal stones (urate or calcium), (c) tophaceous gout, and (d) established gout with chronic kidney disease. A xanthine oxidase inhibitor (allopurinol, febuxostat) is first-line therapy (starting dose of allopurinol 100 mg/day, with gradual upward titration, maximum daily dose 800 mg always adjusted to glomerular filtration rate). The goal of treatment is to maintain the serum uric acid <6 mg/dL or <5 mg/dL in tophaceous gout. If gout is untreated, urate nodules (tophi) under the skin can develop in several areas (fingers, elbows, Achilles tendons), and bony erosions, urate nephropathy, uric acid nephrolithiasis, and heart disease are possible sequelae.

Pseudogout: Most patients only have few attacks that are widely separated in time; thus prophylaxis is not required against pseudogout. For patients with frequent attacks, colchicine at a dose of 0.5 mg twice daily prevents recurrences.

98. Should Interleukin-1β blockade be used for the prevention of gouty attacks?

Interleukin-1β inhibitor (Canakinumab) has been shown to shorten gout attacks. A recent prospective randomized control study showed that during a median follow-up time of 3.7 years although Canakinumab significantly decreased the number of gout attacks it did not affect the patients' uric acid levels [80]. The questions which arise from this study results are (a) what will be the effect of the continuously elevated uric acid levels on other organs like the heart and kidneys and (b) is it cost benefit to administer such an expensive modality when inexpensive measures can have a similar or better therapeutic effect?

99. Which are the current therapeutic uses of colchicine in rheumatic diseases?

- Therapy of acute gout attacks and prophylaxis of recurrent attacks
- Therapy of acute pseudogout attacks and prevention of recurrent attacks

- Familial Mediterranean fever: to induce disease remission, reduce frequency of attacks, and prevent amyloidosis
- Behçet's disease: In mucocutaneous (oral/genital ulcers, erythema nodosum) and joint manifestations
- Neutrophilic dermatoses, especially Sweet's syndrome
- Treatment of acute pericarditis and prevention of recurrent pericarditis [81–85]

100. How effective are oral glucosamines for the treatment of osteoarthritis?

Although widely used, oral glucosamine treatment for osteoarthritis (OA) has been strongly debated for several years, and open trial data are not available. In a recent meta-analysis, it has been shown that any oral glucosamine substance used in patients with clinically or radiographically defined hip or knee OA was no better than placebo for altering pain severity or function restriction neither after short- (3 months) nor after long-term (24 months) follow-up [86].

101. What therapeutic interventions can be used for acute, subacute, and chronic low back pain?

The noninvasive pharmacologic and nonpharmacologic interventions for the treatment of *acute* (<4 weeks), *subacute* (4–12 weeks), and *chronic* (>12 weeks) *low back pain in adults* should include the following:

- Since *acute or subacute* low back pain may improve over time regardless of treatment superficial heat, massage, acupuncture, or spinal manipulation should be proposed by clinicians as initial nonpharmacologic approach. If pharmacologic treatment is anticipated, nonsteroidal anti-inflammatory drugs or skeletal muscle relaxants should be preferred
- Patients with *chronic* low back pain should initially be advised to exercise, take part in multidisciplinary rehabilitation, acupuncture, tai chi, yoga, mindfulness-based stress reduction programs, progressive relaxation, electromyography biofeedback, low-level laser therapy, operant therapy, cognitive behavioral therapy, or spinal manipulation. If this group of patients does not respond adequately to the above interventions, nonsteroidal anti-inflammatory drugs should be used first and thereafter, as second-line treatment, tramadol, or duloxetine. Opioids should be considered only in patients who have not responded to any of the aforementioned treatments and only if the potential benefits prevail over the risks for individual patients [87]

102. Are intradiscal steroids indicated in patients with chronic low back pain associated with acute discopathy?

A prospective randomized double-blind study revealed that intradiscal steroid injection alleviates symptoms for a brief period of time (1 month) [88].

103. Which are the absolute indications for surgical intervention in a patient with herniated intervertebral disc?

Absolute indications for surgery in patients with symptomatic disc herniation include disc herniation causing cauda equina symptoms, progressive muscular weakness and/or sensory deficit of lower extremities, and progressive neurologic deficits despite conservative management.

104. What are the effects of repeated intra-articular triamcinolone used in patients with symptomatic knee osteoarthritis?

In clinical practice, intra-articular corticosteroids are widely considered the most rapidly effective nonsurgical therapeutic modality for knee osteoarthritis and typically provide a substantial post-injection pain relief.

However, it has been shown that in patients with symptomatic knee osteoarthritis repeated (every 3 months) intra-articular triamcinolone results, after two years, in significantly greater cartilage loss without significant reduction in knee pain, compared to intra-articular saline injection. These findings do not support the use of frequently repeated intra-articular corticosteroids for treating patients with symptomatic knee osteoarthritis [89].

105. Which therapeutic modalities are more effective in alleviating pain and improving function in patients with knee osteoarthritis; intra-articular glucocorticoids or physical therapy?

Intra-articular glucocorticoid injections and physical therapy have both been used as non-evidence based therapeutic modalities for knee osteoarthritis. In a recent randomized study patients from the primary care setting in the U.S.A, with osteoarthritis in one or both knees, were randomly assigned in a 1:1 ratio to receive either a glucocorticoid injection or undergo physical therapy. The results of both interventions were assessed at one year using the total score on the Western Ontario and McMaster Universities Osteoarthritis Index (WOMAC). It was shown that patients with knee osteoarthritis who underwent physical therapy had less pain and functional disability at one year than patients who received an intra-articular glucocorticoid injection [90]. Furthermore, another contemporary two-arm, single-blind, parallel-group randomized controlled trial indicates that for patients with mild-to-moderate knee osteoarthritis, it is worth recommending an aquatic cycling training program, as it was shown to substantially alleviate pain and improve knee joint function in these patients [91].

106. Which therapeutic modalities have been recently tested for the management of hand osteoarthritis?

Osteoarthritis of the hand joints produces pain and can limit daily activities. Treatment options are limited and include physical measures like application of cold or warm pads, medicated creams, and administration of paracetamol or nonsteroidal anti-inflammatory medications. A recent placebo-controlled double-blinded study showed that hydroxychloroquine (200–400 mg/day) as an analgesic modality for hand osteoarthritis was not better than placebo [92]. In another contemporary double-blinded, randomized, placebo-controlled study the efficacy of prednisolone 10 mg daily was evaluated in patients with painful hand osteoarthritis. It was found that 6 weeks of prednisolone therapy significantly improved pain and function as well as imaging markers of hand joint inflammation [93].

107. How is pigmented villonodular synovitis (PVNS) treated?

The gold standard for treatment of PVNS is surgical excision with total synovectomy (open or arthroscopic approach). Histology will exclude other causes of synovitis and will show mononuclear cells, macrophages, and multinucleated osteoclast-type giant cells with extensive hemosiderin stores. Hemosiderin deposits reflect the recurrent hemarthrosis in patients with PVNS. Even after surgery, the recurrence rate of PVNS ranges from 20 to 55%. External beam radiation at doses 30 Gy to 50 Gy has demonstrated local control of up to 95% of cases, while when used post-surgically it reduces PVNS recurrence. The use of pexidartinib, a colony-stimulating factor-1 receptor antagonist, was approved by the FDA in August 2019 for use in patients with extensive disease who are not likely to benefit from surgical intervention [94, 95].

108. What is the treatment of fibromyalgia?

The treatment of fibromyalgia demands a multidisciplinary approach that involves physical, pharmacological, and cognitive measures. Current evidence suggests that small doses of tricyclic antidepressants, aerobic exercise, cognitive behavioral therapy, and patient education can be effective in treating fibromyalgia. However, poor compliance of fibromyalgia patients to all these measures is an important issue firstly due to slow or unsatisfactory clinical response and secondly due to inadequate patient education [96].

109. Which are non-pharmacological interventions beneficial for fibromyalgia?

Mild and moderate aerobic exercise performed either in land or in water are effective against pain relief, depressed mood, and poor quality of life in patients with fibromyalgia. Recently, a systematic review and meta-analysis of randomized controlled trials showed that Tai Chi, a discipline involving Chinese martial art, is superior to aerobic exercise programs and conventional therapeutic exercise [97, 98]. Furthermore, transcutaneous electrical nerve stimulation (TENS), in addition to a stable medication regimen, has been shown to reduce pain and fatigue in patients with fibromyalgia [99].

Therapeutic Modalities and Regimens for Osteoporosis

110. What are the general measures for osteoporosis treatment in postmenopausal women not on glucocorticoid therapy?

- Modify the modifiable risk factors (smoking, alcohol, low body weight, sun exposure, calcium/vitamin D3 intake, low physical activity, and amenorrhea)
- Assess fracture risk using dual-energy X-ray absorptiometry (DEXA) scan (T and Z scores) or FRAX tool
- Provide sufficient calcium through diet or supplements: at least 120 mg elemental calcium/day and 800–1000 IU/day vitamin D3 for patients older than 50 years of age

111. Which are the indications for treatment of osteoporosis in postmenopausal women not on glucocorticoid therapy?

- Treat patients with bone mineral density (BMD) T score ≤ -2.5 at femoral neck or spine
- Treat postmenopausal women and men >50 years of age who have osteopenia (T score between −1 and −2.5) and a 10-year probability for hip fracture ≥3% or a 10-year probability for major osteoporotic fracture ≥20% (as assessed by the FRAX tool)
- Start therapy for patients with hip or vertebral fracture
- Monitor BMD every 5 years

112. What is the therapeutic algorithm for the treatment of low bone density or osteoporosis to prevent fractures in men and women?

- Women with known osteoporosis should be offered treatment with bisphosphonates (alendronate, risedronate, and zoledronic acid) to reduce the risk for hip and vertebral fractures. Women who cannot tolerate bisphosphonates and are at high risk for fragility fractures could benefit from subcutaneous administration of denosumab
- Adequate calcium intake is a fundamental aspect of any osteoporosis prevention or treatment. For adults aged 50 years and older, the recommended calcium intake (including diet, plus calcium supplements if necessary when dietary intake is insufficient) is 1200 mg/day. The utility of calcium supplements in increasing bone mass density (BMD) is controversial
- Optimal vitamin D status is essential both in women and in men with osteoporosis. It increases response to bisphosphonate therapy, increases BMD, and prevents fractures. Vitamin D3 supplementation to maintain serum 25-hydroxyvitamin D ≥30 ng/mL in patients with osteoporosis is necessary
- Osteoporotic women should be treated with pharmacologic therapy for 5 years, and during

that time, bone density monitoring is not necessary

- In men with clinically recognized osteoporosis, pharmacologic treatment with bisphosphonates should be offered to reduce the risk for vertebral fracture
- It is *not* recommended to use menopausal estrogen therapy alone or in combination with progesterone or raloxifene for the treatment of osteoporosis in women
- In the case of patients with severe osteoporosis, especially accompanied by fractures or patients who cannot tolerate bisphosphonates or patients who have not responded to other drugs, teriparatide is indicated. Therapy should not exceed 2 years, and it should not be given to patients with bone metastases, Paget's disease, skeletal irradiation, or unexplained increase of serum alkaline phosphatase
- Clinicians should decide whether to treat osteopenic women 65 years of age or older, who are at a high risk for fracture based on a discussion of patient preferences, benefits, harms, and costs of medications [100]

113. In which osteoporotic patients drug holiday of bisphosphonate therapy is indicated?

For oral bisphosphonates, a drug holiday after 5 years of treatment should be considered if fracture risk is no longer high (T score is greater than -2.5, or the patient has remained fracture free), but treatment should be continued up to an additional 5 years if fracture risk remains high. In patients with very high fracture risk a drug holiday should be considered after 6 to 10 years. The duration of bisphosphonate therapy should be carefully monitored since a longer duration of bisphosphonate use has been linked to a higher risk of atypical femur fractures. Nevertheless, the absolute risk of atypical femur fracture is very low as compared with the greater number of fractures that are effectively prevented by bisphosphonates [101]. For zoledronate, a drug holiday should be considered after 3 years in high-risk patients or until fracture risk is no longer high, and treatment should be continued for up to 6 years in very high-risk patients. A bone density re-evaluation is recommended every 1–2 years depending on the bisphosphonate used. If after a drug holiday, assessment shows an increased risk of fracture, patients may benefit from initiating another treatment such as teriparatide or denosumab [102].

114. What is the therapeutic algorithm for the treatment of glucocorticoid-induced osteoporosis in premenopausal women and men <50 years of age?

The therapeutic approach of glucocorticoid-induced osteoporosis differs according to the age group of the patients:

- If there is no fragility fracture, there is no strict recommendation, and prevention is based on clinical judgment and assessment of fracture risk factors
- If there is a fragility fracture, the approach differs:
  - In women without childbearing potential or men aged <50 years:
    If glucocorticoid therapy lasts up to 3 months: alendronate or risedronate (for prednisolone $\geq$5 mg/day) or zoledronic acid (for prednisolone $\geq$7.5 mg/day)
    If glucocorticoid therapy lasts for more than 3 months: alendronate, risedronate, zoledronic acid, or teriparatide, independently of daily prednisolone dose
  - In women with childbearing potential:
    If glucocorticoid therapy lasts up to 3 months: the decision whether to initiate treatment or not should be based on the assessment of fracture risk factors and should be individualized for each patient
    If glucocorticoid therapy lasts for more than 3 months: alendronate, risedronate, zoledronic acid, or teriparatide, if prednisolone $\geq$7.5 mg/day

115. What is the therapeutic algorithm for the treatment of glucocorticoid-induced osteoporosis in postmenopausal women and men >50 years of age?

Initially, in patients with an anticipated glucocorticoid therapy duration of ≥3 months, or prevalent duration of at least 3 months, the patient's risk category should be determined. High-, medium-, and low-risk patient classification are based on an approximation of FRAX using age, sex, race, T score, and the presence of glucocorticoids for the calculation.

- *In low-risk patients*: Treatment should be initiated if prednisolone ≥7.5 mg/day: alendronate, risedronate, or zoledronic acid
- *In medium-risk patients*:
  - If prednisolone <7.5 mg/day: alendronate or risedronate
  - If prednisolone ≥7.5 mg/day: alendronate, risedronate, or zoledronic acid
- *In high-risk patients*:
  - If prednisolone <5 mg/day or treatment duration <1 month: alendronate, risedronate, or zoledronic acid
  - If prednisolone 5 mg/day for ≤1 month or any dose of glucocorticoids used for >1 month: alendronate, risedronate, zoledronic acid, or teriparatide

116. Which are the side effects of bisphosphonates?

Side effects are esophageal irritation (esophagitis) (for the orally administered), osteonecrosis of the jaw, musculoskeletal pains, uveitis (rarely), and atypical femur fractures (subtrochanteric/femur shaft, can be bilateral, often present with a prodromal of thigh pain, typically occurs in patients who have been treated for more than 5 years). Flu-like symptoms (fever, myalgias, and arthralgias) occur in almost 10% of patients after the first intravenous dose of bisphosphonate.

117. In patients with acute osteoporotic compression fracture is vertebroplasty better than sham procedure (placebo surgery)?

Osteoporotic compression fractures are a common cause of morbidity and disability among older patients. Conservative treatment includes rest, back brace, and analgesics. Polymethylmethacrylate (acrylic bone cement) percutaneous injection into compression fractured vertebral bodies, the so-called vertebroplasty, was launched as a therapeutic modality for osteoporotic compression fractures based on observational and not evidence-based studies. A double-blinded controlled trial revealed that vertebroplasty, compared to sham procedure, was not, at 12 months of follow-up, superior for pain control. Thus, vertebroplasty is not recommended for treatment of vertebral fractures given an unclear benefit on overall pain and a potential increased risk of vertebral fractures in adjacent vertebrae [103].

References

1. Park JW, Curtis JR, Moon J, et al. Prophylactic effect of trimethoprim-sulfamethoxazole for pneumocystis pneumonia in patients with rheumatic diseases exposed to prolonged high-dose glucocorticoids. Ann Rheum Dis. 2018;77:644–9.
2. Adwan MH. Drug reaction with eosinophilia and systemic symptoms (DRESS) syndrome and the rheumatologist. Curr Rheumatol Rep. 2017;19:3.
3. Yusuf IH, Ledingham JM, MacPhie E, et al. Monitoring for retinal toxicity in patients taking hydroxychloroquine and chloroquine. Rheumatology (Oxford). 2019;58:3–4.
4. Yamaoka K. Janus kinase inhibitors for rheumatoid arthritis. Curr Opin Chem Biol. 2016;32:29–33.
5. Dougados M, van der Heijde D, Chen Y-C, et al. Baricitinib in patients with inadequate response or intolerance to conventional synthetic DMARDs: results from the RA-BUILD study. Ann Rheum Dis. 2017;76:88–95.
6. Smolen JS, Landewé RBM, Bijlsma JWL, et al. EULAR recommendations for the management of rheumatoid arthritis with synthetic and biological disease-modifying antirheumatic drugs: 2019 update. Ann Rheum Dis. 2020 Jan;22. [Epub ahead of print]

7. Murphy CA, Langrish CL, Chen Y, et al. Divergent pro- and anti-inflammatory roles for IL-23 and IL-12 in joint autoimmune inflammation. J. Exp. Med. 2003;198:1951–7.
8. Oppmann B, Lesley R, Blom B, et al. Novel p19 protein engages IL-12p40 to form a cytokine, IL-23, with biological activities similar as well as distinct from IL-12. Immunity. 2000;13:715–25.
9. Strange A, Capon F, Spencer CC, et al. A genome-wide association study identifies new psoriasis susceptibility loci and an interaction between HLA-C and ERAP1. Nat. Genet. 2010;42:985–9.
10. Reveille JD, Am S, Danoy P, et al. Genome-wide association study of ankylosing spondylitis identifies non-MHC susceptibility loci. Nat Genet. 2020;42:123–7.
11. Filer C, Ho P, Smith RL, et al. Investigation of association of the IL12B and IL23R genes with psoriatic arthritis. Arthritis Rheum. 2008;58:3705–9.
12. McInnes IB, Kavanaugh A, Gottlieb AB, et al. Efficacy and safety of ustekinumab in patients with active psoriatic arthritis: 1-year results of the phase 3, multicentre, double-blind, placebo- controlled PSUMMIT 1 trial. Lancet. 2013;382:780–9.
13. Roberts J, O'Rielly DD, Rahman P. A review of ustekinumab in the treatment of psoriatic arthritis. Immunotherapy. 2018;10:361–72.
14. Schafer P. Apremilast mechanism of action and application to psoriasis and psoriatic arthritis. Biochem Pharmacol. 2012;83:1583–90.
15. Schafer PH, Truzzi F, Parton A, et al. Phosphodiesterase 4 in inflammatory diseases: effects of apremilast in psoriatic blood and in dermal myofibroblasts through the PDE4/CD271 complex. Cell Signal. 2016;28:753–63.
16. McCann FE, Palfreeman AC, Andrews M, et al. Apremilast, a novel PDE4 inhibitor, inhibits spontaneous production of tumour necrosis factor-alpha from human rheumatoid synovial cells and ameliorates experimental arthritis. Arthritis Res Ther. 2010;12:R107.
17. Schafer PH, Parton A, Gandhi AK, et al. Apremilast, a cAMP phosphodiesterase-4 inhibitor, demonstrates anti-inflammatory activity in vitro and in a model of psoriasis. Br J Pharmacol. 2010;159:842–55.
18. Morel J, Constantin A, Baron G, Dernis E, Flipo RM, Rist S, et al. Risk factors of serious infections in patients with rheumatoid arthritis treated with tocilizumab in the French Registry REGATE. Rheumatology (Oxford). 2017;56:1746–54.
19. George MD, Baker JF, Winthrop K, et al. Risk for serious infection with low-dose glucocorticoids in patients with rheumatoid arthritis: a cohort study. Ann Intern Med. 2020 Sep 22. Epub ahead of print.
20. Curtis JR, Xie F, Chen L, et al. The comparative risk of serious infections among rheumatoid arthritis patients starting or switching biological agents. Annals of the Rheumatic Diseases. 2011;70:1401–6.
21. Mori S, Yoshitama T, Hidaka T, et al. Comparative risk of hospitalized infection between biological agents in rheumatoid arthritis patients: a multicenter retrospective cohort study in Japan. PLOS ONE. 2017;12:e0179179.
22. Goodman SM, Springer B, Guyatt G, Abdel MP, Dasa V, George M, et al. 2017 American College of Rheumatology/American Association of Hip and Knee surgeons guideline for the perioperative management of antirheumatic medication in patients with rheumatic diseases undergoing elective total hip or total knee arthroplasty. J Arthroplast. 2017;32:2628–38.
23. George MD, Baker JF, Winthrop KL, et al. Risk of biologics and glucocorticoids in patients with rheumatoid arthritis undergoing arthroplasty: a cohort study. Ann Intern Med. 2019;170:825–36.
24. George MD, Baker JF, Winthrop KL, et al. Immunosuppression and the risk of readmission and mortality in patients with rheumatoid arthritis undergoing hip fracture, abdominopelvic and cardiac surgery. Ann Rheum Dis. 2020;79:573–80.
25. Savarino V, Marabotto E, Zentilin P, et al. Proton pump inhibitors: use and misuse in the clinical setting. Expert Rev Clin Pharmacol. 2018 Nov;11(11):1123–34.
26. Thong BKS, Ima-Nirwana S, Chin KY. Proton pump inhibitors and fracture risk: a review of current evidence and mechanisms involved. Int J Environ Res Public Health. 2019;16:pii: E1571.
27. Bérard A, Zhao JP, Shui I, Colilla S. Leflunomide use during pregnancy and the risk of adverse pregnancy outcomes. Ann Rheum Dis. 2018;77:500–9.
28. Belizna C, Meroni P L, Shoenfeld Y et al. In utero exposure to Azathioprine in autoimmune disease. Where do we stand? Autoimmun Rev. 2020. 102525. [Epub ahead of print]
29. Eudy AM, Siega-Riz AM, Engel SM, et al. Effect of pregnancy on disease flares in patients with systemic lupus erythematosus. Ann Rheum Dis. 2018;77:855–60.
30. Alshawabkeh L, Economy KE, Valente AM. Anticoagulation during pregnancy: evolving strategies with a focus on mechanical valves. J Am Coll Cardiol. 2016;68:1804–13.
31. van Hagen IM, Roos-Hesselink JW, Ruys TP, Merz WM, Goland S, Gabriel H, Lelonek M, Trojnarska O, Al Mahmeed WA, Balint HO, Ashour Z, Baumgartner H, Boersma E, Johnson MR, Hall R. ROPAC Investigators and the EURObservational Research Programme (EORP) Team*. Pregnancy in women with a mechanical heart valve: data of the European society of cardiology registry of pregnancy and cardiac disease (ROPAC). Circulation. 2015;132:132–42.
32. Furer V, Rondaan C, Heijstek MW, et al. 2019 update of EULAR recommendations for vaccination in adult patients with autoimmune inflammatory rheumatic diseases. Ann Rheum Dis. 2020;79:39.
33. Park JK, Lee MA, Lee EY, et al. Effect of methotrexate discontinuation on efficacy of seasonal influenza vaccination in patients with rheumatoid

arthritis: a randomised clinical trial. Ann Rheum Dis. 2017;76:1559–65.
34. Park JK, Lee YJ, Shin K, et al. Impact of temporary methotrexate discontinuation for 2 weeks on immunogenicity of seasonal influenza vaccination in patients with rheumatoid arthritis: a randomized clinical trial. Ann Rheum Dis. 2018;77:898–904.
35. Yokose C, McCormick N, Chen C, et al. Risk of gout flares after vaccination: a prospective case cross-over study. Ann Rheum Dis. 2019;78:1601.
36. Bonanni P, Grazzini M, Niccolai G, Paolini D, Varone O, Bartoloni A, Bartalesi F, Santini MG, Baretti S, Bonito C, Zini P, Mechi MT, Niccolini F, Magistri L, Pulci MB, Boccalini S, Bechini A. Recommended vaccinations for asplenic and hyposplenic adult patients. Hum Vaccin Immunother. 2017;13:359–68.
37. Gossec L, Baraliakos X, Kerschbaumer A, et al. EULAR recommendations for the management of psoriatic arthritis with pharmacological therapies: 2019 update. Ann Rheum Dis. 2020;79:700–12.
38. Bluett J, Sergeant JC, Mac Gregor AJ, et al. Risk factors for oral methotrexate failure in patients with inflammatory polyarthritis: results from a UK prospective cohort study. Arthritis Res Ther. 2018;20:50–60.
39. Murdaca G, Spano F, Contatore M, et al. Immunogenicity of infliximab and adalimumab: what is its role in hypersensitivity and modulation of therapeutic efficacy and safety? Expert Opin Drug Saf. 2016;15:4352.
40. Balsa A, Sanmarti R, Rosas J, et al. Drug immunogenicity in patients with inflammatory arthritis and secondary failure to tumour necrosis factor inhibitor therapies: the REASON study. Rheumatology. 2018;57:688–93.
41. Nakagawa J, Koyama Y, Kawakami A, et al. A novel scoring system based on common laboratory tests predicts the efficacy of TNF-inhibitor and IL-6 targeted therapy in patients with rheumatoid arthritis: a retrospective, multicenter observational study. Arthritis Res Ther. 2017;19:185.
42. Mercer LK, Regierer AC, Mariette X, Dixon WG, Baecklund E, Hellgren K, et al. Spectrum of lymphomas across different drug treatment groups in rheumatoid arthritis: a European registries collaborative project. Ann Rheum Dis. 2017;76:2025–30.
43. Ward MM, Deodhar A, Gensler LS, et al. 2019 Update of the American College of Rheumatology/Spondylitis Association of America/Spondyloarthritis Research and Treatment Network Recommendations for the treatment of ankylosing spondylitis and non-radiographic axial spondyloarthritis. Arthritis & Rheumatology. 2019;71:1599–613.
44. Sveaas SH, Dagfinrud H, Berg IJ, et al. High-Intensity exercise improves fatigue, sleep, and mood in patients with axial spondyloarthritis: secondary analysis of a randomized controlled trial. Phys Ther. 2020;100(8):1323–32.
45. Laskari K, Tzioufas AG, Moutsopoulos HM. Efficacy and long-term follow-up of IL-1R inhibitor anakinra in adults with Still's disease: a case-series study. Arthritis Res Ther. 2011;13:R91.
46. Maria AT, Le Quellec A, Jorgensen C, Touitou I, Rivière S, Guilpain P. Adult onset Still's disease (AOSD) in the era of biologic therapies: dichotomous view for cytokine and clinical expressions. Autoimmun Rev. 2014;13:1149–59.
47. Sakthiswary R, Suresh E. Methotrexate in systemic lupus erythematosus: a systematic review of its efficacy. Lupus. 2014;23:225–35.
48. Kleinmann JF, Tubach F, Le Guern V, Mathian A, Richez C, Saadoun D, et al. International and multidisciplinary expert recommendations for the use of biologics in systemic lupus erythematosus. Autoimmun Rev. 2017;16:650–7.
49. Ioannidis JP, Katsifis GE, Tzioufas AG, Moutsopoulos HM. Predictors of sustained amenorrhea from pulsed intravenous cyclophosphamide in premenopausal women with systemic lupus erythematosus. J Rheumatol. 2002;29:2129–35.
50. Zampeli E, Klinman DM, Gershwin ME, Moutsopoulos HM. A comprehensive evaluation for the treatment of lupus nephritis. J Autoimmun. 2017;78:1–10.
51. Fanouriakis A, Kostopoulou M, Cheema K, et al. 2019 Update of the Joint European League Against Rheumatism and European Renal Association-European Dialysis and Transplant Association (EULAR/ERA-EDTA) Recommendations for the Management of Lupus Nephritis. Ann Rheum Dis. 2020;annrheumdis-2020-216924. Online ahead of print.
52. Fairley JL, Oon S, Saracino AM, Nikpour M. Management of cutaneous manifestations of lupus erythematosus: a systematic review. Semin Arthritis Rheum. 2020;50:95–127.
53. Pengo V, Denas G, Zoppellaro G, et al. Rivaroxaban vs warfarin in high-risk patients with antiphospholipid syndrome. Blood. 2018;132:1365–71.
54. Ordi-Ros J, Sáez-Comet L, Pérez-Conesa M, et al. Rivaroxaban versus Vitamin K antagonist in antiphospholipid syndrome: a non-inferiority randomized trial. Ann Intern Med. 2019;171:685–94.
55. Dufrost V, Risse J, Reshetnyak T, et al. Increased risk of thrombosis in antiphospholipid syndrome patients treated with direct oral anticoagulants. Results from an international patient-level data meta-analysis. Autoimmun Rev. 2018;17:1011–21.
56. Hamulyák EN, Scheres LJ, Marijnen MC, et al. Aspirin or heparin or both for improving pregnancy outcomes in women with persistent antiphospholipid antibodies and recurrent pregnancy loss. Cochrane Database Syst Rev. 2020;5:CD012852.
57. Belizna C. Hydroxychloroquine as an anti-thrombotic in antiphospholipid syndrome. Autoimmun Rev. 2015;14:358–62.
58. Kravvariti E, Koutsogianni A, Samoli E, et al. The effect of hydroxychloroquine on thrombosis prevention and antiphospholipid antibody levels in primary antiphospholipid syndrome: a pilot open label

randomized prospective study. Autoimmun Rev. 2020;19:102491.
59. Pipitone N, Salvarani C. Treatment of inflammatory myopathies. Expert Rev Clin Immunol. 2018;14:607–21.
60. Manoussakis MN, Moutsopoulos HM. Antimalarials in Sjögren's syndrome—the Greek experience. Lupus. 1996;5:S28–30.
61. Moutsopoulos HM, Fragoulis GE, Stone JH. Pathogenesis and clinical manifestations of IgG4-related disease. Up To Date. 2019; Topic 16155 Version 18.0.
62. Saunders P, Tsipouri V, Keir GJ, et al. Rituximab versus cyclophosphamide for the treatment of connective tissue disease associated interstitial lung disease (RECITAL): study protocol for a randomised controlled trial. Trials. 2017;18:275.
63. Narváez J, LLuch J, Alegre Sancho JJ, et al. Effectiveness and safety of tocilizumab for the treatment of refractory systemic sclerosis associated interstitial lung disease: a case series. Ann Rheum Dis. 2019;78:e123.
64. Thompson A, Shea B, Welch V, Fenlon D, Pope JE. Calcium-channel blockers for Raynaud's phenomenon in systemic sclerosis. Arthritis Rheum. 2001;44:1841–7.
65. Matucci-Cerinic M, Denton C, Furst D, Mayes M, Hsu V, Carpentier D, et al. Bosentan treatment of digital ulcers related to systemic sclerosis: results from the RAPIDS-2 randomised, double-blind, placebo-controlled trial. Ann Rheum Dis. 2011;70:32–8.
66. García de la Peña Lefebvre P, Nishishinya MB, Pereda CA, Loza E, Sifuentes Giraldo WA, Román Ivorra JA, et al. Efficacy of Raynaud's phenomenon and digital ulcer pharmacological treatment in systemic sclerosis patients: a systematic literature review. Rheumatol Int. 2015;35(9):1447–59.
67. Roustit M, Giai J, Gaget O, et al. On-demand sildenafil as a treatment for raynaud phenomenon. Ann Intern Med. 2018;169:694–703.
68. Dejaco C, Singh YP, Perel P, et al. 2015 European League Against Rheumatism (EULAR)/American College of Rheumatology (ACR) collaborative recommendations for the management of PMR. Ann Rheum Dis. 2015;74:1799–807.
69. Buttgereit F, Matteson EL, Dejaco C. Polymyalgia rheumatica and giant cell arteritis. JAMA. 2020;324: 993–4.
70. Villiger PM, Adler S, Kuchen S, Wermelinger F, Dan D, Fiege V, et al. Tocilizumab for induction and maintenance of remission in giant cell arteritis: a phase 2, randomised, double-blind, placebo-controlled trial. Lancet. 2016;387:1921–7.
71. Stone JH, Tuckwell K, Dimonaco S, Klearman M, Aringer M, Blockmans D, et al. Trial of tocilizumab in giant-cell arteritis. N Engl J Med. 2017;377:317–28.
72. Singh A, Danda D, Hussain S, et al. Efficacy and safety of tocilizumab in treatment of Takayasu arteritis: a systematic review of randomized controlled trials. Mod Rheumatol. 2020;13:1–8.
73. Koster MJ, Yeruva K, Crowson CS, et al. Efficacy of methotrexate in real-world management of giant cell arteritis: a case-control Study. J Rheumatol. 2019 May;46:501–8.
74. Hočevar A, Ješe R, Rotar Ž, et al. Does leflunomide have a role in giant cell arteritis? An open-label study. Clin Rheumatol. 2019;38:291–6.
75. Cui X, Dai X, Ma L, et al. Efficacy and safety of leflunomide treatment in Takayasu arteritis: case series from the East China cohort. Semin Arthritis Rheum. 2020;50:59–65.
76. Muratore F, Pipitone N, Salvarani C. Standard and biological treatment in large vessel vasculitis: guidelines and current approaches. Expert Rev Clin Immunol. 2017;13(4):345–60.
77. Régnier P, Le Joncour A, Maciejewski-Duval A.Targeting JAK/STAT pathway in Takayasu's arteritis. Ann Rheum Dis. 2020;pii: annrheumdis-2019-216900. [Epub ahead of print]
78. Adler S, Reichenbach S, Gloor A, et al. Risk of relapse after discontinuation of tocilizumab therapy in giant cell arteritis. Rheumatology (Oxford). 2019;58:1639.
79. Walsh M, Merkel AP, Peh C-A, et al. Plasma exchange and glucocorticoids in severe ANCA-associated vasculitis. N Engl J Med. 2020;382:622–31.
80. Solomon DH, Glynn RJ, Mac Fadyen JG. Relationship of Interleukin-1β Blockade with incident gout and serum uric acid levels. Ann Intern Med. 2018;169:535–42.
81. Slobodnick A, Shah B, Krasnokutsky S, Pillinger MH. Update on colchicine, 2017. Rheumatology. 2018;57:4–i11.
82. Slobodnick A, Shah B, Pillinger MH. Colchicine: old and new. Am J Med. 2015;128:461–70.
83. Zhang W, Doherty M, Pascual E, et al. EULAR recommendations for calcium pyrophosphate deposition. Part II: management. Ann Rheum Dis. 2011;70:571–5.
84. Davatchi F, Sadeghi Abdollahi B, Tehrani Banihashemi A, et al. Colchicine versus placebo in Behçet's disease: randomized, double-blind, controlled crossover trial. Mod Rheumatol. 2009;19:542–9.
85. Cacoub PP. Colchicine for treatment of acute or recurrent pericarditis. Lancet. 2014;383:2193.
86. Runhaar J, Rozendaal RM, Middelkoop MV, Bijlsma HJW, Doherty M, Dziedzic KS, et al. Subgroup analyses of the effectiveness of oral glucosamine for knee and hip osteoarthritis: a systematic review and individual patient data meta-analysis from the OA trial bank. Ann Rheum Dis. 2017;76(11):1862–9. pii: annrheumdis-2017-211149.
87. Qaseem A, Wilt TJ, McLean RM, Forciea MA. Clinical guidelines committee of the American College of Physicians. Noninvasive treatments for acute, subacute, and chronic low back pain: a clinical practice guideline from the American College of Physicians. Ann Intern Med. 2017;166:514–30.
88. Nguyen C, Boutron I, Baron G, et al. Intradiscal glucocorticoid injection for patients with chronic low

back pain associated with active discopathy: a randomized trial. Ann Intern Med. 2017;166:547–56.
89. McAlindon TE, LaValley MP, Harvey WF, Price LL, Driban JB, Zhang M, Ward RJ. Effect of intra-articular triamcinolone vs saline on knee cartilage volume and pain in patients with knee osteoarthritis: a randomized clinical trial. JAMA. 2017;317:1967–75.
90. Deyle GD, Allen CS, Allison SC, et al. Physical therapy versus glucocorticoid injection for osteoarthritis of the knee. N Engl J Med. 2020;382:1420–9.
91. Rewald S, Lenssen AFT, Emans PJ, de Bie RA, van Breukelen G, Mesters I. Aquatic cycling improves knee pain and physical functioning in patients with knee osteoarthritis: a randomized controlled trial. Arch Phys Med Rehabil. 2020;101:1288–95.
92. Kingsbury SR, Tharmanathan P, Keding A, et al. Hydroxychloroquine effectiveness in reducing symptoms of hand osteoarthritis. Annals of Internal Medicine. 2018;168:385–96.
93. Kroon FPB, Kortekaas MC, Boonen A, et al. Results of a 6-week treatment with 10 mg prednisolone in patients with hand osteoarthritis (HOPE): a double-blind, randomised, placebo-controlled trial. The Lancet. 2019;394:1993–2001.
94. Ottaviani S, Ayral X, Dougados M, Gossec L. Pigmented villonodular synovitis: a retrospective single-center study of 122 cases and review of the literature. Semin Arthritis Rheum. 2011;40:539–46.
95. Tap WD, Gelderblom H, Palmerini E, et al. Pexidartinib versus placebo for advanced tenosynovial giant cell tumour (ENLIVEN): a randomised phase 3 trial. Lancet. 2019;394:478–87.
96. Cohen H. Controversies and challenges in fibromyalgia: a review and a proposal. Ther Adv Musculoskelet Dis. 2017;9:115–27.
97. Wang C, Schmid CH, Fielding RA, et al. Effect of tai chi versus aerobic exercise for fibromyalgia: comparative effectiveness randomized controlled trial. BMJ. 2018;360:k851.
98. Cheng CA, Chiu YW, Wu D, et al. Effectiveness of Tai Chi on fibromyalgia patients: a meta-analysis of randomized controlled trials. Complement Ther Med. 2019;46:1–8.
99. Dailey DL, Vance CGT, Rakel BA, et al. Transcutaneous electrical nerve stimulation reduces movement-evoked pain and fatigue: a randomized, Controlled Trial. Arthritis Rheumatol. 2019. [Epub ahead of print]
100. Qaseem A, Forciea MA, McLean RM, Denberg TD. Clinical Guidelines Committee of the American College of Physicians. Treatment of low bone density or osteoporosis to prevent fractures in men and women: a clinical practice guideline update from the American college of physicians. Ann Intern Med. 2017;166:818–39.
101. Black DM, Geiger EJ, Eastell R, et al. Atypical femur fracture risk versus fragility fracture prevention with bisphosphonates. N Engl J Med. 2020;383:743–53
102. Camacho PM, Petak SM, Binkley N, et al. American Association of Clinical Endocrinologists/American College of Endocrinology Clinical practice guidelines for the diagnosis and treatment of postmenopausal osteoporosis-2020 update. Endocr Pract. 2020;26:564–70.
103. Firanescu CE, de Vries J, Lodder P, et al. Vertebroplasty versus sham procedure for painful acute osteoporotic vertebral compression fractures (VERTOS IV): randomised sham controlled clinical trial. BMJ. 2018;361:k1551.

Index

H. M. Moutsopoulos, E. Zampeli (eds.), *Immunology and Rheumatology in Questions*,
https://doi.org/10.1007/978-3-030-56670-8

GPSR Compliance

The European Union's (EU) General Product Safety Regulation (GPSR) is a set of rules that requires consumer products to be safe and our obligations to ensure this.

If you have any concerns about our products, you can contact us on ProductSafety@springernature.com

In case Publisher is established outside the EU, the EU authorized representative is:

Springer Nature Customer Service Center GmbH
Europaplatz 3
69115 Heidelberg, Germany

Batch number: 10732809

Printed by Printforce, the Netherlands